Acute Coronary Syndrome

Mun K. Hong and Eyal Herzog (Eds)

Acute Coronary Syndrome

Multidisciplinary and Pathway-Based Approach

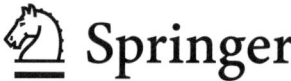 Springer

Mun K. Hong, MD
Cardiac Catheterization Laboratory and
  Interventional Cardiology
Department of Medicine
St. Luke's-Roosevelt Hospital Center
Columbia University College of Physicians and
  Surgeons
New York, NY, USA

Eyal Herzog, MD, FACC
Cardiac Care Unit
St. Luke's-Roosevelt Hospital Center
Columbia University College of Physicians and
  Surgeons
New York, NY, USA

British Library Cataloguing in Publication Data

Acute coronary syndrome
  1. Coronary heart disease
  I. Hong, Mun K.   II. Herzog, Eyal
  616.1'23

ISBN-13: 9781846288685

Library of Congress Control Number: 2007925043

ISBN-13: 978-1-84628-868-5   e-ISBN-13: 978-1-84628-869-2

9 8 7 6 5 4 3 2 1

Springer Science+Business Media
springer.com

Preface

Acute coronary syndrome represents the most urgent cardiac condition requiring an immediate diagnosis and the prompt institution of therapy to save lives and improve long-term quality of life. Recent trials have demonstrated the benefits of various pharmacologic and revascularization strategies. These evidence-based data have provided the basis for AHA/ACC guidelines. However, there is a continuing lack of guideline adherence, adversely affecting patient outcome. In addition, the optimal care of these high-risk patients requires a multidisciplinary approach.

This book is an attempt to provide up to date information on the many aspects of acute coronary syndrome. The authors for each chapter have striven to provide concise review of the current literature and algorithm-based approaches for diagnosis and management of each topic.

This field is rapidly evolving, and there will be many new paradigms with advancing knowledge. The editors hope that despite the dynamic status of the management issues related to acute coronary syndrome, the basic concepts of this book will be valuable to the readers for their patient care.

Mun K. Hong
Eyal Herzog

Contents

Contributors

Aysha Arshad, MD
Division of Cardiology
Department of Medicine
St. Luke's-Roosevelt Hospital
  Center
Columbia University College of
  Physicians and Surgeons
New York, NY, USA

Emad Aziz, DO, MB, ChB
Department of Medicine
St. Luke's-Roosevelt Hospital
  Center
Columbia University College of
  Physicians and Surgeons
New York, NY, USA

Sandhya K. Balaram, MD, PhD
Division of Cardiothoracic Surgery
St. Luke's-Roosevelt Hospital Center
Columbia University College of
  Physicians and Surgeons
New York, NY, USA

Sripal Bangalore, MD, MHA
Department of Cardiology
St. Luke's-Roosevelt Hospital Center
Columbia University College of
  Physicians and Surgeons
New York, NY, USA

Inna Bukharovich, MD
Division of Cardiology
Department of Medicine
St. Luke's-Roosevelt Hospital Center
New York, NY, USA

Farooq A. Chaudhry, MD, FACC,
  FASE
Division of Cardiology
Department of Medicine
St. Luke's-Roosevelt Hospital
  Center
Columbia University College of
  Physicians and Surgeons
New York, NY, USA

Simbo Chiadika, MD
Division of Cardiology
Department of Medicine
St. Luke's-Roosevelt Hospital
  Center
Columbia University College of
  Physicians and Surgeons
New York, NY, USA

Amy Chorzempa, MS, RN, ANP-BC
Division of Cardiology
Department of Medicine
St. Luke's-Roosevelt Hospital Center
Columbia University College of
  Physicians and Surgeons
New York, NY, USA

Randy E. Cohen, MD
Division of Cardiology
Department of Medicine
St. Luke's-Roosevelt Hospital Center
Columbia University College of
  Physicians and Surgeons
New York, NY, USA

Delia Cotiga, MD
Division of Cardiology
Department of Medicine
St. Luke's-Roosevelt Hospital Center
Columbia University College of
  Physicians and Surgeons
New York, NY, USA

David L. Coven, MD, PhD
Department of Cardiology
St. Luke's-Roosevelt Hospital
  Center
Columbia University College of
  Physicians and Surgeons
New York, NY, USA

Matthew Daka, MD
Division of Cardiology
Department of Medicine
St. Luke's-Roosevelt Hospital Center
Columbia University College of
  Physicians and Surgeons
New York, NY, USA

Hossein Eftekhari, MD
Division of Cardiology
Department of Medicine
St. Luke's-Roosevelt Hospital Center
Columbia University College of
  Physicians and Surgeons
New York, NY, USA

Olivier Frankenberger, MD, PhD
Division of Cardiology
Department of Medicine
St. Luke's-Roosevelt Hospital Center
Columbia University College of
  Physicians and Surgeons
New York, NY, USA

Henry H. Greenberg, MD
Division of Cardiology
Department of Medicine
St. Luke's-Roosevelt Hospital Center
Columbia University College of
  Physicians and Surgeons
New York, NY, USA

Khashayar Hematpour, MD
Department of Medicine
St. Luke's-Roosevelt Hospital Center
Columbia University College of
  Physicians and Surgeons
New York, NY, USA

Eyal Herzog, MD, FACC
Cardiac Care Unit
St. Luke's-Roosevelt Hospital
  Center
Columbia University College of
  Physicians and Surgeons
New York, NY, USA

Mun K. Hong, MD
Cardiac Catheterization Laboratory
  and Interventional Cardiology
Department of Medicine
St. Luke's-Roosevelt Hospital
  Center
Columbia University College of
  Physicians and Surgeons
New York, NY, USA

Gregory Janis, MD
Division of Cardiology
Department of Medicine
St. Luke's-Roosevelt Hospital
  Center
Columbia University College of
  Physicians and Surgeons
New York, NY, USA

Elaine B. Josephson, MD
Department of Emergency
  Medicine
St. Luke's-Roosevelt Hospital
  Center
Columbia University College of
  Physicians and Surgeons
New York, NY, USA

Sandeep Joshi, MD
Division of Cardiology
Department of Emergency Medicine
St. Luke's-Roosevelt Hospital
  Center
Columbia University College of
  Physicians and Surgeons
New York, NY, USA

Aslam Khan, MD
Division of Cardiology
Department of Medicine
St. Luke's-Roosevelt Hospital Center
Columbia University College of
  Physicians and Surgeons
New York, NY, USA

Bette Kim, MD
Division of Cardiology
Department of Medicine
St. Luke's-Roosevelt Hospital Center
Columbia University College of
  Physicians and Surgeons
New York, NY, USA

Jayanthi N. Koneru, MD
Division of Cardiology
Department of Emergency Medicine
St. Luke's-Roosevelt Hospital Center
Columbia University College of
  Physicians and Surgeons
New York, NY, USA

Robert Kornberg, MD
Private Practice
RJ Kornberg, MD, PLLC
New York, NY, USA

Atul Kukar, DO
Division of Cardiology
Department of Medicine
St. Luke's-Roosevelt Hospital Center
Columbia University College of
  Physicians and Surgeons
New York, NY, USA

Marrick Kukin, MD
Heart Failure Program
St. Luke's-Roosevelt Hospital
  Center
Columbia University College of
  Physicians and Surgeons
New York, NY, USA

Robert Leber, MD
Division of Cardiology
Department of Medicine
St. Luke's-Roosevelt Hospital Center
Columbia University College of
  Physicians and Surgeons
New York, NY, USA

Michael Lesch, MD
Division of Cardiology
Department of Emergency Medicine
St. Luke's-Roosevelt Hospital Center
Columbia University College of
  Physicians and Surgeons
New York, NY, USA

Kataneh Maleki, MD
Division of Cardiology
Department of Medicine
St. Luke's-Roosevelt Hospital Center
Columbia University College of
  Physicians and Surgeons
New York, NY, USA

Franz Messerli, MD
Division of Cardiology
Department of Medicine
St. Luke's-Roosevelt Hospital Center
Columbia University College of
  Physicians and Surgeons
New York, NY, USA

Nicholas H.E. Mezitis, MD
Division of Endocrinology, Diabetes,
  and Nutrition
St. Luke's-Roosevelt Hospital Center
Columbia University College of
  Physicians and Surgeons
New York, NY, USA

Suneet Mittal, MD
Department of Cardiology
St. Luke's-Roosevelt Hospital Center
Columbia University College of
    Physicians and Surgeons
New York, NY, USA

Dan L. Musat, MD
Department of Cardiology
St. Luke's-Roosevelt Hospital Center
Columbia University College of
    Physicians and Surgeons
New York, NY, USA

Merle Myerson, MD, EdD, FACC
Division of Cardiology
St. Luke's-Roosevelt Hospital Center
Columbia University College of
    Physicians and Surgeons
and
Department of Epidemiology
Mailman School of Public Health of
    Columbia University
New York, NY, USA

Mary O'Sullivan, MD
Department of Pulmonary-Critical
    Care
St. Luke's-Roosevelt Hospital Center
Columbia University College of
    Physicians and Surgeons
New York, NY, USA

Angela Palazzo, MD, FACC
Department of Cardiology
St. Luke's-Roosevelt Hospital Center
Columbia University College of
    Physicians and Surgeons
New York, NY, USA

Gurusher Panjrath, MD
Department of Internal Medicine
St. Luke's-Roosevelt Hospital Center
Columbia University College of
    Physicians and Surgeons
New York, NY, USA

Walter Pierce, MD
Department of Cardiology
St. Luke's-Roosevelt Hospital
    Center
Columbia University College of
    Physicians and Surgeons
New York, NY, USA

Lauren Rosenberg, MD
Division of Cardiology
Department of Medicine
St. Luke's-Roosevelt Hospital Center
Columbia University College of
    Physicians and Surgeons
New York, NY, USA

Alan Rozanski, MD
Division of Cardiology
Department of Medicine
St. Luke's-Roosevelt Hospital
    Center
Columbia University College of
    Physicians and Surgeons
New York, NY, USA

Mark V. Sherrid, MD
Department of Cardiology
St. Luke's-Roosevelt Hospital Center
Columbia University College of
    Physicians and Surgeons
New York, NY, USA

Tina Sichrovsky, MD
Department of Cardiology
St. Luke's-Roosevelt Hospital
    Center
Columbia University College of
    Physicians and Surgeons
New York, NY, USA

Claude Simon, MD, PhD, FACC
Department of Cardiology
St. Luke's-Roosevelt Hospital Center
Columbia University College of
    Physicians and Surgeons
New York, NY, USA

Tseday Sirak, MD, MPH
Department of Cardiology
St. Luke's-Roosevelt Hospital Center
Columbia University College of
    Physicians and Surgeons
New York, NY, USA

Jonathan S. Steinberg, MD
Division of Cardiology
St. Luke's-Roosevelt Hospital Center
Columbia University College of
    Physicians and Surgeons
New York, NY, USA

Daniel G. Swistel, MD
Division of Cardiothoracic Surgery
St. Luke's-Roosevelt Hospital Center
Columbia University College of
    Physicians and Surgeons
New York, NY, USA

Jacqueline E. Tamis-Holland, BA,
    MD, FACC
Division of Cardiology
Department of Medicine
St. Luke's-Roosevelt Hospital Center
Columbia University College of
    Physicians and Surgeons
New York, NY, USA

Seth Uretsky, MD
Department of Cardiology
St. Luke's-Roosevelt Hospital Center
Columbia University College of
    Physicians and Surgeons
New York, NY, USA

Lance W. Weathers, MD
Division of Cardiology
Department of Emergency
    Medicine
St. Luke's-Roosevelt Hospital
    Center
Columbia University College of
    Physicians and Surgeons
New York, NY, USA

Catherine R. Weinberg, MD
Department of Medicine
St. Luke's-Roosevelt Hospital
    Center
Columbia University College of
    Physicians and Surgeons
New York, NY, USA

David M. Wild, MD
Department of Cardiology
St. Luke's-Roosevelt Hospital
    Center
Columbia University College of
    Physicians and Surgeons
New York, NY, USA

Jamshad Wyne, MD
Division of Cardiology
Department of Medicine
St. Luke's-Roosevelt Hospital
    Center
Columbia University College of
    Physicians and Surgeons
New York, NY, USA

1
Acute Coronary Syndrome: Where We Are, How We Got Here, and Where We Are Going

Jayanthi N. Koneru, Lance W. Weathers, and Michael Lesch

Advances in the treatment of acute coronary syndrome (ACS) can justifiably be considered one of the great achievements of modern medicine. The evolution of treatment strategies from "benign neglect" in the early 1900s to an aggressive interventional approach with devices and potent pharmacotherapy in the 2000s represents a remarkable achievement.

The Pre–Coronary Care Unit Era

In the 19th century, animal experiments involving sudden ligation of a major coronary artery and observations from human necropsies led to the conclusion that coronary thrombosis is immediately fatal [1]. In 1901, Krehl reported that coronary thrombosis does not always cause sudden death, that symptoms are more severe when arterial occlusion is sudden as opposed to gradual, and that acute myocardial infarction may be complicated by ventricular aneurysm formation and myocardial rupture [2]. Once it became clear that survival after acute coronary occlusion was possible, attention turned toward treatment. In 1912, Herrick stated that after acute myocardial infarction (AMI), "the importance of absolute rest in bed for several days is clear" [3]. This dictum became the cornerstone for therapy for the next half-century.

In 1928, Parkinson and Bedford published data on 100 AMI patients. They recommended morphine for pain but expressly advised against the use of nitrates because of their hypotensive effect. For survivors of the acute attack, they cautioned that "convalescence will . . . be prolonged and the return to ordinary life [should be] postponed as long as possible" [4].

In 1929, Samuel Levine described a series of 145 AMI patients. He pointed out the frequency of and risk posed by various cardiac arrhythmias and recommended quinidine to treat ventricular tachycardia and intramuscular adrenaline to treat heart block and syncope. Emphasizing the importance of detecting such arrhythmias, Levine suggested that nurses be trained to "follow carefully the rate and rhythm of the apex beat." By use of a stethoscope, arrhythmias could be treated promptly when a physician was not available. This forward-

1

looking recommendation antedated the development of the coronary care unit by a third of a century [5].

Nevertheless, the prescription of bed rest continued to be all-important. In the 1930s and 1940s, there was considerable debate about when in the course of the illness patients could be permitted to sit in a chair, use a commode, ambulate, be discharged from the hospital, and so forth. When Levine and Lown proposed the "armchair treatment" of AMI in 1952, this suggestion was considered radical and provoked heated discussion [6].

By midcentury, it had become clear that AMI was the most common cause of death in the industrialized world; that cardiac rupture was a relatively uncommon complication; that strict limitation of physical activity did not seem to reduce the incidence of this dreaded event; and that long-term bed rest might be associated with the serious complications of venous thrombosis and pulmonary embolism. As a consequence, practice gradually changed. Ambulation was accelerated and convalescence shortened; postinfarction rehabilitation made possible a more rapid return to previous lifestyles and employment.

In 1950, Tinsley Harrison, writing in *Principles of Internal Medicine* [7], recommended that fluids be administered to avoid dehydration and oxygen be administered in the presence of rales and cyanosis. To prevent or relieve coronary spasm, subcutaneous atropine and papaverine followed by sublingual nitroglycerin (glyceryl trinitrate) were advised, as was the routine use of anticoagulants to prevent reinfarction, mural thrombosis, and pulmonary embolism.

In retrospect, therapeutic modalities developed during the first half of the 20th century provided little benefit to patients with AMI, other than for pain relief. Nevertheless, by establishing diagnostic criteria and by elucidating the natural history of the condition, observant physicians set the stage for the dramatic advances that followed.

The Birth of the Coronary Care Unit

The coronary care unit (CCU) was proposed by Desmond Julian in 1961 [8] based on the realization that arrhythmias are the principal cause of early mortality in AMI; the ability to employ continuous ECG monitoring; the development of closed chest defibrillation, and the delegation of the treatment of life-threatening arrhythmias to trained nurses in the absence of physicians. Within 5 years, CCUs reduced the early mortality from AMI from 30% to 15%. Pump failure secondary to extensive myocardial damage emerged as the principal cause of early mortality in AMI. During the 1960s, it became apparent that most AMI deaths are due to cardiac arrhythmias prior to hospitalization. Ambulances equipped with specialized equipment and trained personnel emerged as "mobile CCUs" and have saved many lives [9].

The Challenge of the Limitation of Infarct Size

Residual post–myocardial infarction (MI) left ventricular function emerged as the primary prognostic factor for patients who reached the CCU and did not succumb to arrhythmia. Attention shifted to strategies that would limit infarct size. One such was an attempt to design interventions to alter the balance between oxygen supply and demand in the jeopardized zone. This led to the use of intravenous β-adrenoceptor blockade for the dual purpose of arrhythmia prevention and limiting ischemia-induced myocardial damage [10].

The Debate About the Genesis of the "Culprit Clot" and the Advent of Thrombolysis

The role of coronary thrombosis as a cause of myocardial infarction had been debated for decades. However, long before the debate was settled by Davies [11] in 1985 with his seminal paper about plaque-fissuring; Fletcher et al. [12] and Verstraete [13] proposed the use of thrombolytic therapy of AMI in the 1950s and 1960s. Michael Davies' research on plaque-fissuring has over the years had great impact on the conceptualization of unstable angina and non–ST-elevation myocardial infarction (NSTEMI) because it provided the conceptual framework explaining the sudden destabilization of previously stable angina and provided a unifying theory for unstable angina, NSTEMI, and ST-elevation myocardial infarction (STEMI) in that a single plaque rupture can result in any of the above three syndromes depending upon whether the clot remains totally occlusive or is lysed in part or in whole by the body's intrinsic fibrinolytic mechanisms. In the late 1970s, Chazov and Rentrop and colleagues [14, 15] made the next important advance in the treatment of AMI by performing successful lysis of coronary thrombi with infusion of streptokinase directly into the occluded coronary artery.

Logistical issues prevented the widespread use of this treatment modality. The GISSI and the ISIS trials [16, 17] provided the necessary fillip to overcome this bottleneck, demonstrating that early intravenous administration of streptokinase reduced mortality in patients with ST-segment elevation. Subsequently, tissue-plasminogen activator (t-PA) was proven more effective than streptokinase in opening occluded vessels [18, 19]. However the clinical efficacy of thrombolytic agents is limited largely to patients with ST-segment elevation [20].

Aspirin: Deep Simplicity

Platelets have long been suspected to play a very important role in the development of coronary thrombi. However, this observation was translated into clinical efficacy only after the ISIS-2 trial showed the enormous effectiveness of aspirin—a simple, inexpensive antiplatelet drug—in reducing mortality in AMI [17].

Troponins: Ushering in a New Era in the Laboratory Diagnosis of AMI

In the mid and late 1990s, troponin became the preferred marker for myocardial damage in suspected AMI. Subsequently, the scientific community realized that the high sensitivity of these biomarkers needed to be tempered with the realization that they are not extremely specific for AMI. Nevertheless, troponins are here to stay and since their arrival have played a crucial role not only in the diagnosis of AMI but also in the risk stratification of patients with ACS [21, 22].

Catheter-Based Reperfusion Strategies: Metamorphosis of the Reperfusion Armamentarium

Intraarterial coronary catheterization was used by Andreas Gruentzig to perform the first angioplasty in an awake human in the 1970s [23, 24]. This forever altered the role of a cardiologist in the management of coronary artery disease. In the 1990s, a multitude of studies and meta-analyses demonstrated that primary angioplasty was superior to thrombolysis in the setting of acute ST-elevation MI with regard to mortality and reinfarction rates at 1 month and 6 months postinfarction (PAMI [25], GUSTO-IIB [26], PCAT meta-analysis [27]). Restenosis was a major problem with angioplasty (28% to 47%). The advent of metallic stents has reduced the complications of reocclusion and restenosis (STENT-PAMI trial [28] and CADILLAC [29]). Further reductions in restenosis rates appear to have been achieved by suppressing neointimal proliferation with drug eluting stents (the SIRIUS [30], RAVEL [31, 32], and TAXUS [33] studies).

Explosion of Vascular Biology Research and the Adjuvant Use of Glycoprotein IIb/IIIa Inhibition

Antiplatelet strategies to complement catheter-based reperfusion strategies have been the result of dedicated research in vascular biology and platelet function. The clinical benefit with these strategies was defined by the reduced incidence of death, reinfarction, urgent target vessel revascularization rates, and improved rates of TIMI-3 flow in the target vessel (ADMIRAL and CADILLAC [29]).

Unstable Angina/Non–ST-Elevation Myocardial Infarction and the Debate About the Early Invasive Approach Versus Conservative Approach

The incidence of diagnosed NSTEMI has been steadily increasing. Striking observations over the past two decades regarding the pathophysiology of unstable angina (UA)/NSTEMI include the following: (1) UA and NSTEMI represent a pathophysiologic continuum; (2) the angiographic extent of disease is higher in patients with UA/NSTEMI when compared with those with STEMI; (3) long-term outcomes for both mortality and nonfatal events are actually worse for patients with either UA or NSTEMI compared with STEMI. The two approaches that were traditionally used to treat UA/NSTEMI were the early invasive and the conservative approach. The weight of evidence in 2007 favors the early invasive strategy, particularly in specific high-risk subgroups. However, neither the appropriate timing of angiography nor the precise characterization of the "high-risk subgroup" has yet been established (TACTICS TIMI-18 [34], RITA 3 [35], TIMI IIIB [36], FRISC II [37], and ISAAR-COOL [38] trials).

Risk Stratification and Secondary Prevention

As UA and NSTEMI are increasing in proportion to the incidence of STEMI, risk stratification has gained increasing attention. Because risk stratification is such an integral component in the management decisions of UA/NSTEMI, concerted efforts have been made to identify those patients who benefit from intensive medical treatment. Various markers have been proposed as having prognostic value and incorporated in risk-stratifying algorithms for the management of UA/NSTEMI. The biomarker best validated as a prognostic marker is C- reactive protein [39–41]. The discovery of differences in the nature of the thrombi in NSTEMI and STEMI by technological advances such as angioscopy and intravascular ultrasound (IVUS) has spurred a movement of polymodality medical therapy aimed at lipid lowering [42], platelet antagonism, and reverse remodeling of the heart and its blood vessels.

Future Therapeutic Strategies

Whereas future therapeutic and diagnostic strategies will inevitably be developed, it is manifestly impossible to predict the details. Future research will, however, at a minimum, certainly target the following:

Identification of factors that destabilize previously stable plaque.
Development of diagnostic techniques to identify unstable or unstabilizing plaque.

Development of therapies to transiently and/or permanently stabilize coronary plaques.

Development of newer agents or better paradigms for use of existing anticoagulant/antiplatelet/thrombolytic agents to improve therapeutic efficacy and minimize hemorrhagic complications.

Development of new devices and strategies to define and minimize (eliminate) downstream microvascular occlusion occurring as a result of either disease progression or therapeutic intervention.

References

1. Fye WB. Acute myocardial infarction: a historical summary. In: Gersh BJ, Rahimtoola SH, eds. Acute myocardial infarction. 2nd ed. New York: Chapman and Hall; 1997:1–5.
2. Krehl L. Die Ekrankungen des Herzmuskels und die Nervosen Herzkrankheiten. Vienna: Alfred Holder; 1901.
3. Herrick JB. Certain clinical features of sudden obstruction of the coronary arteries. JAMA 1912;59:2015–2020.
4. Parkinson J, Bedford E. Cardiac infarction and coronary thrombosis. Lancet 1928; 1:4–11.
5. Levine SA. Coronary thrombosis: its various clinical features. Medicine 1929; 8:245–418.
6. Levine SA, Lown B. Armchair treatment of acute coronary thrombosis. JAMA 1952; 148:1365–1369.
7. Harrison TR, Resnik WH. Etiologic aspects of heart disease (including treatment of the different etiologic types). In: Harrison TR, Beeson PB, Resnik WH, Thom GW, Wintrobe MM, eds. Principles of internal medicine. 2nd ed. New York: The Balkiston Co., 1950:1285–1289.
8. Julian DG. Treatment of cardiac arrest in acute myocardial ischemia and infarction. Lancet 1961;ii:840–844.
9. Pantridge JF, Geddes JS. A mobile coronary care unit in the management of myocardial infarction. Lancet 1967;2:271–273.
10. International Collaborative Study Group (ICSG). Reduction of infarct size with the early use of timolol in acute myocardial infarction. N Engl J Med 1984;310:9–15.
11. Davies MJ, Thomas AC. Plaque fissuring—the cause of acute myocardial infarction, sudden ischemic death, and crescendo angina. Br Heart J 1985;53:363–373.
12. Fletcher AP, Sherry S, Alkjaersig H, et al. The maintenance of a sustained thrombolytic state in man. II. Clinical observations on patients with myocardial infarction and other thromboembolic disorders. J Clin Invest 1959;38:1111–1119.
13. Verstraete M. Thrombolytic therapy in recent myocardial infarction. In: Meltzer LE, Dunning AJ, eds. Textbook of coronary care. Amsterdam: Excerpta Medica; 1972: 643–659.
14. Chazov El, Matveeva LS, Mazaev AV, et al. Intracoronary administration of fibrinolysin in acute myocardial infarction. Terapeuticheskds Arkhiv 1976;48:8–19.
15. Rentrop KP, Blanke H, Karsch KR, et al. Acute myocardial infarction: intracoronary application of nitroglycerin and streptokinase. Clin Cardiol 1979;2:354–363.
16. Gruppo Italiano per to Studio della Streptochinasi nell'Infarto Miocardico (GISSI). Effectiveness of intravenous thrombolysic treatment in acute myocardial infarction. Lancet 1986;1:397–402.

17. ISIS-2 (Second International Study of Infarct Survival) Collaborative Group. Randomised trial of intravenous streptokinase, oral aspirin, both, or neither among 17,187 cases of suspected acute myocardial infarction: ISIS-2. Lancet 1988;2: 349–360.

18. The TIMI Study Group. The Thrombolysis in Myocardial Infarction (TIMI) trial. Phase I findings. N Engl J Med 1985;312:932–936.

19. The GUSTO Investigators. An international randomized trial comparing four thrombolysic strategies for acute myocardial infarction. N Engl J Med 1993;329: 673–682.

20. The TIMI IIIB Investigators. Effects of tissue plasminogen activator and a comparison of early invasive and conservative strategies in unstable angina and non-Q wave myocardial infarction. Results of the TIMI IIIB Trial. Circulation 1994;89:1545–1556.

21. Hamm CV, Goldmann BU, Heeschen C, et al. Emergency room triage of patients with acute chest pain by means of rapid testing for cardiac troponin T or troponin I. N Engl J Med 1997;337:1648–1653.

22. Polanczyk CA, Lee TH, Cook EF, et al. Cardiac troponin I as a predictor of major cardiac events in emergency department patients with acute coronary care syndromes. J Am Coll Cardiol 1998;32:8–14.

23. Grüntzig A, Hopff H. Perkutane Rekanalisation chronischer arterieller Verschlüsse mit einem neuen Dilatationskatheter. Dtsch Med Wochenschr 1974;99:2502–2505.

24. Hurst JW. The first coronary angioplasty as described by Andreas Gruentzig. Am J Cardiol 1986;57:185–186.

25. Grines CL, Browne KF, Marco J, et al., for the Primary Angioplasty in Myocardial Infarction Study Group. A comparison of immediate angioplasty with thrombolytic therapy for acute myocardial infarction. N Engl J Med 1993;328:673–679.

26. Armstrong PW, Fu Y, Chang WC, et al., for the GUSTO-IIb Investigators. Acute coronary syndromes in the GUSTO-IIb trial: prognostic insights and impact of recurrent ischemia. Circulation 1998;98:1860–1868.

27. Weaver WD, Simes RJ, Betriu A, et al. Comparison of primary coronary angioplasty and intravenous thrombolytic therapy for acute myocardial infarction: a quantitative review. JAMA 1997;278:2093–2098.

28. Grines CL, Cox DA, Stone GW, et al., for the Stent Primary Angioplasty in Myocardial Infarction Study Group. Coronary angioplasty with or without stent implantation for acute myocardial infarction. N Engl J Med 1999;341:1949–1956.

29. Stone GW, Grines CL, Cox DA, et al. Comparison of angioplasty with stenting, with or without abciximab, in acute myocardial infarction. N Engl J Med 2002;346: 957–966.

30. Moses JW, Leon MB, Popma JJ, et al. Sirolimus-eluting stents versus standard stents in patients with stenosis in a native coronary artery. N Engl J Med 2003;349: 1315–1323.

31. Morice MC, Serruys PW, Sousa JE, et al. A randomized comparison of a sirolimus-eluting stent with a standard stent for coronary revascularization. N Engl J Med 2002;346:1773–1780.

32. Serruys PW, Degertekin M, Tanabe K, et al. Intravascular ultrasound findings in the multicenter, randomized, double-blind RAVEL (RAndomized study with the sirolimus-eluting VElocity balloon-expandable stent in the treatment of patients with de novo native coronary artery Lesions) trial. Circulation 2002;106:798–803.

33. Stone GW, Ellis SG, Cox DA, et al. A polymer-based, paclitaxel-eluting stent in patients with coronary artery disease. N Engl J Med 2004;350:221–231.

34. Cannon CP, Weintraub WS, Demopoulos LA, et al. Comparison of early invasive and conservative strategies in patients with unstable coronary syndromes treated with the glycoprotein IIb/IIIa inhibitor tirofiban. N Engl J Med 2001;344:1879–1887.
35. Fox K, Poole-Wilson P, Henderson R, et al. Interventional versus conservative treatment for patients with unstable angina or non-ST-elevation myocardial infarction: the British Heart Foundation RITA 3 randomised trial. Lancet 2002;360:743–751.
36. Effects of tissue plasminogen activator and a comparison of early invasive and conservative strategies in unstable angina and non-Q-wave myocardial infarction. Results of the TIMI IIIB Trial. Thrombolysis in Myocardial Ischemia. Circulation 1994;89:1545–1556.
37. Invasive compared with non-invasive treatment in unstable coronary-artery disease: FRISC II prospective randomised multicentre study. FRagmin and Fast Revascularisation during Instability in Coronary artery disease Investigators. Lancet 1999;354: 708–715.
38. Neumann FJ, Kastrati A, Pogatsa-Murray G, et al. Evaluation of prolonged antithrombotic pretreatment ("cooling-off" strategy) before intervention in patients with unstable coronary syndromes: a randomized controlled trial. JAMA 2003;290: 1593–1599.
39. Liuzzo G, Biasucci LM, Gallimore JR, et al. The prognostic value of C-reactive protein and serum amyloid A protein in severe unstable angina. N Engl J Med 1994;331:417–424.
40. Morrow DA, Rifai N, Antman EM, et al. C-reactive protein is a potent predictor of mortality independently and in combination with troponin T in acute coronary syndromes: a TIMI 11A substudy. J Am Coll Cardiol 1998;31:1460–1465.
41. Biasucci LM, Liuzzo G, Grillo RL, et al. Elevated levels of C-reactive protein at discharge in patients with unstable angina predict recurrent instability. Circulation 1999;99:855–860.
42. Schwartz GG, Olsson AG, Ezekowitz MD, et al. Effects of atorvastatin on early recurrent ischemic events in acute coronary syndromes. The MIRACL Study: a randomized controlled trial. JAMA 2001;285:1711–1718.

2
The PAIN Pathway for the Management of Acute Coronary Syndrome

Eyal Herzog, Emad Aziz, and Mun K. Hong

Acute coronary syndrome (ACS) subsumes a spectrum of clinical entities, ranging from unstable angina to ST-elevation myocardial infarction [1]. The management of ACS is deservedly scrutinized, as it accounts for 2 million hospitalizations and a remarkable 30% of all deaths in the Unites States each year [2]. Clinical guidelines on the management of ACS, which are based on clinical trials, have been updated and published [3, 4].

Large-scale registries—the NRMI [5], CRUSADE [6], and GRACE [7] registries—have consistently demonstrated a major gap between ACS management guidelines and their practical application in the real world. Accordingly, a major message that emerges from these quality-improvement registries is that there is an urgent need to incorporate the evidence-based guidelines into our daily management of ACS. In an attempt to achieve this goal, we have developed a new pathway for the management of ACS at our institution, St. Luke's Roosevelt Hospital Center (SLRHC), which is a university hospital of Columbia University College of Physicians and Surgeons. The necessity to develop such a pathway at our institution is compelling yet typical of the need at many similar medical centers.

The evidence-based information obtained from the large-scale clinical trials and from the guidelines is increasingly complex. Specifically, it has become exceedingly difficult for all house staff and emergency room staff to grasp all of the subtleties in the management of ACS patients. To address this problem, we have developed a unified pathway for the management of patients presenting with acute chest pain or its equivalent.

The pathway has been designated by the acronym PAIN (priority risk, advanced risk, intermediate risk and negative/low risk), which reflects a patient's most immediate risk stratification upon admission (Fig. 2.1). This risk stratification reflects a patient's 30-day risks for death and myocardial infarction after the initial ACS event.

The PAIN pathway is color-coded (P, red; A, yellow; I, yellow; N, green) and will guide patient management according to a patient's risk stratification. These colors—similar to the road traffic light code—have been chosen as an easy reference for the provider about the sequential risk level of patients with ACS [8].

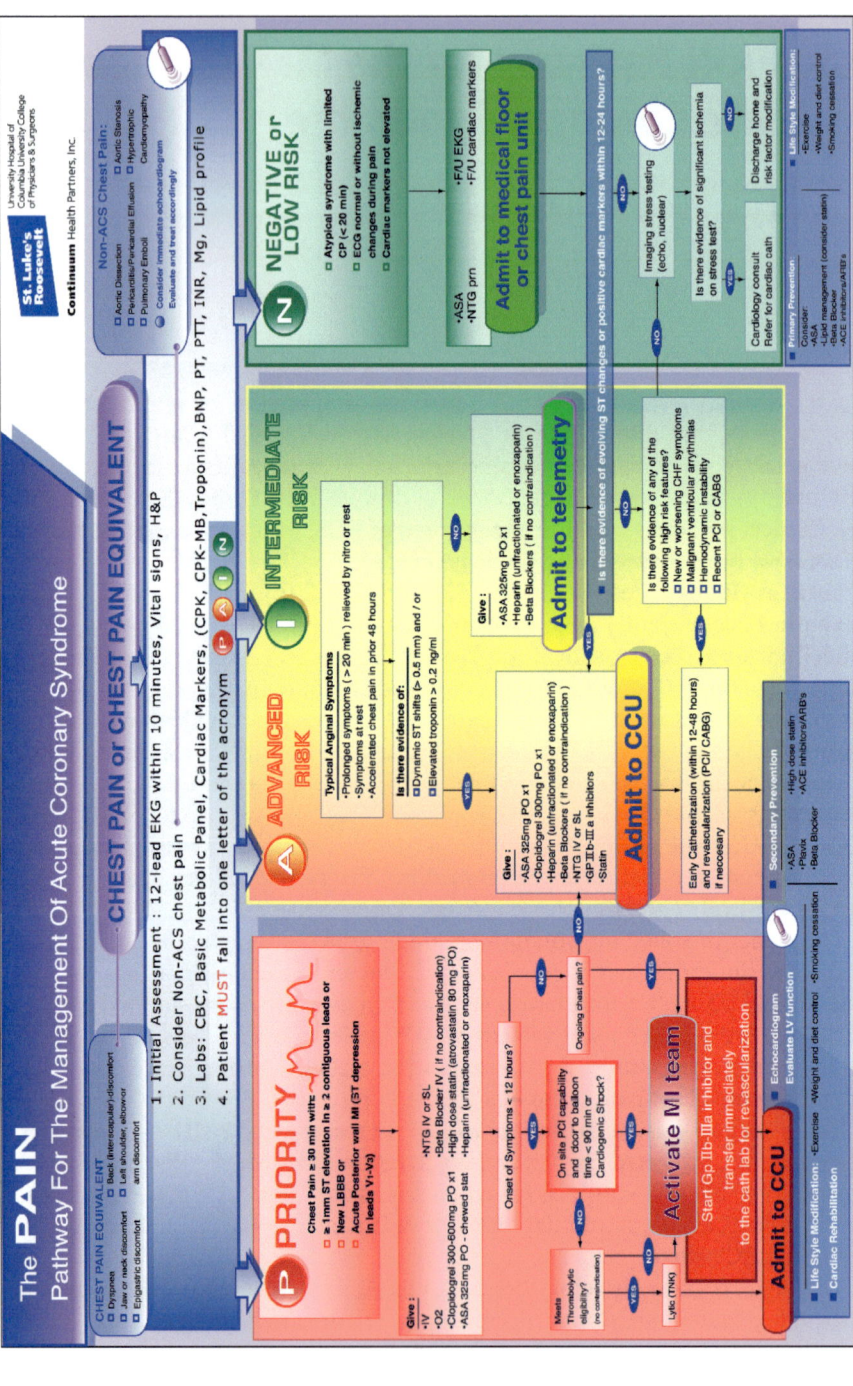

FIGURE 2.1. The PAIN pathway for the management of ACS.

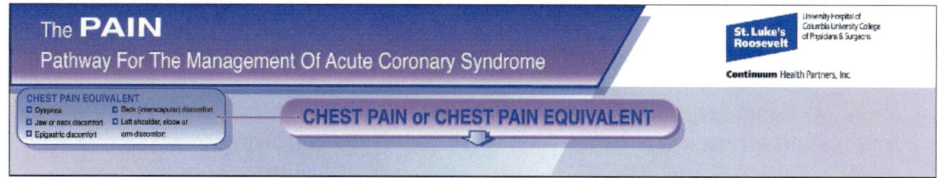

FIGURE 2.2. Chest pain and chest pain equivalent symptoms.

The Goals of the PAIN Pathway and a Road Map to this Acute Coronary Syndrome Book

Initial Assessment of Patients with Chest Pain or Chest Pain Equivalent

Patients who present to emergency departments with chest pain or chest pain equivalent will be enrolled into this pathway.

Figure 2.2 shows the chest pain equivalent symptoms. The initial assessment is seen in Figure 2.3. A detailed description of emergency department assessment is provided in Chapter 5. All patients should have an electrocardiogram (ECG) performed within 10 minutes as well as detailed history and physical exam.

Non-ACS chest pain should be excluded urgently. This includes aortic dissection, pericarditis and pericardial effusion, pulmonary emboli, aortic stenosis, and hypertrophic cardiomyopathy. If any of these emergency conditions is suspected, we recommend obtaining immediate echocardiogram or computed tomography (CT) and to treat accordingly.

Our recommended initial laboratory tests include complete blood count, basic metabolic panel, cardiac markers (to include CPK, CPK-MB, troponin), BNP, PT, PTT, INR, magnesium, and a lipid profile.

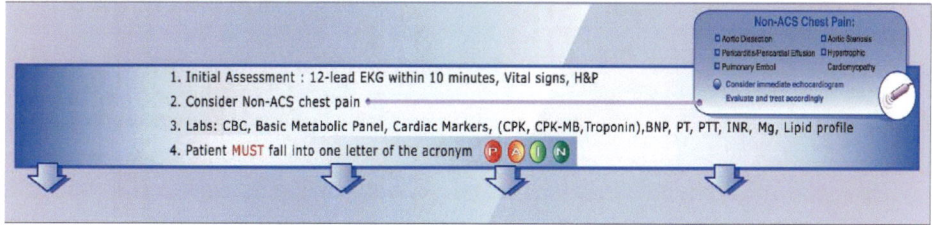

FIGURE 2.3. Initial assessment of patients with chest pain.

Initial Management of PRIORITY Patients (Patients with ST-Elevation Myocardial Infarction)

PRIORITY patients are those with symptoms of chest pain or chest pain equivalent lasting longer than 30 minutes with one of the following ECG criteria for acute myocardial infarction:

1. ST elevation ≥1 mm in two contiguous leads; or
2. New left bundle branch block; or
3. Acute posterior wall myocardial infarction (ST-segment depression in leads V_1-V_3).

The initial treatment of these patients includes obtaining an intravenous line, providing oxygen, treating patients with oral aspirin (chewable 325 mg, stat), clopidogrel (300 mg or 600 mg loading dose), and intravenous beta-blocker (if no contraindication), heparin (unfractionated or enoxaparin), nitroglycerin, and oral high-dose statin (Fig. 2.4). A detailed dosing and the rationale for this management appear in Chapter 6.

The key question for further management of these patients is the duration of the patients' symptoms. For patients whose symptoms exceed 12 hours, presence of persistent or residual chest pain determines the next strategy. If there is no evidence of continued symptoms, these patients will be treated as if they had been risk stratified with the Advanced Risk group.

For patients whose symptoms are less than 12 hours or with ongoing chest pain, the decision for further management is based on the availability of on-site

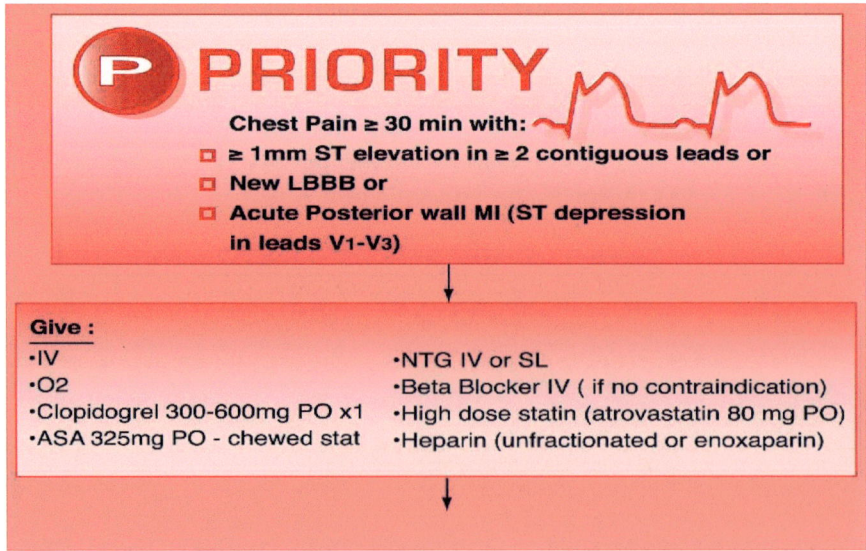

FIGURE 2.4. The initial management of PRIORITY patients (patient with ST-elevation myocardial infarction).

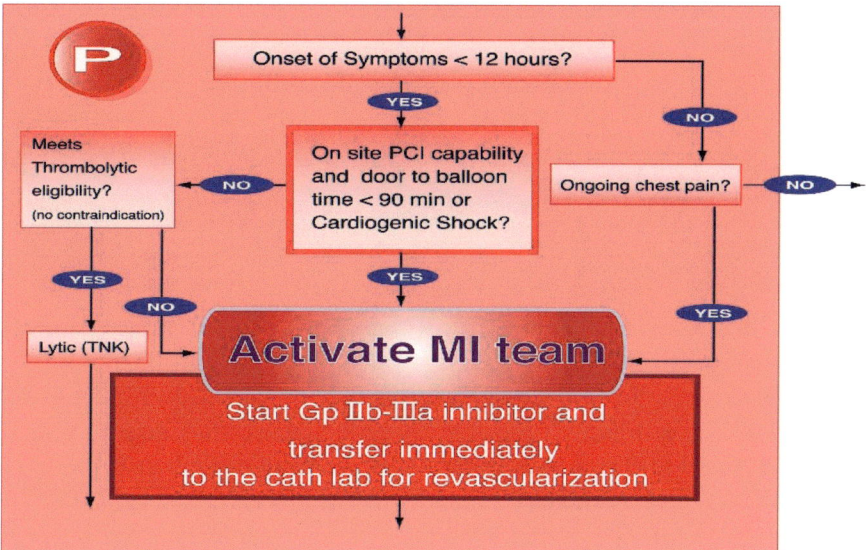

FIGURE 2.5. Advanced management of PRIORITY myocardial infarction patients with expected door to balloon time of less than 90 minutes.

angioplasty (PCI) capability with expected door to balloon time of less than 90 minutes or the presence of cardiogenic shock. A detailed discussion of cardiogenic shock appears in Chapter 13.

Patients with expected door to balloon time of less than 90 minutes should be started on intravenous treatment of glycoprotein IIb/IIIa inhibitors and they should be transferred immediately to the cardiac catheterization lab for revascularization. The myocardial infarction (MI) team is activated for this group of patients (Fig. 2.5).

At our institution, a single call made by the emergency department physician to the page operator activates the MI team, which includes the following health care providers:

1. The interventional cardiologist on-call
2. The director of the cardiac care unit (CCU)
3. The cardiology fellow on-call
4. The interventional cardiology fellow on-call
5. The cath lab nurse on-call
6. The cath lab technologist on-call
7. The CCU nursing manager on-call
8. The senior internal medicine resident on-call.

Activating this group of people has been extremely successful at our institution and has reduced markedly our door to balloon time. These strategies have been recently shown to decrease door to balloon time in the range of 8 to 19 minutes [9].

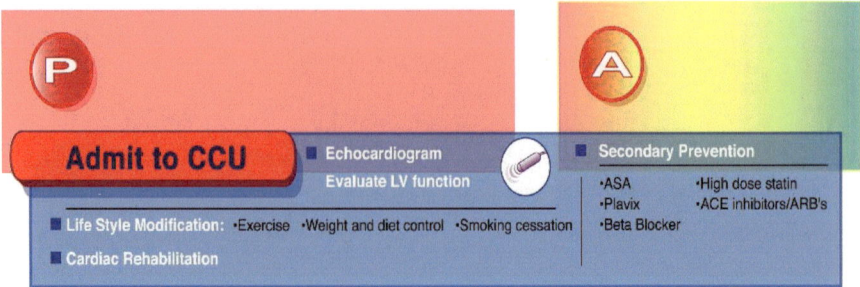

Figure **2.6.** CCU management and secondary prevention for patients with PRIORITY myocardial infarction.

For hospitals with no PCI capability or in situations when door to balloon time is expected to exceed 90 minutes, we recommend thrombolytic therapy if there are no contraindications.

CCU Management and Secondary Prevention for Patients with PRIORITY Myocardial Infarction

Patients with PRIORITY myocardial infarction should be admitted to the CCU (Fig. 2.6). A detailed description of CCU management appears in Chapter 6. All patients should have an echocardiogram to evaluate left ventricle systolic and diastolic function and to exclude valvular abnormality and pericardial involvement (as described in Chapter 14). We recommend a minimum CCU stay of 24 hours to exclude arrhythmia complication (as described in Chapters 16 to 18) or mechanical complication (as described in Chapter 11). For patients with no evidence of mechanical complications or significant arrhythmia, secondary prevention drugs should be started, including aspirin, clopidogrel, high-dose statin, beta-blocker, and angiotensin-converting enzyme (ACE) inhibitor or angiotensin receptor blocker.

Most patients can be discharge within 48 hours with recommendation for lifestyle modification including exercise, weight and diet control, smoking cessation (Chapter 26), and cardiac rehabilitation. Secondary prevention drugs should be continued on discharge as discussed in Chapter 25.

Management of Advanced Risk ACS

Typical anginal symptoms are required to be present in patients, who will enroll into the Advanced Risk or the Intermediate Risk groups. These symptoms include:

1. Prolonged chest pain (>20 minutes) relieved by nitroglycerine or rest;
2. Chest pain at rest; or
3. Accelerated chest pain within 48 hours.

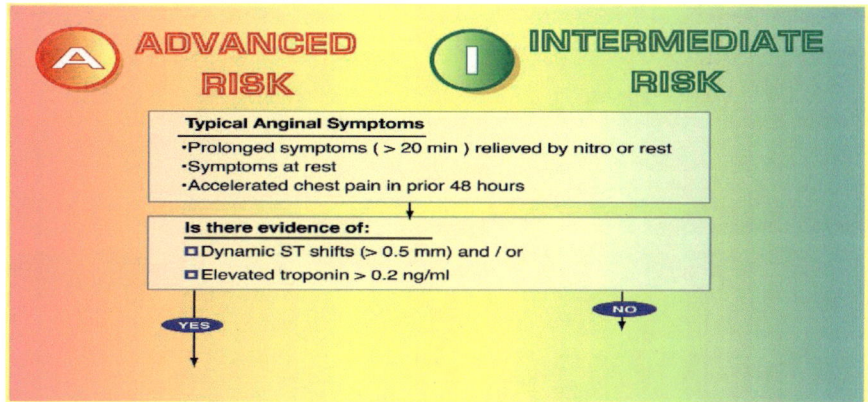

FIGURE 2.7. Risk stratification as Advanced Risk ACS.

In order to qualify for the Advanced Risk group, patients must have either dynamic ST changes on the electrocardiogram (>0.5 mm) and/or elevated troponin (>0.2 ng/mL) (Fig. 2.7).

A detailed description of the management of Advanced Risk patients appears in Chapter 7. We recommend that patients be admitted to the CCU and be treated with aspirin, clopidogrel, heparin, glycoprotein IIb/IIIa inhibitor, beta-blocker, statin, and nitroglycerin if there are no contraindications (Fig. 2.8).

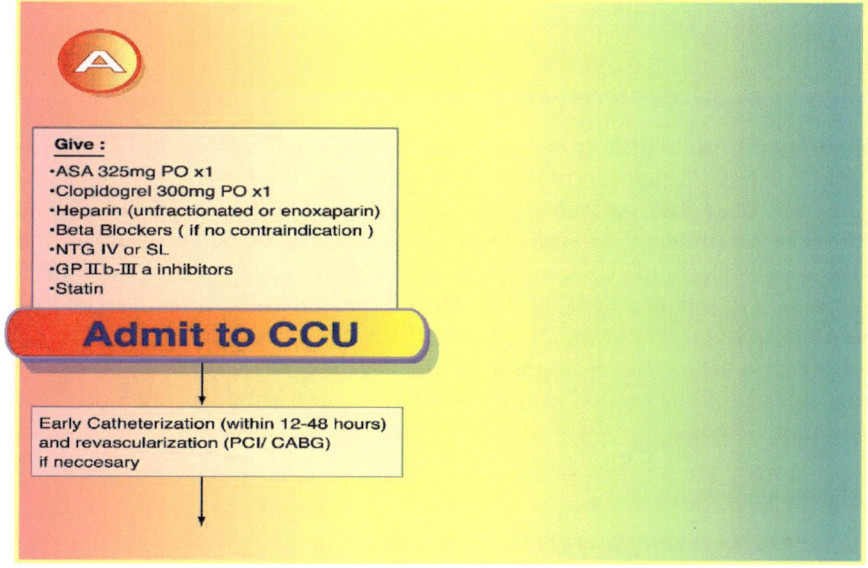

FIGURE 2.8. Management of patients with Advanced Risk ACS.

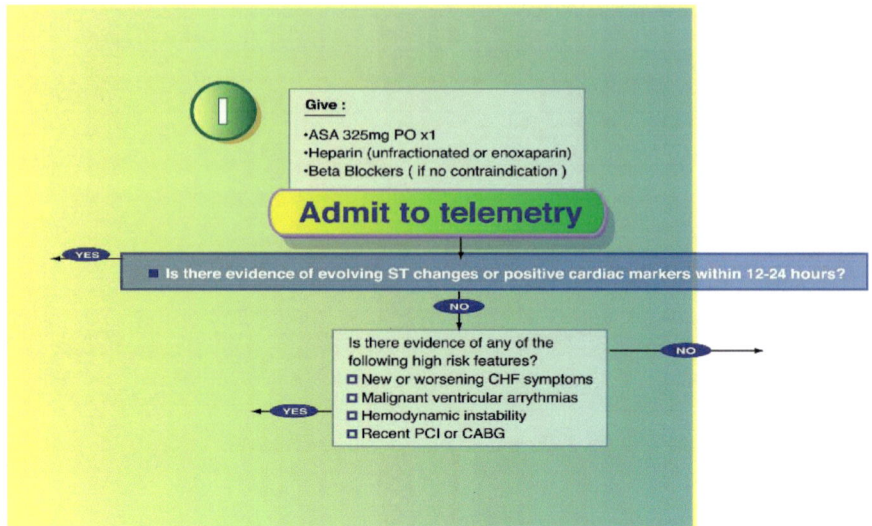

FIGURE 2.9. Management of patients with Intermediate Risk ACS.

These patients should have early cardiac catheterization within 12 to 48 hours and revascularization by PCI or coronary artery bypass surgery (CABG) if necessary. All patients should have an echocardiogram to evaluate left ventricular function. Recommendation for secondary prevention medication, lifestyle modification, and cardiac rehabilitation should be provided similar to the patients in the PRIORITY risk group (Fig. 2.6).

Management of Intermediate Risk Group

Both Intermediate Risk group and Advanced Risk patients present to the hospital with typical anginal symptoms. Compared with the Advanced Risk patients, the Immediate Risk patients *do not* have evidence of dynamic ST changes on the electrocardiogram or evidence of positive cardiac markers (see Chapter 8). These patients should be admitted to the telemetry floor and be given aspirin, heparin, and beta-blocker (Fig. 2.9). We recommend a minimum telemetry stay of 12 to 24 hours. If during this period of time there is evidence of dynamic ST changes on the electrocardiogram or evidence for positive cardiac markers, the patients should be treated as if they had been stratified to the Advanced Risk group.

The Intermediate Risk group patients are assessed again for the following high risk features:

1. New or worsening heart failure symptoms;
2. Malignant ventricular arrhythmias;
3. Hemodynamic instability; or
4. Recent (<6 months) PCI or CABG.

If there is evidence of any of these high-risk features, we recommend to transfer the patient for cardiac catheterization within 12 to 48 hours and for revascularization by PCI or CABG if necessary. Patients with no evidence of high-risk features should be referred for cardiac imaging stress testing (stress echocardiography or stress nuclear test).

Management of Negative or Low Risk Group Patients

These patients have atypical symptoms and do not have significant ischemic ECG changes during pain and do not have elevated cardiac markers.

These patients should be treated only with aspirin and given sublingual nitroglycerin if needed. If a decision was made to admit them to the hospital, they should be admitted to a chest pain unit or to a regular medical floor. They should be followed up for 12 to 24 hours with repeated ECG and cardiac markers (Fig. 2.10). If there is evidence of evolving ST changes on the electrocardiogram or evidence of positive cardiac markers, the patients would be treated aggressively as with the Advanced Risk patients.

If there are no significant ECG changes and all cardiac markers are negative, we recommend cardiac imaging stress testing (by stress echocardiography or stress nuclear test) (Fig. 2.11). Evidence of significant ischemia on any of these stress imaging modalities will be followed by a referral for cardiac catheterization.

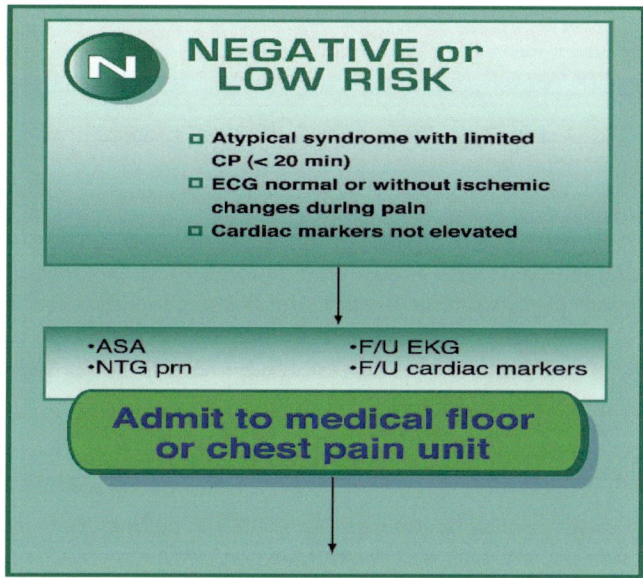

FIGURE 2.10. Initial management of patients with Negative or Low Risk ACS.

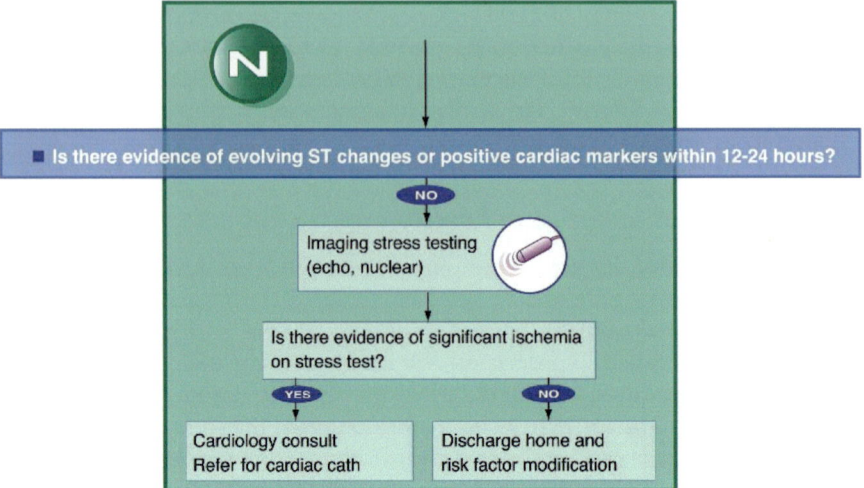

FIGURE **2.11.** Risk stratification of Low Risk patients by using cardiac imaging stress testing.

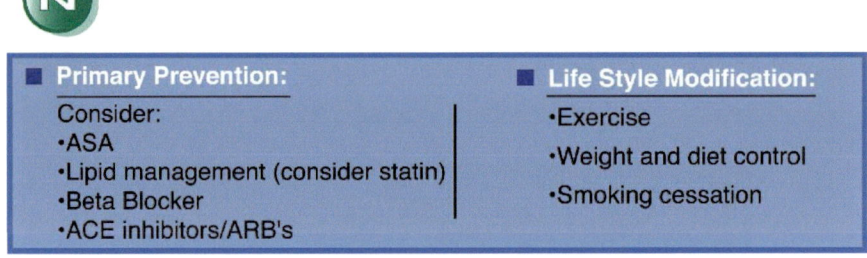

FIGURE **2.12.** Primary prevention for Low Risk patients.

If there is no evidence of significant ischemia on stress testing, the patients will be discharged home with a recommendation for risk-factor modification to include primary prevention medication and lifestyle modification (Fig. 2.12).

In summary, we believe that this comprehensive yet simple pathway will be able to bridge the gap between the complex evidence-based guidelines and practical management of patients with ACS.

References

1. Herzog E, Saint-Jacques H, Rozanski A. The PAIN pathway as a tool to bridge the gap between evidence and management of acute coronary syndrome. Crit Pathways Cardiol 2004;3:20–24.

2. Califf RM. Acute coronary syndromes: ACS essentials. Royal Oak, MI: Physicians' Press; 2003.

3. Braunwald E, Antman EM, Beasley JW, et al. ACC/AHA guidelines update for the management of patients with unstable angina and non-ST elevation myocardial infarction: a report of the American College of Cardiology/American Heart Association Task Force on Practice Guidelines (Committee on the Management of Patients with Unstable Angina). J Am Coll Cardiol 2000;36:970–1062.

4. Antman EM, Anbe DT, Armstrong PW, et al. ACC/AHA guidelines for the management of patients with ST-elevation myocardial infarction. J Am Coll Cardiol 2004;44: 671–719.

5. Spencer FA, Meyer TE, Gore JM, et al. Heterogeneity in the management and outcomes of patients with acute myocardial infarction complicated by heart failure: the National Registry of Myocardial Infarction. Circulation 2002;105:2605–2610.

6. Hoekstra JW, Pollack CV Jr, Roe MY, et al. Improving the care of patients with non-ST-elevation acute coronary syndromes in the emergency department: the CRUSADE initiative. Acad Emerg Med 2002;9:1146–1155.

7. Fox KA, Goodman SG, Klein W, et al. Management of acute coronary syndromes. Variations in practice and outcomes; findings from the Global Registry of Acute Coronary Events (GRACE). Eur Heart J 2002;23:1177–1189.

8. Saint-Jacques H, Burroughs VJ, Watowska J, et al. Acute coronary syndrome critical pathway: chest PAIN caremap—a qualitative research study-provider-level intervention. Crit Pathways Cardiol 2005;4:145–156.

9. Bradley EH, Herrin J, Wang YF, et al. Strategies for reducing the door-to-balloon time in acute myocardial infarction. N Engl J Med 2006;355:2308–2320.

3
Translation of Critical Pathways for Acute Coronary Syndrome into Admission Notes and Discharge Planning

Eyal Herzog, Emad Aziz, and Mun K. Hong

Acute coronary syndrome (ACS) accounts for the majority of admissions to medical and cardiac services in U.S. hospitals. Guidelines for the management of ACS [1, 2] have been published by the American College of Cardiology (ACC) and the American Heart Association (AHA).

We have recently developed and published a unique pathway for the management of ACS [3] at St. Luke's Roosevelt Hospital–Columbia University College of Physician and Surgeons in New York City. Our updated pathway as described in Chapter 2 of this book is designed to optimize care for patients using clinical evidence models and to teach physicians-in-training consensus evaluation and management strategies. To facilitate implementation of our pathway to improve and standardize patient care when appropriate, we have developed user-friendly admission and discharge forms based on these pathways [4]. Residents who rotate through the cardiac care unit, the telemetry and the cardiac medical floors are required to complete these preprinted forms for admission and discharge of patients with ACS. These forms act as a reminder of key points of the pathway, as data collection devices, and most importantly as an agreement or "buy-in" on discharge between patients and their health care providers. The key points of the discharge form include a review of medications, side effects, smoking cessation, exercise, a follow-up appointment, and an understanding that they will be contacted by phone after discharge for follow-up of their condition.

There are two pages to the admission form. The first page (Fig. 3.1) is a general cardiac admission note. It is completed by the admitting resident in lieu of a traditional admission note and serves as a data collection device. The medical intern and the attending physician are required to write the more traditional admission notes. The second page of the admission form (Fig. 3.2) is a composite of admission information based on our chest pain pathway.

This form reproduces the format of the chest pain pathway as described in Chapter 2. It emphasizes the concept of risk stratification of patients presenting with chest pain using the acronym PAIN (priority risk, advanced risk, intermediate risk, and negative/low risk), which reflects the patient's initial risk stratification upon admission. The plan for patient care is dictated by the

St Luke's-Roosevelt Hospital
Advanced Cardiac Admission Protocol

Demographics   Age:_____ Gender:_____
Date:_____   Time of triage:_____
Race: ☐ Black ☐ White ☐ Hispanic ☐ Asian ☐ Others
Primary care physician : _____
Cardiologist (if any) : _____
Admit to: Service: ☐ CCU service   ☐ Medicine Team
　　　　　Floor: ☐ Telemetry ☐ Non Telemetry ☐ CCU
　　　　　　　　 ☐ Teaching | | Non Teaching

History Of Present Illness:

Cardiovascular Risk Factors:
☐ Hypertension (yrs_____)   ☐ Dyslipidemia (yrs_____)
☐ Diabetes (yrs_____)   　　☐ LDL >130mg/dl
☐ Family Hx of early CAD   　☐ HDL<40mg/dl

　Smoking: ☐ Active ☐ Ex-smoker   ☐ Non-Smoker
Others:
• Prior MI   ☐ Yes ☐ No   Date (if yes):_____
• Prior PCI   ☐ Yes ☐ No   Date (if yes):_____
• Prior CABG ☐ Yes ☐ No   Date (if yes):_____
• Known CHF ☐ Yes ☐ No   EF (if yes):_____
• Prior Imaging ☐ Yes ☐ No   Date (if yes):_____
　☐ 2D Echo ☐ Stress Echocardiogram   ☐ Nuclear Test
　Results:_____
　_____
　_____

Past Medical & Surgical History:
PMH:_____
Surgical:_____
Alcohol:_____
Substance abuse:_____

Medications (Home):   (Please enter drug and dose)
☐ Aspirin_____   ☐ Insulin_____
☐ Clopidogrel_____   ☐ Oral hypoglycemics_____
☐ Beta blocker_____   ☐ Anti Retroviral_____
☐ ACEI/ARB_____   ☐ Antibiotics_____
☐ Ca channel blocker___ ☐ Nebulizer/ inhalers_____
☐ Diuretic_____   ☐ Corticosteroids_____
☐ Digoxin_____   ☐ NSAIDS_____
☐ Aldosterone antagonist___ ☐ Statins_____
☐ Others (please specify)_____

Physical Exam: Height:_____ Weight:_____
Vitals: Pulse_____ BP_____ RR_____ Temp_____
HEENT:_____   Extremities_____
Respiratory System:_____
CVS:_____
Abdomen:_____
CNS:_____

Laboratory:
Troponin: 1st_____ 2nd_____ 3rd_____
CPK: 1st_____ 2nd_____ 3rd_____
CK-MB: 1st_____ 2nd_____ 3rd_____
Lipids: LDL_____ HDL_____ Tchols_____
　　　Triglycerides_____

BNP levels: (if Obtained)_____ HBA1c_____ (date)_____
Chest Xray: _____

Electrocardiogram
Rhythm: ☐ Sinus ☐ Sinus Brady ☐ Sinus Tachy ☐ Afib ☐ Aflutter
　　　　☐ Paced ☐ Vtach   ☐ Others_____
AV Conduction: ☐ 1°AVB ☐ 2°AVB ☐ 3°AVB ☐ IVCD
　　　　☐ RBBB ☐ LBBB
Rate: _____   QRS duration_____
Infarct pattern: ☐ STEMI   ☐ NSTEMI
　　　☐ Inferior ☐ Posterior ☐ Anterior ☐ Septal ☐ Lateral
Maximal ST change:_____ elevation/ depression

Hypertrophy: ☐ LAE ☐ RAE ☐ RVH ☐ LVH ☐ LVH with strain
ST T wave changes: (NS = nonspecific)
　　　☐ ST c/w Ischemia ☐ NS ST ☐ NS T
　　　☐ NS ST & T ☐ Early Repolarization
Q Wave: Leads_____

Assessment & Plan:
_____
_____
_____
_____
_____
_____
_____
_____
_____
_____
_____
_____
_____
_____
_____
_____
_____
_____

Resident Name:_____   Beeper No:_____
Signature:_____

Figure 3.1. The first page of the ACS admission form.

category chosen. For example, patients in category A (Advanced Risk) are to be given all the medications corresponding with the section that is coded with "A" including heparin, antiplatelet agents (aspirin, clopidogrel, glycoprotein IIb/IIIa inhibitors), beta-blocker, angiotensin-converting enzyme (ACE) inhibitor, and a statin. In contrast, patients in low risk category "N" are given only aspirin.

St Luke's Roosevelt Hospital

Advanced Cardiac Admission Protocol "ACAP" For Patients With Acute Coronary Syndrome

Chest Pain Risk Stratification

☐ **P**riority   ☐ **A**dvance   ☐ **I**ntermediate   ☐ **N**egative

ST Elevation ACS:

CP (>=30 mins) <u>With:</u>
☐ >= 1mm ST in 2 leads <u>or</u>

☐ New LBBB <u>or</u>

☐ Acute Posterior Wall MI "ST depression in leads V1-V3"

↓

☐ **Activate MI Team**

Typical Anginal Symptoms:
☐ Prolonged Symptoms (>20 min) relieved by NTG or rest
☐ Symptoms at rest
☐ Accelerated chest pain in prior 48 hours

Is there evidence of::
☐ Dynamic ST shifts (>0.5 mm) ➔ NO ➔ **Admit to Telemetry**
☐ Elevated troponin > 0.2 ng/ml

↓

YES

Admit to CCU ◄

☐ Early Catheterization (within 12-48 hours) and revascularization (PCI/CABG)

Is there evidence of any of high risk features?:
☐ New or worsening HF symptoms
☐ Malignant Ventricular Arrhythmias
☐ Hemodynamic Instability
☐ Recent PCI or CABG

☐ Limited CP (<20mins)

☐ EKG normal or without ischemic changes

☐ Cardiac markers not elevated

Plan

Heparins: P A I
☐ UFH (Unfractionated Heparin)
☐ Enoxaprin (1mg/ kg SQ q12h)

Antiplatelet Agents: P A I N

☐ Aspirin (For acute MI first dose 325 mg non enteric coated STAT followed by 75- 325 mg po enteric coated daily)
☐ 81mg ☐ 162 mg ☐ 325 mg
☐ Cannot take aspirin because_____

☐ Clopidogrel (300-600 mg po STAT then 75 mg pc daily) P A
☐ 600 mg ☐ 300 mg ☐ 75 mg
☐ Cannot take because_____

☐ GP IIb/IIIa (Given in conjunction with heparin) P A
☐ Integrilin ☐ Abciximab (prior PCI only)

Nitroglycerine: P A I N
☐ IV
☐ S/L

Beta Blockers: P A I
☐ Metoprolol (25-100 mg) _____ mg po q 12 h
☐ Carvedilol (3.125-25 mg) _____ mg po q 12 h
☐ Cannot take beta blocker because_____
  ☐ Advanced Heart Block ☐ Hypotension ☐ Decompensated CHF
  ☐ Severe Bradycardia ☐ Bronchospastic disease

ACE Inhibitors: P A
☐ Drug_____ mg po (daily/ q12h/ q8h/ q6h)
☐ Cannot take ACEI because_____

Statins: P A
☐ Drug_____ mg po daily
☐ Cannot take statins because_____

Other Medications: _____
_____
_____
_____
_____
_____
_____
_____

FIGURE 3.2. The second page of the admission form for patients with ACS admission based on the PAIN pathway.

The discharge form (Fig. 3.3) has four copies. One is to be given to the patient, the second one to the attending physician, the third one as a permanent part of the medical record, and the last copy used for entry into our database. The purpose of the discharge form is threefold:

1. Summarize all tests and procedures that have been performed during the hospital course.
2. Mandate discharge therapy for ACS patients based on their discharge category according to the acronym PAIN. For example, patients in category P (Priority) are to be given all the medications corresponding with that section

St Luke's Roosevelt Hospital

Cardiology Hospital Summary
For Patients
With Acute Coronary Syndrome

Chest Pain Pathway Discharge Summary

Discharge Category: ☐ **P**riority   ☐ **A**dvance   ☐ **I**ntermediate   ☐ **N**egative

☐ Antiplatelet Agents: **P A I N**
    ☐ Aspirin (75- 325 mg po enteric coated daily)
        ☐ 81mg   ☐ 162 mg   ☐ 325 mg
        ☐ Cannot take aspirin because_____
    ☐ Clopidogrel (75 mg po daily)   **P A**

☐ Beta Blockers: **P A I**
    ☐ Metoprolol (25-100 mg) _____ mg po q 12 h
    ☐ Carvedilol (3.125-25 mg) _____ mg po q 12 h
    ☐ Toprol XL (50-200 mg)_____ mg po daily
    ☐ Cannot take beta blocker because_____
        ☐ Advanced Heart Block   ☐ Hypotension   ☐ Decompensated CHF
        ☐ Severe Bradycardia   ☐ Bronchospastic disease

☐ ACE Inhibitors: **P A**
    ☐ Drug_____mg po (daily/ q12h/ q8h/ q6h)
    ☐ Cannot take ACEI because_____

☐ Statins: **P A**
    ☐ Drug_____mg po daily
    ☐ Cannot take statins because_____

INVESTIGATIONS/ PROCEDURES

☐ **Stress Test:**   Date_____

☐ **2-D Echocardiography:**   Date_____
    Type: ☐ Nuclear   ☐ Stress Echo
    Results_____
_____ EF:_____

☐ **Cardiac Catheterization:**   Date_____
    Intervention_____

I have been treated for chest pain or heart failure. For the quality improvement of the hospital care and to follow up on my own care, I agree to be called in followup over the course of the next year.

Patient's Signature:_____

RN Signature: _____   Date:_____

Housestaff Name:_____

Signature: _____   Date:_____

FIGURE 3.3. The discharge form for patients with ACS based on the PAIN pathway.

that is coded with "P" including antiplatelet agents (aspirin, clopidogrel) beta-blocker, ACE inhibitor, and a statin. If a drug cannot be used, then the reason for this has to be documented.

3. Document clearly medical recommendation for patients. This plan is signed by the patient, the physician, and the nurse. The recommended plan emphasizes the advice given to patients regarding their medical care, including instructions on smoking cessation, diet, and exercise. In signing the recommended plan, patients also give permission for follow-up phone calls from our group.

This signed discharge plan has the potential to optimize discharge planning and improve communication between patients and their health care providers. The explicit nature of this plan, with recommendations mandated according to the critical pathways, will hopefully improve physician adherence to published ACC/AHA guidelines for the management of ACS. In addition to improving standard of care, we believe we can improve patient awareness, compliance, and understanding of their care upon discharge with follow-up telephone calls.

References

1. Braunwald E, Antman EM, Beasley JW, et al. ACC/AHA guideline update for the management of patients with unstable angina and non-ST elevation myocardial infarction: a report of the American College of Cardiology/American Heart Association Task Force on Practice Guidelines (Committee on the Management of Patients with Unstable Angina). J Am Coll Cardiol 2000;36:970–1062.
2. Antman EM, Anbe DT, Armstrong PW, et al. ACC/AHA guidelines for the management of patients with ST-elevation myocardial infarction. J Am Coll Cardiol 2004;44:671–719.
3. Herzog E, Saint-Jacques H, Rozanski A. The PAIN pathway as a tool to bridge the gap between evidence and management of acute coronary syndrome. Crit Pathways Cardiol 2004;3:20–24.
4. Herzog E, Aziz E, Bangalore S, et al. Translation of critical pathways for acute coronary syndrome and for acute heart failure into admission forms and discharge planning. Crit Pathways Cardiol 2005;4:59–63.

4
Epidemiology and Pathophysiology of Acute Coronary Syndrome

Hossein Eftekhari, Inna Bukharovich, Emad Aziz, and Mun K. Hong

Acute coronary syndrome (ACS), one of the life-threatening manifestations of coronary artery disease, ranges from unstable angina, to acute myocardial infarction (non–ST elevation and ST elevation), to sudden cardiac death. The pathophysiology of ACS in the vast majority of cases involves coronary thrombosis overlying a disrupted atherosclerotic plaque [1]. Several autopsy studies have demonstrated that 70% to 80% of coronary thrombi occur at sites where the fibrous cap of coronary artery plaque has ruptured, with extension of the thrombus into the plaque and into the lumen, as well as with propagation of the thrombus upstream from the site of cap rupture [2, 3]. Although it would be preferable to prevent ACS rather than treat it after its occurrence, currently there is no optimal laboratory or imaging modality to predict its timing. Therefore, risk-factor modification is the best approach until reliable, noninvasive tests become available.

Epidemiology

In the United States, more than 13 million patients have coronary artery disease and annually more than 1.1 million patients experience acute myocardial infarction (AMI). Furthermore, 150,000 patients are diagnosed annually with unstable angina [4].

Death due to coronary atherosclerosis accounts for approximately 50% of all cardiac deaths, and 50% of coronary atherosclerosis deaths are sudden [1]. However, the percentages of sudden coronary death caused by disrupted plaques and thrombosis varies between 19% [5] and 81% [6]. Takada et al. examined individuals with old MI who died suddenly during the period from 1998 to 2001. The result of their pathology analysis revealed that sudden deaths were caused by ACS in 55%, fatal arrhythmia in 24%, cardiac pump failure in 14%, and other causes in 6% of cases. These findings signify that a new coronary plaque rupture independent of the old infarct is a major cause of sudden cardiac death with old MI [7]. Based on Centers for Disease Control and Prevention/National Center for Health Statistics (CDC/NCHS) report, 879,000 patients were discharged with initial diagnosis of ACS in 2003 in the United State (767,000 myocardial infarction and 112,000 with unstable angina) [8], and according to the National Heart, Lung, and Blood Institute Framingham Heart Study (NHLBI FHS) report, coronary heart disease comprises more than half of all cardiovascular events in men and women under age 75 [9]. Investigating the data of 7,733 participants in the Framingham Heart Study, Lloyd-Jones et al. demonstrated that the lifetime risks of initial coronary events after age 40 is 49% for men and 32% for women [10]. The NHLBI ARIC (Atherosclerotic Risks in Communities) study also revealed average age-adjusted coronary heart disease incidence rate per 1,000 person-years were 12.5 in white men, 10.6 in black men, 4.0 in white women, and 5.1 in black women [11].

Pathophysiology

Atherosclerosis used to be considered a bland lipid storage disease. According to the conventional theory, fatty streaks (earliest stage of atheroma) evolved into complicated plaques through multiplication of smooth muscle cells within the plaque, which laid down an abundant extracellular matrix. With coronary plaque progression, the arterial lumen narrowed until it impeded flow and caused ACS [12]. However, new advances in vascular biology have demonstrated that atherosclerosis is a systemic immune-mediated inflammatory disease affecting medium-sized and large arteries where various types of cells such as endothelial cells, leukocytes, and intimal smooth muscle cells are involved in its development [13]. It has also been demonstrated that inflammation has a fundamental role in mediating all stages of atherosclerosis from initiation through progression and eventually to its most devastating consequences, such as heart attack and stroke [12, 13]. Additionally, pathology study of atherosclerotic plaques suggests that physical plaque disruption can trigger thrombosis and thus may cause sudden expansion of atherosclerotic plaque and subsequently severe vascular narrowing [14]. Further studies demonstrated that acute thrombosis not only causes acute vascular narrowing but also underlies most acute coronary syndromes [15]. Finally, the concept of gradual progressive growing of atherosclerotic plaque has also been challenged through data that emerged from serial angiographic studies. These data suggested that atherosclerotic plaque progression is a highly unpredictable process and follows a nonlinear course [16].

The Concept of Vulnerable Plaque

In early 1980s, Falk demonstrated that ruptured atherosclerotic plaques were responsible for 40 of 51 recent coronary artery thrombi and 63 larger intimal hemorrhages [17]. He also demonstrated plaque fragments deeply buried in the thrombus overlying the athermanous plaque. In the late 1980s, Muller et al. proposed that the initial step in acute coronary thrombosis is the development

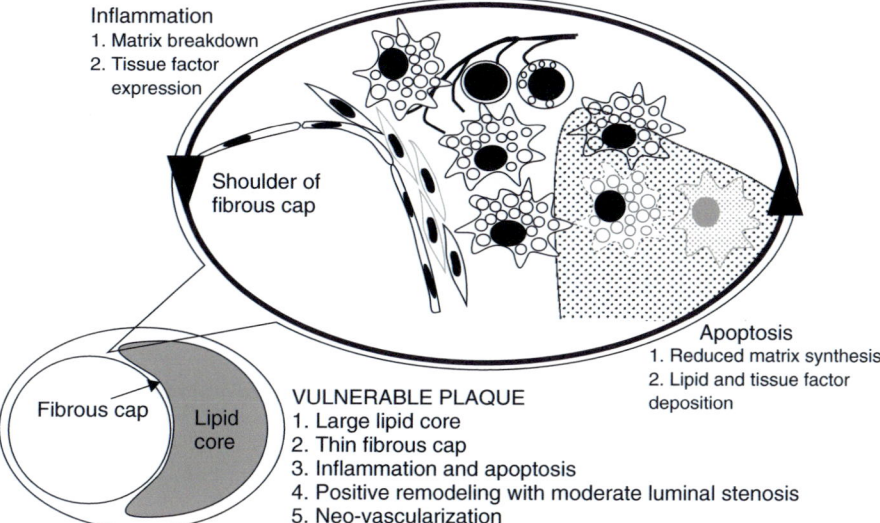

Inflammation
1. Matrix breakdown
2. Tissue factor
   expression

Shoulder of
fibrous cap

Apoptosis
1. Reduced matrix synthesis
2. Lipid and tissue factor
   deposition

Fibrous cap   Lipid
               core

VULNERABLE PLAQUE
1. Large lipid core
2. Thin fibrous cap
3. Inflammation and apoptosis
4. Positive remodeling with moderate luminal stenosis
5. Neo-vascularization

FIGURE 4.1. Components of a vulnerable plaque and a magnified view of the shoulder region with events contributing to plaque rupture. (Reproduced with permission from Shin J, Edelberg JE, Hong MK. Vulnerable atherosclerotic plaque: clinical implications. Curr Vasc Pharmacol 2003;1:183 204.)

of "vulnerable atherosclerotic plaque" [18]. The vulnerable plaques, as a potential precursor of unstable plaques, refer to those coronary atherosclerotic plaques that might become unstable and thus trigger ACS. Structural characteristics of vulnerable plaques include (Fig. 4.1) relatively large volume, positive remodeling, inflammatory cellular infiltrate of fibrous cap, especially at the "shoulder regions" and adventitia, increased neovascularity, central lipid core >40% of the total lesion area, and a thin fibrous cap [19]. These plaques are potentially vulnerable to mechanical stress and/or inflammatory weakening of their collagen structure. However, even today, it is impossible to predict how and when structurally vulnerable plaques may become unstable [20]. This is why detection of plaque vulnerability requires better understanding of the underlying inflammatory, structural, or yet unknown causes of plaque instability [20].

Role of Inflammation and Contribution to Plaque Rupture

Over the past few years, the prominent role of inflammation in atherogenesis and its acute complications have been well appreciated (Fig. 4.2). This new concept has resulted in increased interest in inflammation and immune response as major contributing factors in atherogenesis and ACS [12]. The normal endothelium (atheroprotective) prevents binding of white blood cells. However, in experimental studies, early after initiation of an atherogenic diet, endothelial

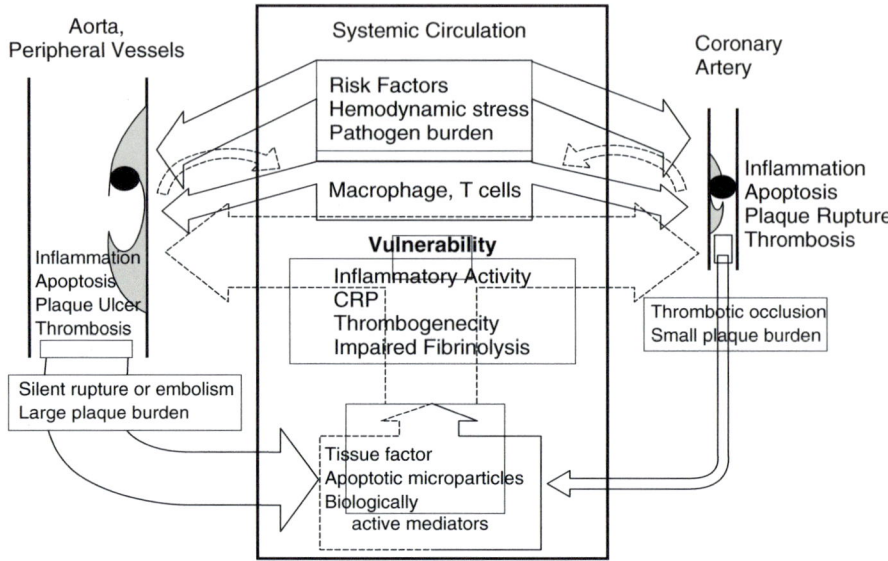

FIGURE 4.2. Potential interaction between the peripheral vascular disease and plaque rupture in coronary arteries. Systemic inflammatory activity is important for the rupture of a coronary artery plaque. It is hypothesized that the atheroma of the aorta and other peripheral vessels affects the vulnerability of the plaques in the coronary arteries through their influence on the circulating blood (*dashed line*, hypothetical interaction). (Reproduced with permission from Shin J, Edelberg JE, Hong MK. Vulnerable atherosclerotic plaque: clinical implications. Curr Vasc Pharmacol 2003;1:183–204.)

cells begin to express on their surface selective adhesion molecules, vascular cell adhesion molecule-1 (VCAM-1), that bind to various classes of leukocytes (monocyte and T lymphocyte) [12]. It has also been demonstrated that at branch points in arteries where the blood flow is disturbed, the endothelium loses its endogenous atheroprotective mechanisms [21]. Additionally, disturbed flow can augment the production of certain leukocyte adhesion molecules (e.g., intercellular adhesion molecule-1 [ICAM-1]) [22]. After adhesion to endothelium, leukocyte penetration into the intima (transmigration) is mediated by different chemoattractant molecules such as monocyte chemoattractant protein-1 (MCP-1), which is responsible for the direct migration of monocytes into the intima at sites of lesion formation [23]. Macrophage colony-stimulating factor (M-CSF), on the other hand, contributes to the differentiation of the blood monocyte into the macrophage, which ingests lipid and subsequently becomes foam cells [24]. Demonstrating the accumulation of activated T lymphocytes early in atheroma formation that persist at the sites of lesion growth and rupture, Mach et al. concluded that they may play an important role in the pathogenesis of atherosclerosis [25]. T cells also elaborate inflammatory cytokines such as γ-interferon and tumor necrosis factor-β that in turn can stimulate macrophages, vascular endothelial cells, and smooth muscle cells [26]. Inflammatory processes are not limited to initiation and evolution of plaque but also significantly contribute in acute thrombotic events. Proteolytic enzymes produced by activated macrophages degrade the collagen, resulting in thinning and weakening of fibrous cap, and leading to plaque rupture. Macrophage production of tissue factor (procoagulant) within atherosclerotic plaques also demonstrates an essential link between arterial inflammation and thrombosis [27]. On the other hand, interferon-γ arising from the activated T lymphocytes in the plaque interferes with collagen synthesis of smooth muscle cells and hence limits their capacity to reinforce the fibrous cap [28]. Vasospasm also contributes to impaired arterial blood flow in the presence of inflammation. This may be due in part to decreased production of nitric oxide. Additionally, augmented release of superoxide anion may annihilate nitric oxide radical, impairing its vasodilator capacity [29]. Nitric oxide in addition to being a vasodilator and platelet aggregation inhibitor has also a direct anti-inflammatory effect by augmenting production of the inhibitor of nuclear factor kappa B (NF-κB), a transcription factor involved in the expression of the genes encoding many proinflammatory functions of vascular wall cells and infiltrating leukocytes [30, 31]. These various findings all highlight the central role of inflammation as a determinant of the biology underlying the acute thrombotic complications of atherosclerosis [15].

Mechanisms of ACS

Coronary artery plaque rupture and subsequent thrombosis are the underlying cause of the majority of acute coronary syndromes [32, 33] and account for about 70% of acute myocardial infarctions and/or sudden coronary deaths (Fig. 4.3). Retrospective autopsy series and a few cross-sectional clinical studies revealed that thrombotic coronary death and acute coronary syndromes are caused by the ruptured plaque in 70% (stenotic, 20%; nonstenotic, 50%), and nonruptured plaques in 30% (erosion, calcified nodule, intraplaque hemorrhage, and unknown) [33–35]. The ruptured plaque represents the main stimulus to both thrombosis and coagulation in several ways, including activation of platelets and coagulation cascade subsequent to contact with collagen in the plaque's extracellular matrix, and tissue factor [36]. Endothelial desquamation (superficial erosion) is known as the second most common underlying cause of ACS, accounting for about 30% of acute coronary thromboses. Such areas of endothelial desquamation form the nidus of a platelet thrombus with subsequent platelet adhesion and activation [37].

Although many episodes of ACS are caused by the disruption or erosion of plaque, other mechanisms that alter myocardial oxygen supply and demand such as vasoconstriction and Prinzmetal angina can occur. In the setting of ACS, vasoconstriction may occur as a response to a mildly dysfunctional endothelium near the culprit lesion or due to the deep arterial damage or plaque disruption. This is usually mediated by platelet-dependent and thrombin-

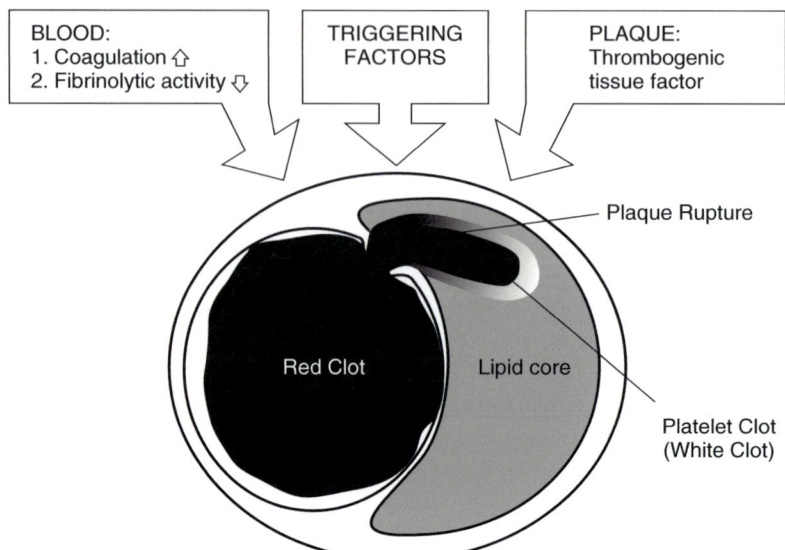

FIGURE 4.3. Rupture of a vulnerable plaque with thrombotic consequences. The plaque rupture exposes the highly thrombogenic lipid core, which in concert with the locally increased thrombogenicity causes the initial white clot (platelet rich) and the occlusive red clot (fibrin and red blood cell rich). (Reproduced with permission from Shin J, Edelberg JE, Hong MK. Vulnerable atherosclerotic plaque: clinical implications. Curr Vasc Pharmacol 2003;1:183–204.)

dependent vasoconstriction. However, in Prinzmetal angina, the site of transient, abrupt spasm is often adjacent to atheromatous plaque. Potential mechanisms of this type of angina include endothelial injury and hypercontractility of smooth muscle.

Transition from Stable Plaque to Vulnerable Plaque

Plaque rupture and endothelial erosion with subsequent thrombus formation are the most frequent causes of ACS [38]. However, intravascular ultrasound (IVUS) study conducted by Rioufol et al. [39] in patients with ACS revealed a high incidence of multiple plaque ruptures in these patients. Likewise, IVUS study by Maehara et al. [40] showed that plaque ruptures occur not only in ACS patients but also in patients with stable angina or asymptomatic ischemia. This finding suggests that the exact mechanisms as well as intrinsic or extrinsic factors contributing to transition of a stable plaque to a vulnerable plaque with or without ruptures are unknown and are likely to be variable among different lesions and patients [41]. Thus, it is not clear why some plaque ruptures lead to clinical syndrome whereas others remain asymptomatic and heal, perhaps leading to disease progression [42]. The transition of a stable plaque into a rupture-prone lesion is linked to the interplay among the fibrous cap thickness, smooth muscle cells, necrotic (lipid) core size, and extent of inflammatory activity [43, 44]. Coronary angioscopy study in patients with unstable angina demonstrated that glistering yellow lesions reflecting increased underlying lipid content were more prone to an acute coronary event compared with white lesions [45]. The lipid core is composed of free cholesterol, cholesterol crystals, and cholesterol esters derived from lipids that have infiltrated the arterial wall and also lipids derived from erythrocyte membrane and the death of foam cells [19, 46]. A large, eccentric lipid core may confer mechanical disadvantage by redistributing circumferential stress to the shoulder regions of the plaque, which contain a larger number of macrophages, T lymphocytes, and a paucity of smooth muscle cells. In nearly 60% of cases, the shoulder region of plaque is the area at which fibrous caps tend to rupture [47–49]. Interestingly, smooth muscle cells contribute to the plaque progression, but for vulnerable plaques, they are the major stabilizer by strengthening the fibrous cap [41].

Histopathology studies have shown that ruptured plaques contain more inflammatory cells than stable plaques. These cells are mostly monocyte macrophages, as well as activated T cells and mast cells that are found adjacent to the sites of cap rupture as well as in the adventitia [50–53]. These inflammatory cells are recruited into the atherosclerotic plaques by adhesion molecules, such as VCAM-1, and chemokines, such as MCP-1. Inflammatory cells can also be recruited inside the atherosclerotic lesion through the adventitial neovasculature, which is enhanced in atherosclerosis. Other factors contributing to recruitment of inflammatory cells and their activation in atherosclerosis include oxidized lipids, cytokines such as M-CSF, increased angiotensin II activity, elevated arterial pressure, diabetes, and chronic infections remote from the arterial wall [19, 54].

Matrix Disintegration Hypothesis of Vulnerable Plaque

It has been hypothesized that depletion of matrix components, especially fibrillar collagens of fibrous cap, caused by an imbalance between its synthesis and degradation leads to fibrous cap thinning. This predisposes the fibrous cap to rupture, either spontaneously or in response to hemodynamic changes or other trigger factors [33, 55]. Matrix metalloproteinases (MMP) are responsible for the matrix degradation. The most intense MMP activity is usually found in the macrophage and the extracellular space around the lipid core [56]. Thus, macrophage activity against oxidized lipoprotein causes serious plaque instability through MMP expression [57–59]. T cells, which tend to localize more at the shoulder region of plaque, also are involved in complex cellular interactions and autoimmune activity against modified lipoprotein [60–63]. The activated T cell–derived cytokine, interferon-γ, inhibits collagen gene expression in smooth muscle cells in vitro, which indirectly suggests that intraplaque activated T cells may inhibit matrix synthesis by producing interferon-γ [19].

Erosion of Plaque and Calcified Nodules

Coronary thrombi have been observed overlying atherosclerotic plaques in about 40% of ACS cases, without rupture of the fibrous cap [64]. Such thrombi occur over plaques with superficial endothelial erosion, which are particularly common in young victims of sudden death, in smokers, and in women [38, 64–66]. Plaques under such thrombi have a proteoglycan-rich matrix rather than a large lipid core, and the prevalence of inflammation is also lower than that found in plaque rupture [65]. The precise mechanisms of thrombosis in this scenario are unknown. It is believed that thrombosis in such case is initiated by enhanced platelet aggregability, depressed fibrinolysis, and increased circulating tissue factor levels [54]. Activated circulating leukocytes may transfer active tissue factor by shedding microparticles and transferring them onto adherent platelets [67, 68]. These circulating sources of tissue factor may contribute to thrombosis at sites of superficial endothelial denudation such as those found in plaque erosion. Furthermore, severe deficiencies of antithrombotic molecules, thrombomodulin, and protein-C receptor in advanced atherosclerotic lesions may also contribute to thrombosis [69].

Potential Triggers for Plaque Rupture

Although vulnerable plaque rupture may occur spontaneously without an obvious triggering factor, it may also follow a particular event, such as extreme physical activity, severe emotional stress, sexual activity, exposure to illicit drugs (cocaine, marijuana, amphetamines), exposure to cold, or acute infection [70–74]. Although plaque rupture often leads to clinical manifestations of an ACS, it may also occur without clinical manifestation (silent plaque rupture). As a major consequence of plaque rupture, thrombus formation is probably regulated by the thrombogenicity of the exposed plaque constituents, severity of underlying stenosis, platelet activation, and also by systemic thrombogenicity and fibrinolytic activity [34]. Lipid-rich plaques having high content of tissue factor may be more thrombogenic than fibrous plaques [75]. The main source of tissue factor is macrophage, which after its apoptosis may impregnate the lipid core with tissue factor–laden microparticles and therefore making the lipid core highly thrombogenic [76]. It has also been shown that atherosclerotic plaques of smokers contain more tissue factor and inflammatory cells than plaques of nonsmokers [77].

References

1. Farb A, Tang AL, Burke AP, et al. Sudden coronary death. Frequency of active coronary lesions, inactive coronary lesions, and myocardial infarction. Circulation 1995; 92:1701–1709.
2. Falk E. Plaque rupture with severe pre-existing stenosis precipitating coronary thrombosis. Characteristics of coronary atherosclerotic plaques underlying fatal occlusive thrombi. Br Heart J 1983;50:127–134.

3. Constantinides P. Atherosclerosis—a general survey and synthesis. Surv Synth Pathol Res 1984;3:477–498.
4. Narula J, Finn AV, Demaria AN. Picking plaques that pop. J Am Coll Cardiol 2005; 45:1970–1973.
5. Warnes CA, Roberts WC. Sudden coronary death: comparison of patients with to those without coronary thrombus at necropsy. Am J Cardiol 1984;54:1206–1211.
6. Davies MJ, Bland JM, Hangartner JR, et al. Factors influencing the presence or absence of acute coronary artery thrombi in sudden ischaemic death. Eur Heart J 1989;10:203–208.
7. Takada A, Saito K, Ro A, et al. Acute coronary syndrome as a cause of sudden death in patients with old myocardial infarction: a pathological analysis. Leg Med (Tokyo) 2003;5(Suppl 1):S292–S294.
8. Thom T, Haase N, Rosamond D, et al. Heart disease and stroke statistics—2006 update: a report from the American Heart Association Statistics Committee and Stroke Statistics Subcommittee. Circulation 2006;113:e85–151.
9. Hurst W. The Heart, arteries and veins. 10th ed. New York: McGraw-Hill; 2002.
10. Lloyd-Jones DM, Wang TJ, Leip EP, et al. Lifetime risk of developing coronary heart disease. Lancet 1999;353:89–92.
11. Jones D. Risk factors for coronary heart disease in African Americans. Arch Intern Med 2002;162:2565.
12. Libby P, Ridker PM, Maseri A. Inflammation and atherosclerosis. Circulation 2002; 105:1135–1143.
13. Falk E. Pathogenesis of atherosclerosis. J Am Coll Cardiol 2006;47(Suppl 1):C7–C12.
14. Davies MJ. Stability and instability: the two faces of coronary atherosclerosis. The Paul Dudley White Lecture, 1995. Circulation 1996;94:2013–2020.
15. Libby P. Current concepts of the pathogenesis of the acute coronary syndromes. Circulation 2001;104:365–372.
16. Yokoya K, Takatsu H, Suzuki T, et al. Process of progression of coronary artery lesions from mild or moderate stenosis to moderate or severe stenosis: a study based on four serial coronary arteriograms per year. Circulation 1999;100:903–909.
17. Falk E. Plaque rupture with severe pre-existing stenosis precipitating coronary thrombosis. Characteristics of coronary atherosclerotic plaques underlying fatal occlusive thrombi. Br Heart J 1983;50:127–134.
18. Muller JE, Tofler GH, Stone PH. Circadian variation and triggers of onset of acute cardiovascular disease. Circulation 1989;79:733–743.
19. Shah PK. Mechanisms of plaque vulnerability and rupture. J Am Coll Cardiol 2003; 41(Suppl S):15S–22S.
20. Maseri A, Fuster V. Is there a vulnerable plaque? Circulation 2003;107:2068–2071.
21. Topper JN, Cai J, Falb D, et al. Identification of vascular endothelial genes differentially responsive to fluid mechanical stimuli: cyclooxygenase-2, manganese superoxide dismutase, and endothelial cell nitric oxide synthase are selectively up-regulated by steady laminar shear stress. Proc Natl Acad Sci U S A 1996;93:10417–10422.
22. Nagel T, Resnick N, Atkinson WJ, et al. Shear stress selectively upregulates intercellular adhesion molecule-1 expression in cultured human vascular endothelial cells. J Clin Invest 1994;94:885–891.
23. Gu L, Okada Y, Clinton SK, et al. Absence of monocyte chemoattractant protein-1 reduces atherosclerosis in low-density lipoprotein-deficient mice. Mol Cell 1998;2: 275–281.

24. Qiao JH, Tripathi J, Mishra NK, et al. Role of macrophage colony-stimulating factor in atherosclerosis: studies of osteopetrotic mice. Am J Pathol 1997;150: 1687–1699.
25. Mach F, Sauty A, Larossi AS, et al. Differential expression of three T lymphocyte-activating CXC chemokines by human atheroma-associated cells. J Clin Invest 1999; 104:1041–1050.
26. Hansson G. The role of the lymphocyte. In: Fuster V, Ross R, Topol E, eds. Atherosclerosis and coronary artery disease. New York: Lippincott-Raven; 1996:557–568.
27. Libby P, Simon DI. Inflammation and thrombosis: the clot thickens. Circulation 2001;103:1718–1720.
28. Libby P, Geng YJ, Aikawa M, et al. Macrophages and atherosclerotic plaque stability. Curr Opin Lipidol 1996;7:330–335.
29. Ohara Y, Peterson TE, Harrison DG. Hypercholesterolemia increases endothelial superoxide anion production. J Clin Invest 1993;91:2546–2551.
30. De Caterina R, Libby P, Peng HB, et al. Nitric oxide decreases cytokine-induced endothelial activation. Nitric oxide selectively reduces endothelial expression of adhesion molecules and proinflammatory cytokines. J Clin Invest 1995;96:60–68.
31. Thurberg BI, Collins T. The nuclear factor-kappa B/inhibitor of kappa B autoregulatory system and atherosclerosis. Curr Opin Lipidol 1998;9:387–396.
32. Fuster V, Badimon L, Badimon JJ, et al. The pathogenesis of coronary artery disease and the acute coronary syndromes (2). N Engl J Med 1992;326:310–318.
33. Falk E, Shah PK, Fuster V. Coronary plaque disruption. Circulation 1995;92:657–671.
34. Davies MJ. A macro and micro view of coronary vascular insult in ischemic heart disease. Circulation 1990;82(Suppl):II38–46.
35. Virmani R, Kolodgie FD, Burke AP, et al. Lessons from sudden coronary death: a comprehensive morphological classification scheme for atherosclerotic lesions. Arterioscler Thromb Vasc Biol 2000;20:1262–1275.
36. Toschi V, Gallo R, Lettino M, et al. Tissue factor modulates the thrombogenicity of human atherosclerotic plaques. Circulation 1997;95:594–599.
37. Faggiotto A, Ross R, Harker L. Studies of hypercholesterolemia in the nonhuman primate. I. Changes that lead to fatty streak formation. Arteriosclerosis 1984;4: 323–340.
38. Davies MJ, Thomas A. Thrombosis and acute coronary-artery lesions in sudden cardiac ischemic death. N Engl J Med 1984;310:1137–1140.
39. Rioufol G, Finet G, Ginon I, et al. Multiple atherosclerotic plaque rupture in acute coronary syndrome: a three-vessel intravascular ultrasound study. Circulation 2002; 106:804–808.
40. Maehara A, Mintz GS, Bui AB, et al. Morphologic and angiographic features of coronary plaque rupture detected by intravascular ultrasound. J Am Coll Cardiol 2002; 40:904–910.
41. Shin J, Edelberg JE, Hong MK. Vulnerable atherosclerotic plaque: clinical implications. Curr Vasc Pharmacol 2003;1:183–204.
42. Fujii K, Kobayashi Y, Mintz GS, et al. Intravascular ultrasound assessment of ulcerated ruptured plaques: a comparison of culprit and nonculprit lesions of patients with acute coronary syndromes and lesions in patients without acute coronary syndromes. Circulation 2003;108:2473–2478.
43. Libby P. Coronary artery injury and the biology of atherosclerosis: inflammation, thrombosis, and stabilization. Am J Cardiol 2000;86:3J–8J.

44. Virmani R, Kolodgie FD, Burke AP, et al. Lessons from sudden coronary death: a comprehensive morphological classification scheme for atherosclerotic lesions. Arterioscler Throm Vasc Biol 2000;20:1262–1275.
45. Uchida Y, Nakamura F, Tomaru T, et al. Prediction of acute coronary syndromes by percutaneous coronary angioscopy in patients with stable angina. Am Heart J 1995;130:195–203.
46. Kolodgie FD, Gold HK, Burke AP, et al. Intraplaque hemorrhage and progression of coronary atheroma. N Engl J Med 2003;349:2316–2325.
47. Heistad DD. Unstable coronary-artery plaques. N Engl J Med 2003;349:2285–2287.
48. Loree HM, Kamm RD, Stringfellow AP, et al. Effects of fibrous cap thickness on peak circumferential stress in model atherosclerotic vessels. Circ Res 1992;71:850–858.
49. Huang H, Virmani R, Younis H, et al. The impact of calcification on the biomechanical stability of atherosclerotic plaques. Circulation 2001;103:1051–1056.
50. Kaartinen M, van der Wal AC, van der Loos CM, et al. Mast cell infiltration in acute coronary syndromes: implications for plaque rupture. J Am Coll Cardiol 1998; 32(3):606–612.
51. Felton CV, Crook D, Davies MJ, et al. Relation of plaque lipid composition and morphology to the stability of human aortic plaques. Arterioscler Thromb Vasc Biol 1997;17:1337–1345.
52. van der Wal AC, Becker AE, van der Loos CM, et al. Site of intimal rupture or erosion of thrombosed coronary atherosclerotic plaques is characterized by an inflammatory process irrespective of the dominant plaque morphology. Circulation 1994; 89:36–44.
53. Laine P, Kaartinen M, Penttila A, et al. Association between myocardial infarction and the mast cells in the adventitia of the infarct-related coronary artery. Circulation 1999;99:361–369.
54. Shah PK. Plaque disruption and thrombosis: potential role of inflammation and infection. Cardiol Rev 2000;8:31–39.
55. Richardson PD, Davies MJ, Born GV. Influence of plaque configuration and stress distribution on fissuring of coronary atherosclerotic plaques. Lancet 1989;2: 941–944.
56. Galis ZS, Sukhova GK, Lark MW, et al. Increased expression of matrix metalloproteinases and matrix degrading activity in vulnerable regions of human atherosclerotic plaques. J Clin Invest 1994;94:2493–2503.
57. Steinberg D, Witztum JL. Lipoproteins and atherogenesis. Current concepts. JAMA 1990;264:3047–3052.
58. Pearson AM. Scavenger receptors in innate immunity. Curr Opin Immunol 1996;8: 20–28.
59. Hansson GK. Cell-mediated immunity in atherosclerosis. Curr Opin Lipidol 1997;8: 301–311.
60. Frostegard J, Wu R, Giscombe R, et al. Induction of T-cell activation by oxidized low density lipoprotein. Arterioscler Thromb 1992;12:461–467.
61. Stemme S, Faber B, Holm J, et al. T lymphocytes from human atherosclerotic plaques recognize oxidized low density lipoprotein. Proc Natl Acad Sci USA 1995;92:3893–3897.
62. Hansson GK, Jonasson L, Seifert PS, et al. Immune mechanisms in atherosclerosis. Arteriosclerosis 1989;9:567–578.
63. Biasucci LM, Liuzzo G, Fantozzi G, et al. Increasing levels of interleukin (IL)-1Ra and IL-6 during the first 2 days of hospitalization in unstable angina are associated with increased risk of in-hospital coronary events. Circulation 1999;99:2079–2084.

64. Farb A, Burke AP, Tang AL, et al. Coronary plaque erosion without rupture into a lipid core. A frequent cause of coronary thrombosis in sudden coronary death. Circulation 1996;93:1354–1363.
65. Virmani R, Burke AP, Farb A. Plaque rupture and plaque erosion. Thromb Haemost, 1999;82(Suppl 1):1–3.
66. Burke AP, Farb A, Malcolm GT, et al. Coronary risk factors and plaque morphology in men with coronary disease who died suddenly. N Engl J Med 1997;336:1276–1282.
67. Rauch U, Bonderman D, Bohrmann B, et al. Transfer of tissue factor from leukocytes to platelets is mediated by CD15 and tissue factor. Blood 2000;96:170–175.
68. Mallat Z, Benamer H, Hugel B, et al. Elevated levels of shed membrane microparticles with procoagulant potential in the peripheral circulating blood of patients with acute coronary syndromes. Circulation 2000;101:841–843.
69. Laszik ZG, Zhou XJ, Ferrell GL, et al. Down-regulation of endothelial expression of endothelial cell protein C receptor and thrombomodulin in coronary atherosclerosis. Am J Pathol 2001;159:797–802.
70. Willich SN, Jimenez AH, Tofler GH, et al. Pathophysiology and triggers of acute myocardial infarction: clinical implications. Clin Invest 1992;70(Suppl 1):S73–78.
71. Willich SN, MacLure M, Mittleman M, et al. Sudden cardiac death. Support for a role of triggering in causation. Circulation 1993;87:1442–1450.
72. Mittleman MA, Lewis RA, MacLure M, et al. Triggering myocardial infarction by marijuana. Circulation 2001;103:2805–2809.
73. Muller JE. Triggering of cardiac events by sexual activity: findings from a case-crossover analysis. Am J Cardiol 2000;86(2A):14F–18F.
74. Peters A, Dockery DW, Muller JE, et al. Increased particulate air pollution and the triggering of myocardial infarction. Circulation 2001;103:2810–2815.
75. Fernandez-Ortiz A, Badimon JJ, Falk E, et al. Characterization of the relative thrombogenicity of atherosclerotic plaque components: implications for consequences of plaque rupture. J Am Coll Cardiol 1994;23:1562–1569.
76. Mallat Z, Hugel B, Ohan J, et al. Shed membrane microparticles with procoagulant potential in human atherosclerotic plaques: a role for apoptosis in plaque thrombogenicity. Circulation 1999;99:348–353.
77. Matetzky S, Tani S, Kangavari S, et al. Smoking increases tissue factor expression in atherosclerotic plaques: implications for plaque thrombogenicity. Circulation 2000;102:602–604.

5
Evaluation in the Emergency Department and Cardiac Biomarkers

Gurusher Panjrath, Elaine B. Josephson, and Eyal Herzog

Coronary artery disease is the leading cause of death in the United States. Approximately 5 million patients present to the emergency department (ED) for chest pain-related complaints every year [1]. In addition, a significant number of patients may present to the ED with atypical symptoms. Early diagnosis and management of acute coronary syndrome (ACS) may lead to a significant reduction in associated morbidity and mortality. ED physicians play an important role in the rapid diagnosis and management of patients with suspected ACS. This provides a diagnostic challenge to the emergency physician. In this chapter, we discuss various presentations of ACS and tools available for rapid diagnosis and immediate management of patients in the ED. In addition, we propose the development of algorithms for the appropriate triage of patients based on severity and diagnosis. We also discuss testing in the ED and prognostic information provided by it and its significance in the subsequent management of the patient.

Chest pain represents one of three most common presenting symptoms by patients in the ED (along with abdominal complaints and fever). Approximately 1.4 million of these patients are admitted for management of unstable angina/non–ST-elevation myocardial infarction (UA/NSTEMI) [1, 2]. The remainder of the patients may still have serious and life-threatening conditions, such as aortic dissection and pulmonary embolism (Table 5.1). It is therefore necessary that a prompt diagnosis be made and that early recognition and treatment be instituted. It has been increasingly recognized that management of conditions constituting ACS has been inconsistent and not concurrent with guidelines. With frequent and important changes occurring in the field based on results of recent clinical trials, it is most appropriate to develop an algorithm-based management strategy that reduces the variability in the management of these patients.

Initial assessment of patients with suspected ACS should incorporate two strategies. The first should be directed toward accurate diagnosis, and the second should involve prognosis and risk of poor outcomes. Initial triage should include a focused history and physical, electrocardiogram (ECG), and measurement of cardiac biomarkers. Based on initial history, physical and ECG patients should be triaged into five categories: Priority, Advanced Risk, Intermediate Risk, Low Risk or Negative, and Non-ACS Chest Pain (see Chapter 2, Fig. 2.1). Patients initially triaged into a particular category may qualify for another category with availability of new results or change in symptoms. For instance, patients entering the intermediate risk category may need to be moved into advanced risk category if there is evidence of high-risk features such as new or worsening congestive heart failure (CHF) symptoms, malignant ventricular arrhythmias, hemodynamic instability, or recent percutaneous intervention or coronary artery bypass graft. Any evolving ST changes or positive cardiac markers within 24 hours will also move a patient into a higher risk category.

Symptoms of ACS may quite often be indistinguishable from certain other emergent as well as benign conditions. ED physicians need to be able to recognize symptoms with the high likelihood of representing ACS [3]. The history including presenting complaint as well as significant risk factors aided by physical exam findings should help the emergency physician to risk-stratify the patient. Other important tools assisting in early and appropriate risk stratification should include an electrocardiogram and cardiac biomarkers. The purpose of risk stratification is not only to identify patients with high likelihood of ACS but also to recognize those patients who have a higher risk of death, recurrent myocardial infarction, or poor outcome. The cardiology team should be immediately involved in management once a patient has been identified with possible ACS.

TABLE 5.1. Differential diagnosis of chest pain mimicking myocardial infarction.

Life-threatening cardiac causes
    Aortic dissection
    Pulmonary embolus
    Perforating ulcer
    Tension pneumothorax
    Boerhaave syndrome (esophageal rupture with mediastinitis)

Non–life-threatening cardiac causes
    Pericarditis
    Brugada syndrome
    Myocarditis
    Vasospastic angina

Non–life-threatening noncardiac causes
    Gastroesophageal reflux (GERD) and spasm
    Chest-wall pain
    Pleurisy
    Peptic ulcer disease
    Panic attack
    Biliary or pancreatic pain
    Cervical disk or neuropathic pain
    Somatization and psychogenic pain disorder

TABLE 5.2. Physical findings suggestive of ACS in a patient with chest pain.

Pulmonary edema
New or worsening mitral regurgitation
S3 gallop
Hypotension
Bradycardia
Tachycardia

Initial History and Physical

Routine questions include onset, type, precipitating factors (exertion, emotion, stress), radiation, nature of discomfort, and frequency of chest pain. Particular attention should be paid to chest pain equivalents such as dyspnea, jaw, neck, epigastric, and upper extremity discomfort. The importance of these symptoms has been increasingly recognized and thus included in the algorithm (see Chapter 2, Fig. 2.2). Other significant information includes age, race, sex, comorbid conditions, and risk factors (smoking, hypertension, dyslipidemia, family history of coronary artery disease and diabetes). Recent cocaine use should also be assessed. This key information can help increase or decrease the pretest likelihood of ACS. While interpreting this information, it is quite essential to keep in mind that women, elderly patients, and certain other subgroups such as diabetics and renal failure patients may present with atypical features (dyspnea, malaise, syncope), which need to be interpreted in the clinical context.

Physical exam should be directed at identifying findings suggestive of ACS as the underlying causative event and patients at high risk of death or poor outcomes. Physical findings that may increase the likelihood of cardiac diagnosis are listed in Table 5.2.

Beyond the utility of aiding diagnosis of ACS, history and physical findings should help investigate any pertinent clues indicative of high risk of bleeding and thus a contraindication to antithrombotic or antiplatelet therapy. History suggestive of recent major bleed, intracranial tumor, major surgery within the previous 2 weeks, or hemorrhagic stroke and supportive finding of fresh gastrointestinal bleeding may be a contraindication for such directed therapy. A rectal exam should be done to test for hemoccult as well, as part of the exam to help identify bleeding risks.

Electrocardiogram

An initial electrocardiogram (ECG) should be obtained on all patients with chest pain within 10 minutes of presentation to the ED (see Chapter 2, Fig. 2.3). Initial ECG findings serves as a powerful risk stratification tool in patients with

TABLE 5.3. ECG findings suggestive of myocardial injury.

ST-segment elevation in two contiguous leads
New-onset left bundle branch block
Hyper/acute T-wave
Transient ST-segment deviation (>0.05 mV) or T-wave inversion (0.2 mV) with symptoms
Fixed Q waves
Abnormal ST-segments or T waves not documented to be new
T-wave flattening or inversion in leads with dominant R waves
Sustained ventricular tachycardia

chest pain [4]. Unfortunately, 55% of initial ECGs may be nondiagnostic. Current American College of Cardiology/American Heart Association (ACC/AHA) guidelines recommend serial ECGs at 5- to 10-minute intervals or continuous 12-lead ST-segment monitoring in patients with nondiagnostic initial ECG in presence of ongoing symptoms and high clinical suspicion for ACS [3, 5]. These recommendations are based on the possibility of evolving changes and instability of the ST segment during ischemia. Despite this, a normal 12-lead ECG often represents a low-risk patient. In contrast, ECG with findings such as new-onset left bundle branch block may suggest need for immediate reperfusion and cardiac catheterization. Similarly, ST-segment depression may imply the risk of development of myocardial infarction in up to 50% of the patients with such findings. Table 5.3 lists ECG findings that should raise suspicion of ischemia-related myocardial injury. To achieve a goal of accurate diagnosis based on ECG interpretation, both ED physicians and nurses should be repeatedly trained for pattern recognition to minimize the chances of missed diagnosis. Subsequent to diagnosis, ECG changes can aid physicians in identifying patients who may have failed successful reperfusion at 1- to 3-hour intervals.

Laboratory Testing and Cardiac Biomarkers

Cardiac biomarkers serve as an important and essential component of initial testing of patients under suspicion of ACS (see Chapter 2, Fig. 2.3). Cardiac biomarkers are intracellular macromolecules that are released into the circulation due to myocardial injury and are available for detection in the peripheral blood. With the advent of point of care testing and improvement in sensitivity and precision of newer assays, biomarkers not only play a role in diagnosis but also add to prognostic data achieved from history, physical, and ECG findings.

Although a perfect biomarker may not be possible, a suitable marker should be found in high concentrations in the cardiac tissue. In addition, it would not be present in other tissues and would be undetectable in the blood of healthy persons. The marker would be released rapidly into the serum after myocardial infarction (MI), and serum concentrations would correspond with extent of injury. The marker should remain elevated long enough to be detected in the interval between symptom onset and ED presentation while falling rapidly enough not to mask reinjury. The assay itself should be inexpensive, rapidly available, and simple enough to perform at any time of day [6].

Emergence of newer and improved biomarkers with better sensitivity for detection of inflammation and necrosis may allow better characterization of the underlying process. Application of a panel of multiple markers may provide substantial knowledge compared with use of single marker [7]. Table 5.4 provides a list of biomarkers in current use and those with possibility of future use in ACS.

Cardiac biomarkers such as troponin (I and T) and CK-MB are the current biomarkers of choice in use for identifying patients with ACS and those at risk for significant complications.

In addition to cardiac biomarkers, standard laboratory testing should be directed at identifying underlying electrolyte abnormalities, coagulation studies, complete blood count, and lipid profile (see Chapter 2, Fig. 2.3). These tests, in addition to unmasking underlying metabolic and hematologic abnormalities causing arrhythmias and demand-supply mismatch due to anemia, also aid in risk stratification of patients with dyslipidemia. Coagulation studies are essential for recognition of bleeding risk, those with underlying prothrombotic states due to coagulation disorders, and for monitoring of anticoagulation levels in patients receiving unfractionated heparin.

Troponin (I and T)

Cardiac troponin I (cTnI) is a very specific marker for myocardial injury. cTnI levels are not detectable until 4 to 6 hours after the initial event and peak at

TABLE 5.4. Biomarkers that have either proven or potential utility in acute coronary syndromes.*

Troponin
CPK / CPK-MB
Myoglobin
Brain natriuretic peptide
High-sensitivity C-reactive protein
Myelopyroxidase
Ischemia-modified albumin
N-terminal pro-brain natriuretic peptide
Placental growth factor
Soluble CD40 ligand
Interleukin-10
Interleukin-6
Monocyte chemoattractant protein-1

*Biomarkers currently in use are set in italics.

TABLE 5.5. Causes of troponin elevation other than ACS.

Trauma (including contusion; ablation; pacing; implantable cardioverter defibrillator (ICD) firings, such as atrial defibrillators, cardioversion, endomyocardial biopsy, cardiac surgery, after-interventional–closure of atrial septal defects)
Congestive heart failure (acute and chronic)
Aortic valve disease and hypertrophic obstructive cardiomyopathy with significant left ventricular hypertrophy
Hypertension
Hypotension, often with arrhythmias
Postoperative noncardiac surgery patients
Renal failure
Critically ill patients, especially with diabetes, respiratory failure
Drug toxicity (e.g., adriamycin, 5 FU, herceptin, snake venoms)
Hypothyroidism
Coronary vasospasm, including apical ballooning syndrome
Inflammatory diseases (e.g., myocarditis, including Parvovirus, B19, Kawasaki disease, smallpox vaccination, or myocardial extension of bacterial endocarditis)

12 to 18 hours but may be elevated up to 1 to 2 weeks after a significant MI. Troponin (I and T) have replaced CK-MB as the predominant marker since redefining of the criteria for acute MI by American College of Cardiology and the European Society of Cardiology. With availability of highly sensitive assays for detection of troponin, revised guidelines require a diagnostic rise and fall in biomarkers in addition to symptoms or ECG changes significant for ischemia. Unfortunately, unstable angina cannot be included or excluded on the basis of any currently available biomarker. Serum troponin I should be measured in all patients under suspicion of ACS. While interpreting elevations in troponin I, it is essential to remember that troponin I can be elevated in conditions other than ACS, such as sepsis, congestive heart failure, pulmonary embolism, tachyarrhythmia, and myocarditis [8]. Table 5.5 lists conditions other than ACS that may be associated with elevated troponin levels. Hence, minimal elevations in troponin I in the absence of chest pain or ECG changes but with other abnormalities such as sepsis or renal failure should not be considered ACS. However, recent evidence demonstrates that even the minimal elevation in troponin I in these patients is a poor long-term prognostic marker [9].

CK-MB

CK-MB is one of the three creatine kinase (CK) isoenzymes. Creatine kinase consists of two subunits, B (predominant in brain tissue) and M (predominant in muscle tissue). Combinations of these two subunits results in three CK isoenzymes: CK-BB, CK-MB, and CK-MM. Although CK in cardiac tissue is 85%

CK-MM and 15% CK-MB, cardiac tissue is the most abundant source of CK-MB. CK-MB is the cardiac marker of choice for the purpose of estimating the size and extent of confirmed acute MI. It is detectable in the circulation at 4 to 6 hours after myocardial injury and peaks at 12 to 24 hours. Compared with cTnI, it returns to baseline within 2 to 3 days. This makes CK-MB useful in the detection of reinfarction. Serial CK-MB values provide the information we need for quantifying the infarction. CK-MB is also present in skeletal muscle, and thus an elevated level can be seen in conditions involving skeletal muscle injury or breakdown, such as vigorous exercise, trauma, muscular dystrophies, myositis, and rhabdomyolysis.

B-type Natriuretic Peptide

B-type natriuretic peptide (BNP) is useful in heart failure and signifies poor outcomes in patients with ACS. A strong association between elevations in BNP as well as N-terminal (NT)-proBNP levels and mortality has been shown in patients with ACS. BNP is released from myocytes mainly in response to increases in ventricular wall stress. Myocardial injury resulting in systolic dysfunction, impaired ventricular relaxation, and stunned myocardium, thereby causing increased preload and release of BNP has been proposed as the underlying mechanism of release of BNP and NT-proBNP in patients with ACS.

BNP is a useful adjunct to the multimarker panel currently in use for patients presenting to the ED with chest pain. It may be an aid in diagnosis in patients with NSTEMI and nondagnostic levels of CK-MB, troponin I, or both. BNP provides valuable prognostic information pertaining to mortality, which is independent of risk indicators, such as older age, renal insufficiency, and left ventricular dysfunction [10]. A biphasic pattern of NT-proBNP has been demonstrated after anterior MI. Whereas elevated NT-proBNP levels on admissions are frequently observed, the second peak portents poor outcomes [6].

Myoglobin

Myoglobin is a small cytoplasmic protein present in muscle. Myoglobin of cardiac origin enters the coronary circulation through capillaries during cellular infarction. This allows its detection in the peripheral circulation much earlier than other markers of cardiac injury. Elevations in serum myoglobin levels can be seen as early as 1 to 4 hours after symptom onset. It reaches peak concentration at 6 to 9 hours and returns to baseline in 18 to 24 hours. Because of its rapid rise and fall, myoglobin offers a potential for early detection of myocardial injury during ACS. Diagnostic value of myoglobin is improved if measured serially after the onset of symptoms. A 100% increase in measured level at 2 hours after onset of symptoms results in 95% sensitivity and specificity for acute MI compared with a single elevated value. Pitfalls for use of myoglobin include its presence in high concentrations in skeletal muscle, thus making it relatively nonspecific for myocardial injury, and its dependence on renal function for clearance from the peripheral circulation. However, it may be valuable as an early marker of acute MI and aid in early exclusion of patients without myocardial injury when combined with more specific cardiac markers, such as troponin and CK-MB. When measured within 3 hours of chest pain onset, the sensitivity of myoglobin has been reported to be as low as 24% and as high as 81%, with specificity ranging from 76% to 96%. At 6 hours from chest pain onset, the sensitivity and specificity ranges increase to 55% to 100% and 76% to 98%, respectively. Unfortunately, the testing strategy still appears to fail to detect 5% to 10% of patients with acute MI, limiting the value of a negative test result.

Practical Approach

It is noteworthy that absence of detectable biomarkers on presentation of a patient to the ED, particularly within 6 hours of onset of chest pain, should not exclude ACS. As discussed before, serial testing should be performed [11]. The biomarkers should be tested at baseline, 6- to 9-hour, and 12- to 24-hour intervals to exclude myocardial injury. If troponins are elevated in patients without a clinical picture or electrocardiographic evidence of ischemia, other causes of troponin elevation should be considered. Point of care testing in the ED helps in rapid decision making. However, due to lack of sensitivity in point of care devices compared with a central laboratory, patients with small level of elevation of troponin may be missed.

Initial Treatment in the Emergency Department

Patients with chest pain and possible ACS need to be evaluated efficiently as discussed before. Once they have been triaged into appropriate category, supportive care should be instituted to relieve symptoms and maintain oxygenation if required. All patients should be on continuous monitoring until further data become available. Further conservative versus invasive strategy should be based on predefined criteria based on ACC/AHA guidelines and should be modified for capabilities and setup of individual hospitals. Emergent cardiac catheterization should be arranged for patients in the Priority category. Advanced Risk category patients should also be considered for early cardiac catheterization (within 12 to 24 hours). In centers or situations where the door to balloon time exceeds 90 minutes, patients in the Priority Risk category should receive immediate thrombolytic therapy (if not contraindicated). Patients falling into the Negative category should be admitted to noncardiology teams or to chest pain units for observation and undergo exercise testing with radionuclide or echocardiographic imaging. Patients without any findings can be safely discharged home with follow-up with a cardiologist. Table 5.6 lists the medicines routinely used by ED physicians and highlights key points in their use.

TABLE 5.6. Initial pharmacological agents.

Agent	Dosage	Key points
Pain management		
Nitrates	Nitroglycerin 0.4 mg sublingual as needed	Maintain systolic blood pressure over 90 mm Hg
		Do not reduce mortality in patients with acute MI Intravenous nitroglycerin is recommended in the first 24 hours for patients with STEMI
	Topical nitroglycerin paste every 6 hours (6-hour paste-free window every 24 hours)	
	Intravenous nitroglycerine at 10 μg/min and titrate up to 200 μg/min	Careful assessment during the use of nitrates in patients with inferior and right ventricular infarction is required to prevent severe hypotension as a result of decreased preload
		Contraindicated in patients with recent phosphodiesterase-5 inhibitors use (risk for severe and prolonged hypotension)
Morphine	Morphine sulfate 2 to 4 mg IV every 5 minutes as needed	
Antiplatelet therapy		
ASA	325 mg PO initial dose followed by 81 OR 162 mg PO daily	Use of aspirin and clopidogrel in combination should be considered for all patients with ACS falling in priority and advanced categories
Clopoidogrel	300 to 600 mg PO loading dose followed by 75 mg PO daily	Contraindications: Bleeding, known triple vessel disease or strong suspicion that patient may require coronary artery bypass grafting (CABG)
		Benefit of reduced early ischemic events and morbidity should be taken into account for majority of patients while deciding to hold clopidogrel for possible CABG
		Pretreatment with aspirin and clopidogrel reduces periprocedural MI, death, and other complications of urgent PCI
Beta-blockers		
IV + PO metoprolol	25 to 50 mg PO q6 hours for 48 hours, then 100 mg PO q12 hours OR 5 mg IV over 1–2 minutes, repeat every 5 minutes for total initial dose 15 mg; followed by 25 to 50 mg PO q6 hours for 48 hours, then 100 mg PO q12 hours	Indicated in all patients with ACS Exception: Decompensated severe heart failure, cardiogenic shock, severe reactive airway disease, or signficant bradycardia (less than 50 beats/min)
IV + PO atenolol	50 to 100 mg PO daily OR 5 mg IV, repeated in 5 minutes, then followed by 50 to 100 mg PO daily	Oral initiation of beta-blockers therapy is appropriate in low risk patients Metoprolol is a preferable agent
IV esmolol	Loading dose, 500 mcg/kg IV bolus over 1 minute followed by maintenance dose	Ultrashort-acting beta-blocker IV esmolol

(Continued)

Table **5.6.** *Continued*

Agent	Dosage	Key points
ACE inhibitor		
Lisinopril	5 mg PO daily; titrate to maximum tolerated dose	If ACE cannot be administered, ARB should be given
Captopril	6.25 mg PO followed by 12.5 mg PO q8 hours; titrate to maximum tolerated dose	ACEI inhibitor is contraindicated in significant hypotension, clinically relevant azotemia, serum creatinine greater than 2.4 mg/dL, bilateral renal artery stenosis, or any hypersensitivity to ACE inhibitor
Antithrombotic agent		
IV unfractionated heparin	60–70 units/kg IV bolus followed by 12–15 units/kg/hr infusion	Achieve an activated partial thromboplastin time (aPTT) of 1.5 to 2.0 times control
Low-molecular-weight heparin		
Enoxaparin	1 mg/kg subcutaneous q12 hours	Use of enoxaparin should be considered over heparin unless contraindicated
		Enoxaparin should preferably not be used in patient with reduced glomerular filtration rate and dose should be adjusted for age >75
Glycoprotein IIb/IIIa inbitors		
Efptifibatide	180 mcg/kg bolus IV followed by 2 mcg/kg/min infusion	Priority and advanced risk patients
		Hemodynamically unstable patients undergoing revascularization
		Indicated in refractory ischemia despite ASA, clopidogrel and heparin
		Eptifibatide needs dose reduction in renal failure patients
Tirofiban	0.4 mcg/kg/min bolus IV for 30 minutes followed by 0.1 mcg/kg/min infusion	
Abciximab	0.25 mg/kg bolus IV (over 5 minutes) followed by 0.125 mcg/kg/min infusion	

IV, intravenous; PO, by mouth.

Conclusion

Hospitals should develop protocols to be followed by ED physicians and the cardiology team. These directives and pathways should be based on guidelines and in agreement with all the health care providers, including physicians and nursing staff. Quality improvement initiatives need to be undertaken [12]. Systematic review and feedback should be provided to all the parties involved, including emergency room and cardiology staff, laboratory personnel, and pharmacy staff. Improvement in diagnostic or laboratory tests turnaround time should be addressed for availability of data in a timely and consistent fashion.

Application of a multiteam approach combined with quality improvement measures and regular training of personnel will result in improvement in care and timely management of patients with ACS in the ED.

References

1. Nourjah P. National hospital ambulatory medical care survey: 1997 emergency department summary. Hyattsville, MD: National Center for Health Statistics; 1999:304.
2. National Center for Health Statistics. Detailed diagnosis and procedures: national hospital discharge survey, 1996. Hyattsville, MD: National Center for Health Statistics; 1998:13.
3. Gibler WB, Cannon CP, Blomkalns AL, et al. Practical implementation of the guidelines for unstable angina/non-ST-segment elevation myocardial infarction in the emergency department. Ann Emerg Med 2005;46:185–197.
4. Savonitto S, Ardissino D, Granger CB, et al. Prognostic value of the admission electrocardiogram in acute coronary syndromes. JAMA 1999;281:707–713.
5. Antman EM, Anbe DT, Armstrong PW, et al. ACC/AHA guidelines for the management of patients with ST-elevation myocardial infarction—executive summary: a report of the American College of Cardiology/American Heart Association Task Force on Practice Guidelines (Writing Committee to Revise the 1999 Guidelines for the Management of Patients With Acute Myocardial Infarction). Circulation 2004;110:588–636.
6. Maisel AS, Braunwald E. Cardiac biomarkers: a contemporary status report. Nature Clinical Practice Cardiovascular Medicine 2006;3:24–34.
7. Morrow DA, Braunwald E. Future of biomarkers in acute coronary syndromes: moving toward a multimarker strategy. Circulation 2003;108:250–252.
8. Jaffe AS. Elevations in cardiac troponin measurements: false false-positives. Cardiovasc Tox 2001;1:87–92.
9. Aviles RJ, Askari AT, Lindahl B, et al. Troponin T levels in patients with acute coronary syndromes, with or without renal dysfunction. N Engl J Med 2002;346:2047–2052.
10. De Lemos JA, Morrow DA, Bentley JH, et al. The prognostic value of B-type natriuretic peptide in patients with acute coronary syndromes. N Engl J Med 2001;345:1014–1021.
11. Newby LK, Christenson RH, Ohman EM, et al. Value of serial troponin T measures for early and late risk stratification in patients with acute coronary syndromes. The GUSTO IIa Investigators. Circulation 1998;98:1853–1859.
12. French WJ. Trends in acute myocardial management: use of the National Registry of myocardial infarction in quality improvement. Am J Cardiol 2000; 85:5B–9.

6
Diagnosis and Treatment of ST-Segment Elevation Myocardial Infarction

Matthew Daka, Emad Aziz, Robert Leber, and Mun K. Hong

ST-segment elevation myocardial infarction (STEMI) represents the Priority group of the PAIN pathway. This diagnosis should be promptly ascertained and the proper treatment algorithm (see Chapter 2, Figs. 2.1 and 2.4 to 2.6) immediately applied to maximize the preservation of ischemic myocardium at risk and minimize the acute and late morbidity/mortality [1, 2].

The American College of Cardiology/American Heart Association (ACC/AHA) guidelines on STEMI [3] suggest that all patients presenting to the emergency department (ED) with a history of chest pain or symptoms suggestive of STEMI should undergo the following:

1. Triaged through a predetermined, institution-specific chest pain protocol such as our PAIN pathway. The protocol should include several diagnostic possibilities. We suggest the top six to be the following with pertinent diagnostic tests:
   - Acute coronary syndrome (unstable angina, non–ST-segment elevation myocardial infarction [NSTEMI], and STEMI): 12-lead electrocardiogram (ECG) and cardiac biomarkers.
   - Acute aortic dissection: urgent computed tomography (CT) angiogram or transesophageal echocardiography.
   - Acute pulmonary embolism: chest x-ray, urgent helical CT or ventilation-perfusion scan.
   - Tension pneumothorax: physical examination and chest x-ray.
   - Acute perforation of peptic ulcer or esophageal tear or rupture: pneumomediastinum on chest x-ray for pneumomediastinum or air under the diaphragm.
   - Acute pericarditis: history and 12-lead ECG, a normal coronary angiogram, and transthoracic echocardiogram.
2. Placed on a cardiac monitor with a defibrillator on standby. A 12-lead ECG should be performed and interpreted by an experienced physician within 10 minutes of ED arrival.
3. If STEMI is present, the decision to establish reperfusion either by primary angioplasty (PCI), the preferred revascularization option [4], or fibrinolytic

therapy should be made within 20 minutes of ED arrival. The goal is to achieve a door to needle time for fibrinolytics within 30 minutes or a door to balloon time for primary PCI within 90 minutes of arrival to the ED [3]. These goals should not be understood as the ideal times for reperfusion but rather the longest times that should be considered acceptable for effective reperfusion therapy.

4. During this time, a focused history and physical examination should be performed, the aim of which is to:

- Assess risk factors of coronary artery disease (CAD) and other history to exclude the potentially lethal differential diagnoses listed above.
- Perform a quick but thorough review of exclusion criteria for fibrinolytic treatment if STEMI is confirmed and if the patient is in a non–primary PCI center.
- Identify the subset of patients with signs of left ventricular decompensation, organ hypoperfusion and/or shock, or other complications, such as mechanical complications of STEMI (see Chapter 11) so that these high-risk patients can be transferred quickly to the cardiac catheterization laboratory in a primary PCI capable center.

Immediately after the diagnosis of STEMI, the patients should also receive oxygen and adjunct pharmacology (see Chapter 5).

Reperfusion

The current ACC/AHA guidelines for the treatment of STEMI recommend that a reperfusion strategy, based on either pharmacological management with a fibrinolytic agent or mechanical management with PCI, should be implemented as soon as possible after arrival in the ED (class I-A recommendation) [1]. Factors affecting the choice of reperfusion therapy include time between onset of chest pain and presentation, access to a skilled facility capable of primary PCI, and patient characteristics at presentation.

Timing Is Important for Selecting Reperfusion Strategy

The ACC/AHA STEMI guidelines appear to favor fibrinolytic therapy over PCI when symptom duration is ≤3 hours, as the likelihood of fresh thrombus amenable to fibrinolytic agent is high, especially if there is an anticipated delay of >1 hour from needle insertion to balloon inflation. However, in cases where the anticipated delay is <1 hour between needle insertion and balloon inflation, PCI is still preferred given its safety over thrombolysis associated with approximately 1% intracranial hemorrhage [4]. PCI is the favored strategy when there is a delay between symptom onset and presentation (>3 hours) and when PCI can be performed in a timely manner with a door to balloon time goal of ≤90 minutes. The following is a synopsis from the ACC/AHA STEMI guidelines [1] (Table 6.1).

TABLE 6.1. Criteria for selecting reperfusion therapy.

If presentation is <3 hours and there is no delay to an invasive strategy, there is no preference to either strategy; however:	
An invasive strategy is generally preferred if:	Fibrinolysis is generally preferred if:
1. Late presentation (>3 hours since symptom onset)	Early presentation (<3 hours from symptom onset) and delay to invasive strategy

2. Skilled PCI lab available with surgical backup [5]:
  • Operator experience: >75 primary PCI cases/year
  • Team experience: >36 primary PCI cases/year
	Invasive strategy is not an option:
	  • Cath lab is occupied/not available
	  • Vascular access difficulties
	  • No access to skilled PCI lab

3. Medical contact to balloon or door to balloon time <90 minutes	Delay to invasive strategy:
	  • Prolonged transport
	  • Door to balloon time >90 minutes

4. <1 hour delay vs. time to fibrinolytic therapy with a fibrin-specific agent
5. High risk STEMI:
  • Cardiogenic shock
  • Killip class III or IV
6. Contraindications to fibrinolysis, including increased risk of bleeding and ICH
7. Diagnosis of STEMI is in doubt
	• <1 hour delay vs. immediate fibrinolytic therapy with a fibrin-specific agent

ICH, intracranial hemorrhage

Fibrinolytic Therapy

It is well-known that time from onset of symptoms to fibrinolytic therapy is an important predictor of MI size and patient outcome [6]. The efficacy of fibrinolytic agents in lysing thrombus diminishes with the passage of time [7]. Fibrinolytic therapy administered within the first 2 hours (especially the first hour) can occasionally abort MI and dramatically reduce mortality [8, 9]. The National Heart Attack Alert Working Group recommends that EDs strive to achieve a 30-minute door to needle time to minimize treatment delays [10]. Prehospital fibrinolysis by skilled EMS personnel reduces treatment delays by up to 1 hour and reduces mortality by 17% [11].

Contraindications to Fibrinolytic Therapy in STEMI

Absolute contraindications:

1. Any prior intracranial hemorrhage.
2. Known structural cerebral vascular lesion (arteriovenous malformations, aneurysms, etc.).
3. Known malignant intracranial neoplasms (primary or metastatic).
4. Ischemic stroke within 3 months except acute ischemic stroke within 3 hours.
5. Suspected aortic dissection.

6. Active bleeding or bleeding diathesis (excluding menses).
7. Significant closed-head or facial trauma within 3 months.

Relative contraindications:

1. History of chronic, severe, poorly controlled hypertension.
2. Severe uncontrolled hypertension on presentation (systolic blood pressure [SBP] >180 mm Hg or diastolic blood pressure [DBP] >110 mm Hg).
3. History of prior ischemic stroke greater than 3 months, dementia, or known intracranial pathology not covered under absolute contraindications.
4. Traumatic or prolonged (greater than 10 minutes) CPR.
5. Major surgery within the last 3 weeks
6. Recent internal bleeding (within 2 to 4 weeks).
7. Noncompressible vascular punctures.
8. Pregnancy.
9. Active peptic ulcer
10. Current use of anticoagulation: the higher the international normalized ratio (INR), the higher the risk of bleeding.
11. For streptokinase/anistreplase: prior exposure (more than 5 days ago) or prior allergic reaction to these agents.

Prerequisites for Superiority of PCI over Fibrinolysis

The current STEMI guidelines [1] indicate that the benefit of PCI over fibrinolytic reperfusion pertains to primary PCI performed in a skilled facility with cardiothoracic surgical backup and by experienced interventionalists. Requirements for a skilled facility and experienced interventionalist are as follows: (1) an annual total of 400 PCI procedures by the facility (at least 36 primary PCI); and (2) an operator that performs 75 PCI procedures annually (at least 11 primary PCI).

The suggested relationship between PCI-capable centers and improved outcomes is illustrated by findings from a retrospective analysis of 1997 Medicare claims data demonstrating that the need for coronary artery bypass graft (CABG) surgery after PCI occurred more frequently (2.25% vs. 1.55%; $P < 0.001$) when the procedure was performed by inexperienced staff (>60 vs. <30 cases per year) and that the risk of 30-day mortality was higher (4.29% vs. 3.15%; $P < 0.001$) for patients treated at low-volume PCI centers (<80 vs. >160 Medicare cases per year) [5].

Why Primary PCI Should Be the Preferred, Standard Reperfusion Strategy for STEMI

1. Primary PCI results in substantially better rates of normal flow in the culprit artery compared with treatment with fibrinolytic agents (TIMI grade 3: 74% to 93% [12, 13] vs. 60% to 63% [14–16]). Fibrinolysis fails to restore blood

flow completely in 30% to 40% of patients with STEMI, and analyses of random-ized clinical trials comparing primary PCI and fibrinolysis have shown improved clinical outcomes with primary PCI [4, 17].

2. For primary PCI compared with fibrinolytic therapy, compelling data from randomized trials suggest lower rates of adverse events [4]:
- Mortality (5.0% vs. 7.0%)
- Nonfatal reinfarction (3.0% vs. 7.0%)
- Hemorrhagic stroke and intracranial hemorrhage (0.05% vs. 1.0%).

3. Fibrinolytic therapy, albeit widely available, is limited by early and late reocclusion of the infarct-related artery:
- The incidence of reocclusion after successful fibrinolysis increases over time as shown in a series of studies [18–20]. It is up to 25% to 30% within months of STEMI [21, 22]. Reocclusion rate after fibrinolysis is 28% at 3 months [22] and 25% at 1 year [19]. Reocclusion of a previ-ously patent artery is a cause of increased in-hospital mortality and is also detrimental to the long-term recovery of left ventricular function [23].

On the other hand, coronary stenting virtually eliminates vascular recoil, and multiple studies have shown low reocclusion rates between 0% and 6% on follow-up angiography ranging from 6.2 days to 7.7 months after angioplasty with stent placement for STEMI [24–28].

4. Emergent cardiac catheterization enables an anatomic risk stratification strategy:
- A subset of patients will have severe three-vessel or left main disease or anatomic features unfavorable for PCI and may be candidates for urgent or emergency CABG. These patients will be missed if a fibrinolytic strategy is used.
- Another subset of patients will have spontaneously reperfused coronary arteries or may have acute pericarditis or other nonthrombotic causes of ST-segment elevation, such as epicardial or microvascular spasm or Tako-Tsubo cardiomyopathy [29]. These patients can be treated medically and conservatively, avoiding the risks of fibrinolytic therapy.
- Additionally, identification of high-risk patients by cardiac catheteriza-tion, such as those with concomitant valvular disease, may facilitate addi-tional strategies that will improve outcome, whereas low-risk patients may be eligible for early hospital discharge.

5. Primary PCI is superior to fibrinolytic therapy in high-risk patients such as those with anterior wall myocardial infarction, cardiogenic shock, or conges-tive heart failure:
- Primary PCI in patients with anterior STEMI reduces mortality compared with fibrinolytic therapy although there is no difference in patients with non–anterior STEMI [30, 31].
- Patients with cardiogenic shock treated with coronary revascularization experienced an absolute 9% reduction in 30-day mortality compared with those managed with medical stabilization [32].

- In NRMI-II, patients with CHF had a 33% relative risk reduction with primary PCI compared with a 9% relative risk reduction with fibrinolytic therapy [33].

Strategies to Minimize the Door to Balloon Time

There are many strategies to reduce the door to balloon time, and a recent report by Bradley et al. [34] suggests practical ways to achieve this important goal. In their survey of hospitals and review of 28 different strategies, six of them were found to significantly reduce the door to balloon time. They included the following, many of which we have already in place at our institution (see Chapter 2):

1. ED physicians activate the catheterization laboratory or the MI team (reducing 8.2 minutes).
2. A single call to a central page operator activates the catheterization laboratory or the MI team (13.8-minute reduction).
3. ED physicians activate the catheterization laboratory or the MI team while the patient is being transported by the ambulance to the hospital (saving 15.4 minutes).
4. The on-call staff is expected to arrive in the catheterization laboratory within 20 minutes after being paged (reducing 19.3 minutes vs. >30 minutes).
5. The on-call interventionalist stays in the hospital for these emergencies (14.6-minute reduction).
6. A collaborative feedback is provided between the ED and the catheterization laboratory (8.6-minute reduction).

Most of these strategies can be implemented without undue stress on the system, except for the attending interventionalist taking the call in the hospital. These reductions in precious minutes are especially important when many patients still present late after the onset of their symptoms.

Transfer to Primary PCI Center

The balance of risk/benefit between the transfer of patients for PCI and more immediate treatment with fibrinolytic therapy remains uncertain. If the expected door to balloon time exceeds the expected door to needle time by more than 60 minutes, fibrinolytic treatment with a fibrin-specific agent such as tenecteplase (TNK) should be considered unless it is contraindicated. This is particularly important when symptom duration is less than 3 hours but is less important with longer symptom duration, when less ischemic myocardium can be salvaged. The CAPTIM trial [35] showed lower mortality with prehospital fibrinolysis than with primary PCI, and the PRAGUE-2 trial [36] showed lower mortality with primary PCI after interhospital transfer than with on-site fibrinolysis. In these two trials, PCI was superior to fibrinolysis when symptom duration was greater than 2 to 3 hours but not when symptom duration was shorter.

Also, the DANAMI-2 trial (<u>Dan</u>ish Trial in <u>A</u>cute <u>M</u>yocardial <u>I</u>nfarction), conducted in Denmark, found that patients treated at facilities without interventional cardiology capabilities had better composite outcomes when the patients were transferred for PCI within 2 hours of presentation than with pharmacological reperfusion treatment at the local hospital [37]. Importantly, the mean time to treatment was delayed only 44 minutes. Whether these results could be replicated elsewhere is not known.

Conclusion on Reperfusion Strategy

Given the logistical issues, it is not possible to say definitively that a particular reperfusion approach is for all patients, in all clinical settings, at all times of day. The most important recommendation is that a reperfusion therapy should be selected immediately for all patients with suspected STEMI. The appropriate and timely use of any reperfusion therapy is likely more important than the type of therapy, as "time is muscle" and the latter determines the long-term outcome.

Other Therapeutic Options

Facilitated PCI

Facilitated PCI is defined as PCI after an initial treatment with a pharmacological regimen such as full-dose fibrinolysis, half-dose fibrinolysis, a glycoprotein (GP) IIb/IIIa inhibitor, or a combination of reduced-dose fibrinolytic therapy and a platelet GP IIb/IIIa inhibitor. Facilitated PCI should be differentiated from primary PCI without fibrinolysis or GP IIb/IIIa inhibitor therapy, from primary PCI with a GP IIb/IIIa inhibitor started at the time of PCI, and from rescue PCI after unsuccessful fibrinolysis. Potential advantages include earlier time to reperfusion, improved patient stability, greater procedural success rates, higher thrombolysis in myocardial infarction (TIMI) flow rates, and improved survival. However, studies have not demonstrated any benefit in reducing infarct size or improving outcomes compared with primary PCI [38]. Facilitated PCI is a class IIb recommendation, not evidence-based, by the ACC/AHA STEMI guidelines.

Rescue PCI

Rescue (also known as salvage) PCI is defined as PCI within 12 hours after failed fibrinolysis for patients with continuing or recurrent myocardial ischemia. Rescue PCI has resulted in higher rates of early infarct artery patency, improved regional infarct-zone wall motion, and greater freedom from adverse in-hospital events than with a deferred PCI strategy or medical therapy. The Randomized Evaluation of Rescue PCI with Combined Utilization End Points (RESCUE) trial demonstrated a reduction in rates of in-hospital death and a combined end point of death and CHF that was maintained up to 1 year after study entry for patients presenting with anterior STEMI who failed fibrinolytic therapy when PCI was performed within 8 hours after the onset of symptoms [39]. Improvement in TIMI grade flow from ≤2 to 3 may offer additional clinical benefit. Similar data are not available for patients with non–anterior STEMI.

Delayed PCI and the Open Artery Hypothesis

Should stable, high-risk STEMI patients with persistent, complete occlusion of the infarct-related artery presenting outside the currently accepted period for myocardial salvage of 12 hours receive only optimal medical therapy or should they, in addition, undergo PCI of the infarct-related artery? The answer to this question is still unclear. The "open artery hypothesis" asserts that the restoration of antegrade flow in the infarct-related artery days, weeks, or even several months after myocardial infarction would improve long-term outcome and survival even if left ventricular function did not improve. Two pivotal trials led to this assertion: the Western Washington trial [40] in which fibrinolytic therapy, using streptokinase, improved survival without improving left ventricular function, and the Second International Study of Infarct Survival (ISIS-2 trial), in which streptokinase improved mortality even in patients receiving it between 13 and 24 hours after the onset of STEMI [41]. The open artery hypothesis is also strongly supported by several nonrandomized, retrospective studies [42–44]. However, the recently published results of the multicenter, randomized Open Artery Trial (OAT Trial) did not corroborate the open artery hypothesis [45]. The OAT trial, which randomized 2,166 patients with total occlusion of the infarct-related artery within 3 to 28 days after STEMI and mean left ventricular ejection fraction below 50% to optimal medical therapy alone or optimal medical therapy with PCI, showed no reduction in major cardiovascular events (death, reinfarction, or heart failure) during a mean follow-up of up to 4 years. There was a statistically non-significant trend toward excess reinfarction in the PCI cohort. In patients presenting late after STEMI, rigorous selection criteria that include demonstrating a large area of myocardium at risk and ascertainment of myocardial viability using noninvasive tests may be necessary before PCI of the infarct-related artery is undertaken.

The Role of Serum Cardiac Biomarkers in the Diagnosis of STEMI

Although serum cardiac biomarkers (troponin I and T, creatine kinase [CK], CK-MB, and myoglobin) are useful for confirming diagnosis, estimating infarct size, and provide useful prognostic information in STEMI patients (see Chapter 5 for further details), initiation of reperfusion strategy should never be delayed while awaiting the results of cardiac biomarker assay. The amount of cardiac biomarker released is a sign of the extent of myocardial necrosis/damage and provides prognostic information, but also the kinetics of release of these biomarkers may serve as a noninvasive assessment of successful reperfusion after fibrinolytic therapy [46].

Earlier detection of CK-MB or cardiac troponins in less than 6 hours from the onset of definite chest pain in STEMI patients suggest an acute ischemic/ occlusive episode that precedes patients' reference chest pain. STEMI patients with troponin T elevation less than 6 hours after chest pain onset have a higher mortality [47]. Myoglobin, found in both cardiac and skeletal muscle, can be detected 2 hours after the onset of STEMI albeit not cardiac specific. Though not widely used, the rapid release kinetics of myoglobin makes it an attractive biomarker for the early diagnosis of reperfusion.

Drugs used to treat STEMI patients are discussed in detail in Chapters 8 and 9.

References

1. Berger PB, Ellis SG, Holmes DR Jr, et al. Relationship between delay in performing direct coronary angioplasty and early clinical outcome in patients with acute myocardial infarction: results from the Global Use of Strategies to Open Occluded Arteries in Acute Coronary Syndromes (GUSTO-IIb) trial. Circulation 1999;100: 14–20.
2. Cannon CP, Gibson CM, Lambrew CT, et al. Relationship of symptom-onset-to-balloon time and door-to-balloon time with mortality in patients undergoing angioplasty for acute myocardial infarction. JAMA 2000;283:2941–2947.
3. Antman EM, Anbe DT, Armstrong PW, et al. ACC/AHA guidelines for the management of patients with ST-elevation myocardial infarction: a report of the American College of Cardiology/American Heart Association Task Force on Practice Guidelines (Committee to Revise the 1999 Guidelines for the Management of Patients with Acute Myocardial Infarction). Circulation 2004;110:e82–292.
4. Keeley EC, Boura JA, Grines CL. Primary angioplasty versus intravenous thrombolytic therapy for acute myocardial infarction: a quantitative review of 23 randomised trials. Lancet 2003;361:13–20.
5. McGrath PD, Wennberg DE, Dickens JD Jr, et al. Relation between operator and hospital volume and outcomes following percutaneous coronary interventions in the era of the coronary stent. JAMA 2000;284:3139–3144.
6. Boersma E, Maas AC, Deckers JW, et al. Early thrombolytic treatment in acute myocardial infarction: reappraisal of the golden hour. Lancet 1996;348:771–775.
7. Zeymer U, Tebbe U, Essen R, et al. Influence of time to treatment on early infarct-related artery patency after different thrombolytic regimens. ALKK-Study Group. Am Heart J 1999;137:34–38.
8. Appleby P, Baigent C, Collins R, et al. Indications for fibrinolytic therapy in suspected acute myocardial infarction: collaborative overview of early mortality and major morbidity results from all randomised trials of more than 1000 patients. Fibrinolytic Therapy Trialists' (FTT) Collaborative Group. Lancet 1994;343:311–322.
9. Weaver WD, Cerqueira M, Hallstrom AP, et al. Prehospital-initiated vs hospital-initiated thrombolytic therapy. The Myocardial Infarction Triage and Intervention Trial. JAMA 1993;270:1211–1216.

10. Emergency department: rapid identification and treatment of patients with acute myocardial infarction. National Heart Attack Alert Program Coordinating Committee, 60 Minutes to Treatment Working Group. Ann Emerg Med 1994;23:311–329.

11. Morrison LJ, Verbeek PR, McDonald AC, Sawadsky BV, Cook DJ. Mortality and prehospital thrombolysis for acute myocardial infarction: a meta-analysis. JAMA 2000;283:2686–2692.

12. A clinical trial comparing primary coronary angioplasty with tissue plasminogen activator for acute myocardial infarction. The Global Use of Strategies to Open Occluded Coronary Arteries in Acute Coronary Syndromes (GUSTO IIb) Angioplasty Substudy Investigators. N Engl J Med 1997;336:1621–1628.

13. Grines CL, Cox DA, Stone GW, et al. Coronary angioplasty with or without stent implantation for acute myocardial infarction. Stent Primary Angioplasty in Myocardial Infarction Study Group. N Engl J Med 1999;341:1949–1956.

14. The effects of tissue plasminogen activator, streptokinase, or both on coronary-artery patency, ventricular function, and survival after acute myocardial infarction. The GUSTO Angiographic Investigators. N Engl J Med 1993;329:1615–1622.

15. Bode C, Smalling RW, Berg G, et al. Randomized comparison of coronary thrombolysis achieved with double-bolus reteplase (recombinant plasminogen activator) and front-loaded, accelerated alteplase (recombinant tissue plasminogen activator) in patients with acute myocardial infarction. The RAPID II Investigators. Circulation 1996;94:891–898.

16. Cannon CP, Gibson CM, McCabe CH, et al. TNK-tissue plasminogen activator compared with front-loaded alteplase in acute myocardial infarction: results of the TIMI 10B trial. Thrombolysis in Myocardial Infarction (TIMI) 10B Investigators. Circulation 1998;98:2805–2814.

17. Weaver WD, Simes RJ, Betriu A, et al. Comparison of primary coronary angioplasty and intravenous thrombolytic therapy for acute myocardial infarction: a quantitative review. JAMA 1997;278:2093–2098.

18. Neuhaus KL, von Essen R, Tebbe U, et al. Improved thrombolysis in acute myocardial infarction with front-loaded administration of alteplase: results of the rt-PA-APSAC patency study (TAPS). J Am Coll Cardiol 1992;19:885–891.

19. White HD, French JK, Hamer AW, et al. Frequent reocclusion of patent infarct-related arteries between 4 weeks and 1 year: effects of antiplatelet therapy. J Am Coll Cardiol 1995;25:218–223.

20. Wilson SH, Bell MR, Rihal CS, et al. Infarct artery reocclusion after primary angioplasty, stent placement, and thrombolytic therapy for acute myocardial infarction. Am Heart J 2001;141:704–710.

21. Meijer A, Verheugt FW, Werter CJ, et al. Aspirin versus coumadin in the prevention of reocclusion and recurrent ischemia after successful thrombolysis: a prospective placebo-controlled angiographic study. Results of the APRICOT Study. Circulation 1993;87:1524–1530.

22. Takens BH, Brugemann J, van der Meer J, et al. Reocclusion three months after successful thrombolytic treatment of acute myocardial infarction with anisoylated plasminogen streptokinase activating complex. Am J Cardiol 1990;65:1422–1424.

23. Nijland F, Kamp O, Verheugt FW, et al. Long-term implications of reocclusion on left ventricular size and function after successful thrombolysis for first anterior myocardial infarction. Circulation 1997;95:111–117.

24. Antoniucci D, Santoro GM, Bolognese L, et al. A clinical trial comparing primary stenting of the infarct-related artery with optimal primary angioplasty for acute

myocardial infarction: results from the Florence Randomized Elective Stenting in Acute Coronary Occlusions (FRESCO) trial. J Am Coll Cardiol 1998;31:1234–1239.

25. Antoniucci D, Valenti R, Buonamici P, et al. Direct angioplasty and stenting of the infarct-related artery in acute myocardial infarction. Am J Cardiol 1996;78: 568–571.

26. Kastrati A, Pache J, Dirschinger J, et al. Primary intracoronary stenting in acute myocardial infarction: long-term clinical and angiographic follow-up and risk factor analysis. Am Heart J 2000;139:208–216.

27. Rodriguez A, Bernardi V, Fernandez M, et al. In-hospital and late results of coronary stents versus conventional balloon angioplasty in acute myocardial infarction (GRAMI trial). Gianturco-Roubin in Acute Myocardial Infarction. Am J Cardiol 1998;81:1286–1291.

28. Suryapranata H, van't Hof AW, Hoorntje JC, et al. Randomized comparison of coronary stenting with balloon angioplasty in selected patients with acute myocardial infarction. Circulation 1998;97:2502–2505.

29. Kurisu S, Sato H, Kawagoe T, et al. Tako-tsubo-like left ventricular dysfunction with ST-segment elevation: a novel cardiac syndrome mimicking acute myocardial infarction. Am Heart J 2002;143:448–455.

30. Stone GW, Grines CL, Browne KF, et al. Influence of acute myocardial infarction location on in-hospital and late outcome after primary percutaneous transluminal coronary angioplasty versus tissue plasminogen activator therapy. Am J Cardiol 1996;78:19–25.

31. Henriques JP, Zijlstra F, van't Hof AW, et al. Primary percutaneous coronary intervention versus thrombolytic treatment: long term follow up according to infarct location. Heart 2006;92:75–79.

32. Hochman JS, Sleeper LA, Webb JG, et al. Early revascularization in acute myocardial infarction complicated by cardiogenic shock. SHOCK Investigators. Should We Emergently Revascularize Occluded Coronaries for Cardiogenic Shock. N Engl J Med 1999;341:625–634.

33. Wu AH, Parsons L, Every NR, Bates ER. Hospital outcomes in patients presenting with congestive heart failure complicating acute myocardial infarction: a report from the Second National Registry of Myocardial Infarction (NRMI-2). J Am Coll Cardiol 2002;40:1389–1394.

34. Bradley EH, Herrin J, Wang Y, et al. Strategies for reducing the door-to-balloon time in acute myocardial infarction. N Engl J Med 2006;355:2308–2320.

35. Bonnefoy E, Lapostolle F, Leizorovicz A, et al. Primary angioplasty versus prehospital fibrinolysis in acute myocardial infarction: a randomised study. Lancet 2002;360:825–829.

36. Widimsky P, Budesinsky T, Vorac D, et al. Long distance transport for primary angioplasty vs immediate thrombolysis in acute myocardial infarction. Final results of the randomized national multicentre trial—PRAGUE-2. Eur Heart J 2003;24: 94–104.

37. Andersen HR, Nielsen TT, Rasmussen K, et al. A comparison of coronary angioplasty with fibrinolytic therapy in acute myocardial infarction. N Engl J Med 2003; 349:733–742.

38. Keeley EC, Boura JA, Grines CL. Comparison of primary and facilitated percutaneous coronary interventions for ST-elevation myocardial infarction: quantitative review of randomized trials. Lancet 2006;367:579–588.

39. Ellis SG, da Silva ER, Heyndrickx G, et al. Randomized comparison of rescue angioplasty with conservative management of patients with early failure of thrombolysis for acute anterior myocardial infarction. Circulation 1994;90:2280–2284.

40. Kennedy JW, Ritchie JL, Davis KB, et al. Western Washington randomized trial of intracoronary streptokinase in acute myocardial infarction. N Engl J Med 1983;309:1477–1482.

41. ISIS-2 (Second International Study of Infarct Survival) Collaborative Group. Randomised trial of intravenous streptokinase, oral aspirin, both, or neither among 17,187 cases of suspected acute myocardial infarction: ISIS-2. Lancet 1988;2: 349–360.

42. Cigarroa RG, Lange RA, Hillis LD. Prognosis after acute myocardial infarction in patients with and without residual anterograde coronary blood flow. Am J Cardiol 1989;64:155–160.

43. Lange RA, Cigarroa RG, Hillis LD. Influence of residual antegrade coronary blood flow on survival after myocardial infarction in patients with multivessel coronary artery disease. Coron Artery Dis 1990;1:59–63.

44. Lamas GA, Flaker GC, Mitchell G, et al. Effect of infarct artery patency on prognosis after acute myocardial infarction. Circulation 1995;92:1101–1109.

45. Hochman JS, Lamas GA, Buller CE, et al., for the Occluded Artery Trial Investigators. Coronary intervention for persistent occlusion after myocardial infarction. N Engl J Med 2006;355:2395–2407.

46. Alpert JS, Thygesen K, Antman E, et al. Myocardial infarction redefined—a consensus document of The Joint European Society of Cardiology/American College of Cardiology Committee for the redefinition of myocardial infarction. J Am Coll Cardiol 2000;36:959–969.

47. Ohman EM, Armstrong PW, White HD, et al. Risk stratification with a point-of-care cardiac troponin T test in acute myocardial infarction. GUSTOIII Investigators. Global Use of Strategies To Open Occluded Coronary Arteries. Am J Cardiol 1999; 84:1281–1286.

7
Diagnosis and Treatment of Non–ST-Segment Elevation Myocardial Infarction

Jacqueline E. Tamis-Holland, Sandeep Joshi, Angela Palazzo, and Sripal Bangalore

Acute coronary syndrome (ACS) is a spectrum of clinical events ranging from unstable angina (UA) to acute myocardial infarction (AMI). AMI includes both non–ST-segment elevation myocardial infarction (NSTEMI) and ST-segment elevation myocardial infarction (STEMI). UA and NSTEMI have similar pathophysiologic and clinical presentations. Often they are difficult to distinguish on initial appearance and are frequently grouped together as one clinical syndrome. However, NSTEMI portends an increased risk due to an elevation in cardiac biomarkers reflecting myocardial necrosis. NSTEMI is a highly prevalent and life-threatening manifestation of ACS accounting for more than 1.2 million patient hospitalizations in the United States alone [1] and is a major cause of morbidity and mortality in the Western world.

Pathophysiology

ACS occurs when there is an imbalance between myocardial oxygen supply and demand. In NSTEMI, the most common cause for this imbalance is thrombus formation at the site of an atherosclerotic plaque, resulting in *incomplete* vessel occlusion or *transient* total occlusion. Atherosclerotic plaques are composed of cellular debris and a lipid core with an overlying fibrous cap. Disruption of the fibrous cap will expose the lipid core to the arterial lumen, providing a substrate for platelet aggregation and activation at the disrupted endothelial surface. Fibrinogen bridges the activated platelets by binding to two glycoprotein (GP) IIb/IIIa receptors, resulting in the formation of a platelet-fibrin hemostatic plug, which then propagates into either an occlusive or nonocclusive thrombus [2]. In NSTEMI, this thrombus does not completely occlude the arterial lumen and antegrade flow remains intact. Clumps of activated platelets or components of the disrupted plaques can propagate down the arterial tree. These microemboli may result in myocardial necrosis and are presumed to be responsible for the release of biochemical markers of AMI associated with NSTEMI [2]. Alternate mechanisms for NSTEMI are less common. These include (1) smooth muscle cell spasm with transient obstruction; (2) moderate or severe atherosclerosis, with a concomitant increase in myocardial oxygen demand such as that seen with hemodynamically unstable hypotension or anemia; (3) inflammatory diseases of the blood vessels (vasculitis), resulting in vessel damage, with intimal thickening and arterial narrowing; and (4) secondary conditions that may be extrinsic to the coronary vessels, including embolic events as a result of left atrial myxoma, atrial fibrillation, paradoxical emboli, valvular vegetations, or clot.

Diagnosis

It is important to have a high index of suspicion when evaluating patients with chest pain or suspected ACS so that an early diagnosis can be made and appropriate care can be initiated (see Chapter 2, Figs. 2.1, 2.7, and 2.8). It is recommended that patients with suspected ACS be placed in a location with continuous electrocardiogram (ECG) monitoring and close observation until the diagnosis is made or discounted. This evaluation should consist of assessing both the likelihood of ACS and the patients' risk for subsequent cardiac events, as initial medical therapy and subsequent hospital management will be determined by these factors.

History and Physical Examination

Angina is typically described as chest discomfort, frequently referred to as chest "tightness," "squeezing," or "grabbing" that occurs with increased activity and is relieved with rest. In cases of NSTEMI, these symptoms are generally prolonged and not relieved with rest or nitroglycerin. Accompanying symptoms may include left arm or jaw pain, profound diaphoresis, nausea or dyspnea and epigastric pain. Although the presence of sharp, pleuritic or atypical chest pain, or chest pain that is reproduced by palpation of the sternum is less consistent with angina, the diagnosis of NSTEMI in such cases may still be considered if the index of suspicion is otherwise high. The quality of pain, albeit helpful, should not entirely make or discount a diagnosis of NSTEMI. Supporting information may include a prior history of atherosclerotic heart disease (ASHD) or MI, as well as the presence or absence of risk factors such as hypertension, tobacco use, diabetes mellitus, hyperlipidemia, and a family history of premature ASHD.

The physical examination often does not provide additional information in the diagnosis of NSTEMI, but it can be helpful in the assessment of complications of infarction. Alternative etiologies for the patient's presenting symptoms may be suggested by physical findings and comorbidities, including chronic obstructive pulmonary disease (COPD), infection, or peripheral vascular disease, which can alter the approach to invasive treatment.

Electrocardiogram

The ECG is essential to the diagnosis, risk stratification, and treatment of patients with ACS. The American College of Cardiology/American Heart Association (ACC/AHA) guidelines recommend that an ECG be performed within 10 minutes of presentation of ongoing chest pain [3, 4]. Dynamic ST-segment changes including ST-segment depressions or transient ST-segment elevations ≥1 mm or deep T-wave inversions ≥2 mm support the diagnosis of cardiac ischemia or infarction. The presence of a normal ECG does not exclude the possibility of NSTEMI as a small percentage of patients with a normal ECG but typical symptoms can go on to develop infarction [5]. The presence of a normal or nondiagnostic ECG does provide prognostic information. Patients with a documented infarction and a nondiagnostic ECG have been shown to have a lower risk of long-term complications when compared with patients with dynamic ECG changes [6, 7].

Biochemical Cardiac Markers

Cardiac markers are intracellular macromolecules that are released into the bloodstream when myocardial necrosis is present. Cardiac biomarkers should be obtained on all patients presenting with a suspected NSTEMI. The biochemical markers include the cardiac troponins (troponin T and troponin I), creatine kinase MB (CK-MB), and myoglobin. Assays measuring the cardiac troponins I and T are extremely sensitive and very specific; thus, they are the marker of choice for assessing myocardial necrosis. If troponin measurements are unavailable, then the CK-MB should be measured. Serum myoglobin measurements are highly sensitive but less specific for the detection of early cardiac necrosis and are only useful when used in conjunction with CK-MB or the cardiac troponins. The biochemical markers of necrosis are often not detectable until several hours after symptom onset. Therefore, it is recommended that cardiac enzyme levels be obtained on admission and at 6 to 9 and 12 to 24 hours.

Risk Stratification

Risk stratification of patients with NSTEMI is essential for assessing both short- and long-term risk, to individualize patient care, and to provide the most appropriate management options. Certain therapies have been shown to be more effective in patients who are at higher risk, whereas a less aggressive approach may be used in low-risk patients. Risk assessment is based on a compilation of the patient's clinical history, physical examination, ECG, and biochemical markers. Various systems have been proposed to facilitate clinicians in estimating a patient's risk profile.

The Thrombolysis in Myocardial Infarction (TIMI) risk score for NSTEMI and unstable angina is a 7-point system that can be used to predict a patient's risk for death, nonfatal myocardial infarction, or severe ischemia requiring urgent revascularization at 2 weeks after the initial presentation [8]. Variables analyzed include (1) age >65 years; (2) prior known coronary stenosis of >50%; (3) the presence of at least three coronary artery disease risk factors; (4) elevated cardiac enzymes; (5) ST-segment deviation on ECG; (6) recurrent angina prior to presentation; and (7) aspirin use within the last week.

The Agency for Health Care Policy and Research (AHCPR) guidelines for unstable angina use a simple estimate of cardiac risk to estimate outcome [9]. Low-risk patients include those patients with a normal ECG and without rest or nocturnal chest pain. High-risk patients are those with evidence of extensive myocardial infarction or compromise, including ongoing chest pain, pulmonary edema or rales, S3 gallop, murmur of new mitral regurgitation, hypotension, or dynamic ST changes. Intermediate-risk patients are those patients who fall between the two spectrums described. In a prospective study of patients with angina, 30-day mortality was 0% for low-risk patients, 1.2% for intermediate-risk patients, and 17% for high-risk patients.

Elevated cardiac troponin levels provide prognostic information during ACS. NSTEMI patients with elevated troponins have a higher incidence of death or subsequent AMI when compared with those patients without elevated troponin [10]. The risk increases proportionally with the quantity of troponin detected [11, 12]. In addition, patients with elevated cardiac troponins have been shown to greatly benefit from certain treatments such as GP IIb/IIIa inhibitors and low-molecular-weight heparins and from interventional procedures for revascularization [13–15].

Treatment

Anti-ischemic Agents

Oxygen

Oxygen is administered to patients with NSTEMI to provide symptomatic relief of dyspnea and to maintain oxygen saturations above 90% in hypoxic patients. The routine use of supplemental oxygen has not been shown to affect outcome in patients with NSTEMI.

Nitrates

Nitroglycerin is a potent venodilator. It predominately exerts its effect by reducing preload, which results in a reduction in wall stress and myocardial oxygen demand. It may also have some direct effect on coronary artery vascular tone, although this mechanism is less well defined. The reduction in preload is helpful in treating patients with heart failure. Therefore, nitroglycerin is given to patients with NSTEMI for relief of ongoing chest pain, treatment of refractory hypertension, or congestive heart failure (CHF). It is especially useful in cases where vasospasm is suspected. Nitroglycerin is initially given sublingually and subsequently administered intravenously if there is no response. The routine use of nitroglycerin in the absence of angina-like symptoms or CHF is not recommended as it does not appear to affect outcome [16, 17]. Nitroglyc-erin should be withheld in patients with suspected right ventricular infarction or hypotension, as the reduction in preload may exacerbate these conditions.

Beta-Blockers

Beta-blockers decrease myocardial contractility and slow heart rate, which results in decreased myocardial oxygen demand. Although there are limited studies examining the early use of beta-blockers in the NSTEMI patient, studies of patients with STEMI have demonstrated a reduction in mortality and recur-rent myocardial infarction when early intravenous beta-blockers are adminis-tered [18, 19]. Therefore, the ACC/AHA guidelines recommend that in the absence of a contraindication, beta-blockers should be initiated to all patients early in the setting of NSTEMI [3, 4]. In higher risk patients, they should be given as an intravenous bolus, followed by oral dosing. Beta-blockers should be withheld in patients with important contraindications to their use, including active heart failure, hemodynamic instability, severe bradycardia or high-grade AV block, and significant COPD.

Calcium Channel Blockers

These agents decrease the influx of calcium ions across the cardiac smooth muscle membranes resulting in smooth muscle cell relaxation. They are gener-ally classified into two groups: dihydropyridine calcium channel antagonists (amlodipine, nifedipine) and non-dihydropyridine calcium channel antago-nists (such as verapamil and diltiazem). Dihydropyridine calcium channel antagonists predominantly have an affect on peripheral smooth muscle relax-ation while non-dihydropyridines result in a reduction in myocardial contrac-tility and atrioventricular (AV) nodal conduction. All of these agents have some coronary vasodilator properties. Because of the uncertain benefit regarding the routine use of calcium channel blockers in the setting of patients with coronary artery disease [20, 21], their use is reserved for patients with suspected coronary artery spasm as the etiology for the infarction or in patients with refractory hypertension requiring multiple agents.

Morphine Sulfate

Morphine sulfate, a potent anxiolytic as well as an analgesic agent, also has beneficial hemodynamic effects such as vasodilation. It is predominately used for control of refractory angina or treatment of CHF. A recent report from the CRUSADE Initiative, a nonrandomized, retrospective observational registry enrolling patients with NSTEMI, revealed a higher mortality in patients given any intravenous morphine within the first 24 hours of presentation. The use of morphine was associated with increased in-hospital mortality (odds ratio of 1.41) even after matching on propensity score for treatment [22]. Although this is a nonrandomized trial, this finding warrants some caution with the use of morphine in NSTEMI patients, especially its hypotensive effects.

Antiplatelet Therapy

Aspirin

Aspirin irreversibly inhibits platelet cyclooxygenase-1, resulting in a reduction in thromboxane A_2 and a decrease in platelet activation and aggregation. Studies evaluating aspirin use in patients with ACS have been consistent in demonstrating benefit [23, 24]. As a result, the ACC/AHA guidelines recommend that all patients with NSTEMI receive aspirin on initial presentation [3, 4]. An initial dose of 162 to 325 mg should be given and continued indefinitely if ASHD is present. There are infrequent contraindications to aspirin use, including active bleeding or severe peptic ulcer disease, or aspirin allergy. Aspirin allergy is rare, and anyone reporting an allergy to aspirin should be questioned further to verify the accuracy of this statement. Individuals who are truly intolerant of aspirin should be treated with clopidogrel. Alternately, they may be considered for aspirin desensitization.

ADP Receptor Antagonists

Clopidogrel and ticlopidine are thienopyridines that exert inhibitory effects on platelet activation and aggregation through noncompetitive blockage of the platelet adenosine diphosphate (ADP) receptor. Ticlopidine has been associated with serious hematologic disorders and it is not routinely used for the treatment of coronary heart disease unless there is a contraindication to the use of clopidogrel.

Unlike aspirin, clopidogrel has a delayed release profile and may take several days to achieve a full antiplatelet effect. Therefore, it is often given as a loading dose of 300 mg to 600 mg followed by a daily dose of 75 mg. The CURE study demonstrated that the addition of clopidogrel to aspirin in patients with unstable angina or NSTEMI resulted in a 20% reduction in cardiovascular outcomes at 1 year [25]. This benefit was noted in both high-risk and low-risk patients. Clopidogrel has been associated with a higher risk for major bleeding, in particular among patients undergoing coronary artery bypass surgery (CABG) within 5 days of drug discontinuation [25]. The ACC/AHA guidelines recommend the use of clopidogrel plus aspirin in hospitalized patients with NSTEMI who are managed either with an early interventional or medical approach and are not at high risk for bleeding [4]. Therapy with clopidogrel should be continued for at least 1 month after MI and preferably up to 9 to 12 months [26, 27]. A lower dose of aspirin (75 to 100 mg) is recommended when concomitant clopidogrel is administered.

Glycoprotein IIb/IIIa Inhibitors

Activation of the GP IIb/IIIa receptor on the platelet surface is the final common pathway to platelet aggregation. There are several agents currently available that antagonize the GP IIb/IIIa receptor. These agents include tirofiban, eptifibatide, and abciximab. Tirofiban is a synthetic nonpeptide that competitively inhibits the GP IIb/IIIa receptor. Because of its reversible binding, tirofiban has a short half-life with a return of platelet activity within 3 to 4 hours after the discontinuation of the drug [28]. Eptifibatide is a synthetic peptide that competitively inhibits the GP IIb/IIIa receptor. This agent has a pharmacokinetic profile similar to tirofiban, with a short half-life and a return of normal platelet activity within 3 to 4 hours of drug discontinuation [29]. Abciximab, a Fab fragment of a murine antibody, has not been proved to be of benefit in the initial medical stabilization of patients with UA/NSTEMI [30] and therefore the ACC/AHA has not recommended its use as initial "upstream" therapy in this setting.

Both tirofiban and eptifibatide have been shown to decrease the likelihood of adverse outcomes among high-risk patients with UA/NSTEMI [29, 31, 32]. The benefit of these agents is particularly notable for patients with elevated troponin levels, high TIMI risk scores, or a planned early invasive strategy. These agents have been associated with a tendency toward increased bleeding and thrombocytopenia, although the rates of major bleeding do not appear to be significantly increased. In view of this information, these agents are recommended by the ACC/AHA for high-risk patients scheduled for planned PCI. Low-risk patients who are likely to receive a conservative approach to therapy are less likely to benefit from this therapy [3, 4].

Antithrombotic Therapy

Antithrombotic agents prevent thrombus propagation by inhibiting components of the coagulation cascade and by inhibiting thrombin activity. Unfractionated heparin (UFH) is a glycosaminoglycan composed of heterogeneous chains with different molecular weights and anticoagulation activity. UFH exerts its anticoagulation effect via its interaction with antithrombin III. Because of its ability to bind to plasma proteins and cells, the use of UFH can result in a wide variation in therapeutic response, hence monitoring of the activated partial thromboplastin time (aPTT) is required. A weight-adjusted intravenous loading dose is followed by a continuous infusion. Optimal dosing includes an initial bolus of 60 to 70 U/kg to a maximum of 5,000 units, followed by a 12 to 15 U/kg infusion. Subsequent dosing should be weight based and aimed to achieve an aPTT of 50 to 70 seconds [3, 4]. UFH has been widely used in the setting of UA/NSTEMI. Several studies have shown that the early administration of UFH either alone or in combination with aspirin is associated with a lower rate of recurrent myocardial infarction and ischemia [33, 34].

Low-molecular-weight heparins (LMWHs) are derived via cleavage of UFH to yield smaller chains with different molecular weights and anticoagulation properties. LMWHs are more effective than UFH in catalyzing the inhibition of factor Xa by antithrombin III than in the inactivation of thrombin. Because LMWHs have a reduced binding affinity to proteins or cells, there is a more predictable dose-response relationship with a longer half-life than UFH. As a result, there is no required laboratory monitoring of activity and more convenient subcutaneous administration. LMWHs have been demonstrated to be of greater benefit than UFH in certain high-risk patients [35, 36]. Accumulating data have shown that LMWHs can be given safely and effectively to UA/NSTEMI patients in conjunction with GP IIb/IIIa inhibitors undergoing PCI therapy [37]. The ACC/AHA recommends that patients with NSTEMI be given anticoagulation with UFH or LMWHs in addition to antiplatelet therapy with aspirin and/or clopidogrel [3, 4].

Additional Medical Therapies

Angiotensin-Converting Enzyme Inhibitors

Angiotensin-converting enzyme (ACE) inhibitors have been shown to reduce morbidity and mortality among patients presenting with ACS who have signs or symptoms of left ventricular dysfunction or heart failure [38, 39]. In the absence of contraindications, ACE inhibitors should be administered to all patients with NSTEMI complicated by CHF or left ventricular dysfunction. An ACE inhibitor may be considered as routine care in all post-ACS patients as well [3, 4] and should be initiated within 24 hours of presentation.

Statin Therapy

The 3-hydroxy-3 methylglutaryl (HMG) coenzyme A reductase inhibitors or statins predominately exert their effects by lowering low-density lipoprotein (LDL) cholesterol and triglycerides and raising high-density lipoprotein (HDL) cholesterol. The degree to which they improve cardiovascular outcomes, however, is out of proportion to their LDL-lowering effects, and it is likely that statins have other "pleiotropic effects" on atherosclerosis. These include stabilization of the atherosclerotic plaque, inhibition of thrombogenicity, and improvement in endothelial function [40]. Statins are predominately used in the chronic setting for the primary or secondary prevention of cardiovascular events. More recently, they have been introduced in the acute setting. Data suggest that the early aggressive use of high-dose statins in patients with ACS results in decreased plaque progression and decreased cardiovascular events [41–43]. Therefore, all patients admitted with NSTEMI should be considered for high-dose statin therapy initiated during hospitalization unless there is a contraindication [4].

The Role of Early Revascularization

After initial medical stabilization, the patient with NSTEMI can be considered for various management options, including an initial strategy of aggressive medical therapy (early conservative strategy) versus an intended invasive approach (early invasive strategy). In the conservative strategy, the patient is medically treated with optimal anti-ischemic and antiplatelet/anticoagulant regimens. Once stabilized, the patient is referred for noninvasive stress-imaging tests (i.e., stress echo or stress nuclear studies) for risk stratification. In this approach, invasive testing and revascularization are reserved for those patients with a complicated postinfarction course, including CHF or arrhythmias, spontaneous ischemia despite maximal medical therapy, or significant ischemia on imaging studies. In an early invasive strategy, patients are also initially medically stabilized with aggressive medical therapy. Subsequently, all patients without contraindications are referred for early catheterization and revascularization with PCI or CABG as indicated.

Most contemporary studies examining these two approaches have favored an early invasive strategy. In the TACTICS TIMI-18, RITA-3, and FRISC II studies, catheterization and revascularization with CABG or PCI resulted in a significant reduction in clinical end points, including death, recurrent myocardial infarction, and rehospitalization for ACS [44–46]. The benefit was most notable among patients with elevated troponin levels or a high TIMI risk score. The most recent study to look at these strategies among NSTEMI patients failed to demonstrate a benefit to an early invasive approach and, in fact, suggested a higher risk of recurrent infarction in those patients assigned to an initial invasive therapy [47]. Differences in study design and end point definitions may explain some of the variability in outcomes for these studies. Nonetheless, the latter study suggests that in a contemporary era of aggressive medical therapy, stable patients could be medically treated and referred for invasive testing as clinically indicated and still have an acceptably good outcome. Recently, a meta-analysis of seven large contemporary trials, including the four aforementioned studies, demonstrated a significant mortality benefit from an early invasive approach [48]. Therefore, based on this body of evidence, the ACC/AHA recommends that high-risk patients with UA or NSTEMI without any contraindications to angiography or revascularization be treated with an early invasive approach [4]. Patients without high-risk features can be considered with either a conservative or invasive strategy as clinically appropriate.

Prognosis

Prior to the introduction of guideline-based therapies, patients with NSTEMI had the least favorable prognosis when compared with patients with other forms of ACS. Mortality rates exceeded even those for patients with STEMI, and the incidence of recurrent infarction was high [49]. With the introduction of aggressive medical therapies and advanced catheter-based interventions, subsequent cardiac events have improved dramatically. Clinical trials have reported mortality rates as low as 2% in-hospital and 3% to 4% at 1 year of follow-up [48], although epidemiologic studies have demonstrated higher events with in-hospital mortality averaging 8% [50]. Mortality is affected by aggressiveness of therapy, with lower rates among patients treated with guideline recommended therapies [50, 51].

Despite these recommendations, patients are not always optimally managed. It is important that physicians are constantly reminded of the need to provide patients with guideline recommended care. The CRUSADE program is a national quality improvement initiative that is designed to increase the practice of evidence-based medicine for patients diagnosed with unstable angina or NSTEMI incorporating the ACC/AHA guidelines as the standard for care [52]. This and other initiatives will help to educate the physician and other health care workers caring for the patient with NSTEMI in an effort to optimize outcomes.

References

1. Patel MR, Chen AY, Peterson ED, et al. Prevalence, predictors, and outcomes of patients with non-ST-segment elevation myocardial infarction and insignificant coronary artery disease: results from the Can Rapid risk stratification of Unstable angina patients Suppress ADverse outcomes with Early implementation of the ACC/AHA Guidelines (CRUSADE) initiative. Am Heart J 2006;152:641–7.
2. Davies MJ. The pathophysiology of acute coronary syndromes. Heart 2000;83: 361–366.
3. Braunwald E, Antman EM, Beasley JW, et al. ACC/AHA guidelines for the management of patients with unstable angina and non ST segment elevation myocardial infarction. A report of the American College of Cardiology/American Heart Association Task Force on Practice Guidelines (Committee on the Management of Patients with Unstable Angina). J Am Coll Cardiol 2000;36:970–1062.
4. Braunwald E, Antman EM, Beasley JW, et al. ACC/AHA 2002 guideline update for the management of patients with unstable angina and non-ST segment elevation myocardial infarction: a report of the American College of Cardiology/American Heart Association Task Force on Practice Guidelines (Committee on the Management of Patients with Unstable Angina). Circulation 2002;106: 1893.
5. Rouan GW, Lee TH, Cook EF, et al. Clinical characteristics and outcome of acute myocardial infarction in patients with initially normal or nonspecific electrocardiograms (a report from the Multicenter Chest Pain Study). Am J Cardiol 1989;64: 1087–1092.
6. Cannon CP, McCabe CH, Stone PH, et al. The electrocardiogram predicts one-year outcome of patients with unstable angina and non-Q wave myocardial infarction: results of the TIMI III registry ECG ancillary study. Thrombolysis in Myocardial Ischemia. J Am Coll Cardiol 1997;30:133–140.
7. Welch RD, Zalenski RJ, Frederick PD, et al. Prognostic value of a normal or nonspecific initial electrocardiogram in acute myocardial infarction. JAMA 2001;286: 1977–1984.
8. Antman EM, Cohen M, Bernink PJ, et al. The TIMI risk score for unstable angina/non ST-segment elevation MI; a method for prognostication and therapeutic decision making. JAMA 2000;284:835–842.
9. Katz DA, Griffith JL, Beshansky JR, et al. The use of empiric clinical data in the evaluation of practice guidelines for unstable angina. JAMA 1996;276:1568–1574.
10. Pettijohn JL, Doyle T, Spiekerman AL, et al. Usefulness of positive troponin-T and negative creatine kinase levels in identifying high-risk patients with unstable angina pectoris. Am J Cardiol 1997;80:510–511.

11. Antman EM, Tanasijevic MJ, Thompson B, et al. Cardiac-specific troponin-I levels to predict the risk of mortality in patients with acute coronary syndromes. N Engl J Med 1996;335:1342–1349.

12. Lindahl B, Venge P, Wallentin L. Relation between troponin T and the risk of subsequent cardiac events in unstable coronary artery disease. The FRISC study group. Circulation 1996;93:1651–1657.

13. Newby LK, Ohman EM, Christenson RH, et al. Benefit of glycoprotein IIb/IIIa inhibition in patients with acute coronary syndromes and troponin t-positive status: the paragon-B troponin T substudy. Circulation 2001;103:2891–2896.

14. Hamm CW, Heeschen C, Goldmann B, et al. Benefit of abciximab in patients with refractory unstable angina in relation to serum troponin T levels. c7E3 Fab Antiplatelet Therapy in Unstable Refractory Angina (CAPTURE) Study Investigators. N Engl J Med 1999;340:1623–1629.

15. Heeschen C, Hamm CW, Goldmann B, et al. Troponin concentrations for stratification of patients with acute coronary syndromes in relation to therapeutic efficacy of tirofiban. PRISM Study Investigators. Platelet Receptor Inhibition in Ischemic Syndrome Management. Lancet 1999;354:1757–1762.

16. ISIS-4: a randomized factorial trial assessing early oral captopril, oral mononitrate, and intravenous magnesium sulfate in 58,050 patients with suspected acute myocardial infarction. ISIS-4 (Fourth International Study of Infarct Survival) Collaborative Group. Lancet 1995;345:669–685.

17. GISSI-3: Effects of lisinopril and transdermal glyceryl trinitrate singly and together on 6-week mortality and ventricular function after acute myocardial infarction. Gruppo Italiano per lo Studio della Sopravvivenza nell'infarto Miocardico. Lancet 1994;343:1115–1122.

18. Randomized trial of intravenous atenolol among 16027 cases of suspected acute myocardial infarction: ISIS-1. First International Study of Infarct Survival Collaborative Group. Lancet 1986;2:57–66.

19. Roberts R, Rogers WJ, Mueller HS, et al. Immediate versus deferred beta-blockade following thrombolytic therapy in patients with acute myocardial infarction. Results of the Thrombolysis in Myocardial Infarction (TIMI) II-B. Circulation 1991;83(2): 422–437.

20. Gibson RS, Boden WE. Calcium channel antagonists: friend or foe in postinfarction patients? Am J Hypertens 1996;9:172s–176s.

21. Theroux P, Taeymans Y, Morissette D, et al. A randomized study comparing propranolol and diltiazem in the treatment of unstable angina. J. Am Coll Cardiol 1985; 5:717–722.

22. Meine TJ, Roe MT, Chen AY, et al. Association of intravenous morphine use and outcomes in acute coronary syndromes: results from the CRUSADE Quality Improvement Initiative. Am Heart J 2005;149:1043–1049.

23. Cairns JA, Gent M, Singer J, et al. Aspirin, sulfinpyrazone, or both in unstable angina. Results of a Canadian multicenter trial. N Engl J Med 1985;313:1369–1375.

24. Yusuf S, Wittes J, Friedman L. Overview of results of randomized clinical trials in heart disease. II. Unstable angina, heart failure, primary prevention with aspirin and risk factor modification. JAMA 1988;260:2259–2263.

25. The Clopidogrel in Unstable Angina to Prevent Recurrent Events Trial Investigators. Effect of Clopidogrel in addition to Aspirin in patients with acute coronary syndromes without ST segment elevation. N Engl J Med 2001;345:494–502.

26. Mehta SR, Yusuf S, Peters RJ, et al. Effects of pretreatment with clopidogrel and aspirin followed by long-term therapy in patients undergoing percutaneous coronary intervention: the PCI-CURE study. Lancet 2001;358:527–533.

27. Steinhubl SR, Berger PB, Mann JT III, and the CREDO investigators. Early and sustained dual oral antiplatelet therapy following percutaneous coronary intervention: a randomized controlled trial. JAMA 2002;288:2411–2420.

28. The RESTORE Investigators. Effects of platelet glycoprotein IIb/IIIa blockade with tirofiban on adverse cardiac events in patients with unstable angina or acute myocardial infarction undergoing coronary angioplasty. Circulation 1997;96:1445–1453.

29. Inhibition of platelet glycoprotein IIb/IIIa with eptifibatide in patients with acute coronary syndromes. The PURSUIT Trial Investigators. Platelet glycoprotein IIb/IIIa in unstable angina: receptor suppression using int therapy. N Engl J Med 1998;339:436–443.

30. Simoons ML; GUSTO IV-ACS Investigators. Effect of glycoprotein IIb/IIIa receptor blocker abciximab on outcome in patients with acute coronary syndromes without early coronary revascularization: the GUSTO IV-ACS randomized trial. Lancet. 2001;357:1915–1924.

31. Platelet Receptor Inhibition in Ischemic Syndrome Management (PRISM) Study Investigators. A comparison of aspirin plus tirofiban with aspirin plus heparin for unstable angina. N Engl J Med 1998;338:1498–5056.

32. Huynh T, Theroux P, Snapinn S, et al. Effect of platelet glycoprotein IIb/IIIa receptor blockade with tirofiban on adverse cardiac events in women with unstable angina/non-ST-elevation myocardial infarction (PRISM-PLUS Study). Am Heart J 2003;146: 668–673.

33. Risk of myocardial infarction and death during treatment with low dose aspirin and intravenous heparin in men with unstable coronary artery disease. The RISC Group. Lancet 1990;336:827–830.

34. Theroux P, Ouimet H, McCans J, et al. Aspirin, heparin, or both to treat acute unstable angina. N Engl J Med 1988;319:1105–1111.

35. Antman EM, Cohen M, Radley D, et al. Assessment of the treatment effect of enoxaparin for unstable angina/non-Q wave myocardial infarction. TIMI IIb-ESSENCE meta-analysis. Circulation 1999;100:1602–1608.

36. Bijsterveld NR, Peters RJ, Murphy SA, et al. Recurrent cardiac ischemic events early after discontinuation of short-term heparin treatment in acute coronary syndromes: results from the Thrombolysis in Myocardial Infarction (TIMI) 11B and Efficacy and Safety of Subcutaneous Enoxaparin in Non-Q-Wave Coronary Events (ESSENCE) studies. J Am Coll Cardiol 2003;42:2083–2089.

37. Ferguson JJ, Califf RM, Antman EM, and the SYNERGY Trial Investigators. Enoxaparin vs. unfractionated heparin in high-risk patients with non-ST-segment elevation acute coronary syndromes managed with an intended early invasive strategy: primary results of the SYNERGY randomized trial. JAMA 2004;292:45–54.

38. Tokmakova MP, Skali H, Kenchaiah S, et al. Chronic kidney disease, cardiovascular risk, and response to angiotensin-converting enzyme inhibition after myocardial infarction: the Survival And Ventricular Enlargement (SAVE) study. Circulation 2004;110:3667–3673.

39. Borghi C, Bacchelli S, Esposti DD, et al. Effects of the administration of an angiotensin-converting enzyme inhibitor during the acute phase of myocardial infarction in patients with arterial hypertension. SMILE Study Investigators. Survival of Myocardial Infarction Long-term Evaluation. Am J Hypertens 1999;12:665–672.

40. Treasure CB, Klein JL, Weintraub WS, et al. Beneficial effects of cholesterol-lowering therapy on the coronary endothelium in patients with coronary artery disease. New Engl J Med 1995;332:481–487.
41. Cannon CP, Braunwald E, McCabe CH, and the Pravastatin or Atorvastatin Evaluation and Infection Therapy—Thrombolysis in Myocardial Infarction 22 Investigators. Intensive versus Moderate Lipid Lowering with Statins after Acute Coronary Syndromes. N Engl J Med 2004:350:1495–1504.
42. Nissen SE, Murat TE, Schoenhagen P, et al. Effect of intensive compared with moderate lipid-lowering therapy on progression of coronary atherosclerosis: a randomized controlled trial. JAMA 2004;291:1071–1080.
43. Hulten E, Jackson JL, Douglas K, et al. The effect of early, intensive statin therapy on acute coronary syndrome: a meta-analysis of randomized controlled trials. Arch Intern Med 2006;166:1814–1821.
44. Fragmin and Fast Revascularisation during Instability in Coronary Artery Disease (FRISC II) Investigators. Invasive compared with non-invasive treatment in unstable coronary artery disease: FRISC II prospective randomized multicenter study. Lancet 1999;354:708–715.
45. Cannon CP, Weintraub WS, Demopoulos LA, and TACTICS (Treat Angina with Aggrastat and Determine Cost of Therapy with an Invasive or Conservative Strategy)—Thrombolysis in Myocardial Infarction 18 Investigators. Comparison of early invasive and conservative strategies in patients with unstable coronary syndromes treated with the glycoprotein IIb/IIIa inhibitor tirofiban. N Engl J Med 2001;344: 1879–1887.
46. Fox KA, Poole-Wilson P, Clayton TC, et al. 5-year outcome of an international strategy in non-ST elevation acute coronary syndrome: the British Heart Foundation RITA 3 randomized trial. Lancet 2005;366:914–920.
47. de Winter RJ, Windhausen F, Cornel JH, and the Invasive versus Conservative Treatment in Unstable Coronary Syndromes (ICTUS) Investigators. Early invasive versus selectively invasive management for acute coronary syndromes. N Engl J Med 2005; 353:1095–1104.
48. Bavry AA, Kumbhani DJ, Rassi AN, et al. Benefit of early invasive therapy in acute coronary syndromes: a meta-analysis of contemporary randomized clinical trials. J Am Coll Cardiol 2006;48:1319–1325.
49. Edlavitch SA, Crow R, Burke GL, et al. Secular trends in Q wave and non-Q wave acute myocardial infarction. The Minnesota Heart Survey. Circulation 1991;83: 492–503.
50. Peterson ED, Pollack CV Jr, Roe MT, et al. Early use of glycoprotein IIb/IIIa inhibitors in non–ST-elevation acute myocardial infarction: observations from the National Registry of Myocardial Infarction 4. J Am Coll Cardiol 2003;42;45–53.
51. Ryan JW, Peterson ED, Chen AY, et al. Optimal timing of intervention in non–ST-segment elevation acute coronary syndromes: insights from the CRUSADE (Can Rapid risk stratification of Unstable angina patients Suppress ADverse outcomes with Early implementation of the ACC/AHA guidelines) Registry. Circulation 2005;112;3049–3057.
52. Ticoci, P, Peterson ED, Roe MT, et al. Patterns of guideline adherence and care delivery for patients with unstable angina and non-ST segment elevation myocardial infarction (from the CRUSADE Quality Improvement Initiative). Am J Cardiol 2006;98:S30–S35.

8
Diagnosis and Treatment of Unstable Angina

Aslam Khan, Robert Kornberg, and David L. Coven

Stable angina pectoris is defined as chest pain that is substernal, brought on by exertion, and relived with rest or nitroglycerin. The pain usually radiates to the left arm, jaw, or back. Unstable angina (UA) is angina pectoris that is either occurring at rest, new in onset, or increasing in intensity. New-onset unstable angina is severe angina (Canadian Cardiovascular Society class III [Table 8.1] or greater) that is less than 1 month old. Crescendo angina is angina increasing in intensity, duration, or frequency to at least Canadian Cardiovascular Society (CCS) class III. Rest angina is angina occurring at rest and usually lasting greater than 20 minutes [1]. By definition, UA patients have negative cardiac biomarkers (troponins, creatine kinase [CK]-MB) with or without ST changes. Because of the similar pathophysiology between UA and non–ST-segment elevation myocardial infarction (NSTEMI), their treatment often overlaps. When following this treatment algorithm, it is important to remember that patients with UA tend to be at lower risk of major adverse outcomes than those patients with NSTEMI.

Significance

It is estimated that approximately 1.2 million Americans were diagnosed with acute coronary syndrome (ACS) in 2006. About 25% of these ischemic episodes were due to UA [2]. Appropriate management initially lowers mortality (1.7% at 30 days) in patients with UA compared with NSTEMI or ST-segment elevation myocardial infarction (STEMI). However, these patients tend to have a higher long-term mortality after the event [3]. Thus, it is critical to appropriately identify patients with UA and treat them aggressively.

Diagnosis of Unstable Angina (Step 1)

Due to the various clinical presentations of ACS, it may be challenging to diagnose early when evidence of myocardial injury may not be apparent. Other serious nonischemic cardiovascular symptoms must be ruled out (e.g., aortic

TABLE 8.1. Canadian Cardiovascular Society Angina Grading System.

Class	Description of stage
I	"Ordinary physical activity does not cause . . . angina," such as walking or climbing stairs. Angina occurs with strenuous, rapid, or prolonged exertion at work or recreation.
II	"Slight limitation of ordinary activity." Angina occurs on walking or climbing stairs rapidly; walking uphill; walking or stair climbing after meals; in cold, in wind, or under emotional stress; or only during the few hours after awakening. Angina occurs on walking >2 blocks on the level and climbing >1 flight of ordinary stairs at a normal pace and under normal conditions
III	"Marked limitations of ordinary physical activity." Angina occurs on walking 1 to 2 blocks on the level and climbing 1 flight of stairs under normal conditions and at a normal pace.
IV	"Inability to carry on any physical activity without discomfort—anginal symptoms may be present at rest."

Source: Braunwald E, Mark DB, Jones RH, et al. Unstable angina: diagnosis and management. AHCPR Publication No. 94-0602. Rockville, MD: Agency for Health Care Policy and Research and the National Heart, Lung, and Blood Institute, US Public Health Service, US Department of Health and Human Services; 1994.

dissection). Less serious cardiac and noncardiac conditions must also be excluded (e.g., pericarditis or gastritis). Traditional risk factors increase the likelihood of coronary artery disease (CAD) but not of acute ischemia [4, 5]. Thus, in making the diagnosis of ACS, these factors should not be the only

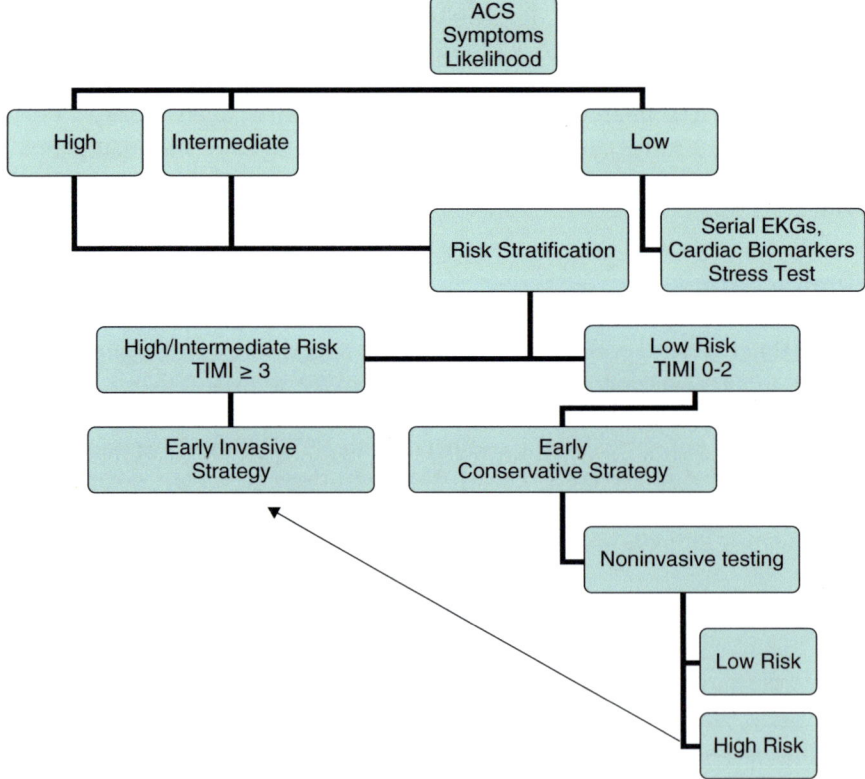

FIGURE 8.1. Triage of patients with unstable angina based on TIMI risk scores.

TABLE 8.2. The likelihood that a patient's symptoms represent ACS.

High likelihood
1. Chest or left arm pain or discomfort as chief symptom reproducing prior documented angina.
2. Known history of coronary artery disease, including myocardial infarction.
3. Transient mitral regurgitation, hypotension, diaphoresis, pulmonary edema.
4. New, or presumably new, transient ST-segment deviation (≥ 0.05 mV) or T-wave inversion (≥ 0.2 mV) with symptoms.
5. Elevated cardiac biomarkers (troponin I, troponin T, or CK-MB).

Intermediate likelihood
1. Absence of any of the high-likelihood characteristics.
2. Chest or left arm pain as chief complaint.
3. Age >70 years.
4. Male sex.
5. Diabetes mellitus.
6. Peripheral vascular disease.
7. Old ST/T wave changes or fixed Q waves.
8. Negative biomarkers.

Low likelihood
1. Absence of any of the intermediate- or high-likelihood characteristics.
2. Recent cocaine use.
3. Reproducible chest pain.
4. Flat/inverted T waves in leads with dominant R waves.
5. No ST changes.
6. Negative cardiac biomarkers.

Source: Braunwald E, Mark DB, Jones RH, et al. Unstable angina: Diagnosis and management. AHCPR Publication No. 94-0602. Rockville, MD: Agency for Health Care Policy and Research and the National Heart, Lung, and Blood Institute, US Public Health Service, US Department of Health and Human Services; 1994.

variable used in the algorithm. Instead, it has been proved that combination of history, physical exam, electrocardiogram (ECG), and serum biomarkers results in a greater predictor of ACS [6]. This brings us to step 1 in the algorithm (Fig. 8.1). Using these subjective and objective findings, the practitioner should categorize the patient into high, intermediate, or low likelihood that his or her symptoms represent ACS (Table 8.2) (see Chapter 2, Fig. 2.1) [7]. High-likelihood patients not only are more likely to have ACS but also carry an increased risk for adverse outcomes. On the other end of the spectrum are patients with low likelihood of ACS; they should be appropriately identified and followed up with serial ECGs and cardiac biomarkers and noninvasive stress testing (see Chapter 2, Fig. 2.10) [8].

Risk Stratification (Step 2)

Once a patient has been identified as having UA (high- or intermediate-likelihood symptoms represent ACS), it becomes key to appropriately categorize him or her in terms of expected outcomes (see Chapter 2, Fig. 2.7). Certain presenting clinical features (risk factors) of the patient have been identified as independent future predictors of poor outcomes. These risk factors are multiple

TABLE **8.3.** TIMI risk score.

Risk factors	Points
Age ≥65 years	1
≥3 CAD risk factors (FHx, HTN, ↑ Chol, DM, active smoker)	1
Known CAD (stenosis ≥50%)	1
ASA use in past 7 days	1
Recent (≤24 hours) severe angina	1
↑ Cardiac markers	1
ST deviation ≥0.5 mm	1
Risk score (0–2, low risk; 3–7, high risk)	Total points

Source: Antman EM, Cohen M, Bernink PJ, et al. The TIMI risk score for unstable angina/non-ST elevation MI: a method for prognostication and therapeutic decision making. JAMA 2000;284:835–842.
FXx, family history; HTN, hypertension; ↑Chol, hypercholesterolemia; DM, diabetes mellitus.

and range from age, sex, diabetes to heart rate, systolic blood pressure, and presence of arrhythmias at presentation [9, 10]. Combined risk assessment scores have been developed that integrate all the preceding factors and, based on the score, stratify patients into low- or high-risk categories [11–13]. In subsequent studies, these scores have been proven to be accurate in predicting outcomes at 30 days and 1 year [14–18]. However, the main drawback of some of these scores is that they may be too complex, requiring computer computations, to calculate at bedside. Antman et al. have developed a 7-point "TIMI risk score" (Table 8.3). This score is not only simple to use but also has been validated in several studies. This score takes into account seven risk factors assigning each 1 point. The score is then calculated by the sum of the risk factors. With a score less than 3, the patient is thought to be low risk for major adverse events. When the score is ≥3, the patient is at high risk for such events and requires more aggressive management.

Early Invasive Versus Early Conservative Strategy (Step 3)

After risk stratification, we come to step 3 of the pathway. In patients with UA/NSTEMI, two strategies are possible: a routine invasive strategy where all patients undergo coronary angiography shortly after admission (≤48 hours) and, if indicated, coronary revascularization; or a conservative strategy where medical therapy alone is used initially with selection of patients for angiography based on clinical symptoms or noninvasive evidence of persistent myocardial ischemia. Several large-scale clinical trials have been conducted to evaluate which strategy is superior. Earlier trials failed to demonstrate an improvement in outcomes with the routine use of an early invasive strategy [19, 20]. These studies were conducted before the common use of intracoronary stents and glycoprotein IIb/IIIa inhibitors, and this factor is thought to be the primary reason for the lack of benefit seen with an invasive approach [21]. Subsequent studies reevaluated the potential benefits of these two strategies, investigating glycoprotein IIb/IIIa inhibitors and coronary stents. Data from these trials showed a clear benefit of invasive approach in patients at intermediate or higher risk for negative outcome [18, 22]. Patients who are at low risk for adverse outcomes (TIMI risk ≤2) may be managed medically with results equal to that of the invasive therapy group [18].

It is with these low-risk patients that further treatment diverges based on prognostic factors delineated during stress testing (see Chapter 9). At 24 to 48 hours after these low-risk patients are stabilized medically, they should undergo noninvasive testing [23]. An imaging study is recommended (i.e., echocardiogram) to assess left ventricular function. These patients should also undergo either an exercise or pharmacological stress test to evaluate for any residual zones of ischemia despite maximal medical therapy. If provocable ischemia is documented or high-risk features are present (Table 8.4), there is a benefit of revascularizing this cohort of patients [24]. Moreover, if patients initially deemed to be low risk develop certain high-risk clinical indicators (Table 8.5), they should undergo coronary angiography. Patients without any high-risk features may be discharged home after stabilization on appropriate preventative medical regimen (see Chapter 2, Fig. 2.12).

TABLE 8.4. Noninvasive test results predicting high risk for adverse outcomes.

Exercise electrocardiographic testing
Abnormal horizontal or downsloping ST-segment depression with
   Onset at heart rate <120 beats/min or ≤6.5 METs
   Magnitude ≥2.0 mm
   Postexercise duration of ≥6 minutes
   Depression in multiple leads
Abnormal systolic blood pressure response
   With sustained decrease of >10 mm Hg or flat blood pressure response ≤130 mm Hg, associated with
      abnormal electrocardiogram
Other
   Exercise-induced ST-segment elevation
   Ventricular tachycardia

Radionuclide myocardial perfusion imaging
Abnormal myocardial tracer distribution in more than one coronary artery region at rest or with stress or an
   anterior defect that reperfuses
Abnormal myocardial distribution with increased lung uptake
Cardiac enlargement

Left ventricular imaging
Stress radionuclide ventriculography
   Exercise EF ≤50%
   Rest EF ≤35%
   Fall in EF ≥10%

Stress echocardiography
   Rest EF ≤35%
   Wall motion score index >1

Source: Zipes DP, Lippy P, Braunwald E, eds. Braunwald's heart disease. 7th ed. Philadelphia: Elsevier Saunders; 2005:1261.
METs, metabolic equivalent; EF, ejection fraction.

TABLE **8.5.** Clinical indicators of high risk of adverse events.

Recurrent angina/ischemia at rest or with low-level activities despite intensive anti-ischemic medical therapy
Decreased left ventricular systolic function (e.g., EF less than 0.40 on noninvasive study)
Hemodynamic instability
Sustained ventricular tachycardia
PCI within 6 months
Prior CABG
High-risk findings on noninvasive stress testing
Recurrent angina/ischemia with CHF symptoms, an S3 gallop, pulmonary edema, worsening rales, or new or worsening MR

METs, metabolic equivalent; EF, ejection fraction.

Medications

Medicines used to treat UA fall into two categories: antiplatelet/antithrombotic and anti-ischemic (see also Chapters 5 and 7). Antiplatelet/antithrombotic agents prevent thrombus/clot formation; they usually do not dissolve already formed clot. Anti-ischemic medications work by either increasing oxygen supply to the myocardium or by decreasing myocardial oxygen demand.

Antiplatelet/Antithrombotic Medications

Aspirin

Aspirin (ASA) is one of the key medications in the treatment armamentarium for UA. The data for the use of ASA is compelling. It has been shown to reduce mortality by 50% in several clinical trials [25, 26]. By acetylating the cyclooxygenase enzyme, ASA inhibits the formation of thromboxane A_2, a potent platelet activator, thus inhibiting one of the first steps in the formation of a platelet plug. When a patient with UA is identified, they should be treated with 162 to 325 mg ASA [27, 28]. This dose should be administered to the patient as chewable baby ASA. This allows for rapid absorption of the drug through the buccal mucosa into the bloodstream. Once a patient has been given the loading dose, they can be treated with a reduce dose of ASA (81 mg). This low-dose therapy is just as effective as higher doses and is associated with fewer complications [29, 30]. ASA should be continued indefinitely after an event.

Clopidogrel

This agent works by inhibiting the adenosine diphosphate (ADP) receptor on platelets. This inhibition prevents platelet activation and aggregation. There is strong evidence for the addition of clopidogrel to ASA on admission in the management of patients with UA and NSTEMI, in whom either a noninterventional or interventional approach is intended [31]. There is a question of how long this medication should be continued. For patients in the noninvasive group, the drug should be continued for approximately 9 to 12 months, whereas in the early invasive group, clopidogrel should be continued for 1 months in those with bare metal stents and much longer in those with drug-eluting stents [32].

Heparin

Unfractionated heparin (UFH) works by binding to antithrombin and greatly enhancing its activity. Antithrombin inhibits formation of fibrin from fibrinogen, thus preventing one of the final steps in clot formation. It prevents thrombus propagation but does not aid in dissolution of existing thrombi. When combined with aspirin, UFH has been shown to further reduce the risk of death and future myocardial infarctions [26, 33]. Patients receive a bolus of 60 U/kg and are then started on $12\,U\,kg^{-1}\,h^{-1}$ drip. Patients' partial thromboplastin time (PTT) should be checked every 6 hours for 18 hours, then daily thereafter [34]. The goal of therapy is to keep the PTT between 50 to 70 seconds [35]. UFH should be continued for approximately 2 to 5 days after the event in the conservative arm. It is usually stopped immediately after an intervention in the invasive group.

Low-Molecular-Weight Heparin

Low-molecular-weight heparin (LMWH) has the benefit of predictable anticoagulation activity; thus, it does not need routine PTT monitoring. It works similar to UFH; however, LMWH has an increased anti–factor Xa activity. This increased upstream blockade in the coagulation pathway allows for a more efficient inhibition of thrombin formation. Furthermore, its high bioavailability allows LMWH to be administered subcutaneously twice daily. Several trials have been performed comparing UFH and LMWH in UA/NSTEMI. Enoxaparin is the LMWH with the most data to support its use in UA. Enoxaparin has been proven to be superior to UFH [16, 17]. However, this benefit was mainly seen in patients with intermediate to high risk of adverse events (TIMI risk ≥3). There are also mixed data about whether enoxaparin remains superior to UFH when these agents are combined with IIb/IIIa inhibitors [36–38]. Overall, enoxaparin is a safe and effective alternative to unfractionated heparin. It is dosed at 1 mg/kg subcutaneously and may be given even just prior to percutaneous coronary intervention (PCI); however, most interventionalists prefer to hold the medication the morning of the procedure [39]. Its use is restricted in the obese patient population and in those with renal failure.

Glycoprotein IIb/IIIa Inhibitors

Glycoprotein (GP) IIb/IIIa inhibitors block the final step in clot formation—the cross-linking of fibrin across two platelets. Three agents are available commercially: abciximab, eptifibatide, and tirofiban. Eptifibatide and tirofiban have been shown to reduce mortality in patients with UA/NSTEMI in both conserva-tive and early invasive groups, whereas abciximab is reserved for patients undergoing PCI [40–42]. It is important to remember that GP IIb/IIIa inhibitors should be used in patients at high risk for adverse cardiac events that are under-going PCI or are managed conservatively because contraindications to PCI exist [43]. Due to its long half-life, abciximab is stopped 1 hour after PCI. Eptifibatide and tirofiban are continued for approximately 12 to 24 hours after PCI and 48 to 72 hours in medically managed patients. Administration for all these medica-tions requires a weight-based bolus followed by an infusion drip. Because these agents are often used in conjunction with ASA, clopidogrel, or heparin, there is a risk of major bleeding.

Anti-Ischemic Medications

Beta Blockers

Beta-blockers inhibit sympathetic activity on the myocardium. This leads to decreased heart rate and contractility (negative chronotropic and inotropic activity), thus decreased myocardial oxygen demand. Evidence outlining the efficacy of beta-blockers in UA is limited at best. However, data extrapolated from other forms of ACS show a benefit with beta-blockers [1]. Routine admin-istration of intravenous (IV) followed by oral beta-blockers at the initial pre-sentation of ACS should be avoided [44]. This is because the gains seen in preventing death and ventricular fibrillation are nullified with cardiogenic shock. It is prudent to wait until the patient has become stable and then treat with oral beta-blockers. No trials have been done to show the optimal duration of long-term oral therapy with beta-blockers in patients with UA. Thus, espe-cially in the high-risk group, beta-blocker therapy should be carried out indefinitely.

Nitrates

Nitrates work by causing venous and arterial dilatation, thus reducing preload, afterload, and myocardial oxygen demand. No survival benefit has been shown with nitrates [45, 46]. However, they are excellent for relieving symptoms of ischemia. Patients should be treated with 0.4 mg sublingual tablets of nitroglyc-erin given 5 minutes apart over 15 minutes. If this fails to relieve pain, patients should be administered IV nitroglycerin starting at 10 μg/min titrated up every 5 minutes until symptomatic improvement or until systolic blood pressure less than 100 mm Hg is reached. Nitrates should be avoided in patients who have taken sildenafil in the past 24 hours, as this can exacerbate and prolong the effects of nitroglycerin leading to hypotension and even death.

Calcium Channel Blockers

Calcium channel blockers are also effective in reducing blood pressure and heart rate. They can be used if ischemia persists despite maximal beta-blocker therapy or if beta-blockers are contraindicated. Diltiazem should be avoided in patients with left ventricular dysfunction, and nifedipine should not be administered unless the patient has been pretreated with beta-blockers.

Other Medications

Morphine

Morphine can be administered 1 to 5 mg IV in patients with ongoing chest pain despite nitrate therapy. No mortality benefit is seen with this agent (see Chapter 7 regarding potentially increased mortality). Nonetheless, morphine is effective at reducing anxiety and pain associated with acute ischemia. One should watch for hypotension with morphine use especially if concomitant nitrate therapy is being used.

Angiotensin-Converting Enzyme Inhibitors

There seems to be no benefit of early (<24 hours) short-term treatment with angiotensin-converting enzyme (ACE) inhibitors in patients with UA, and it may be actually harmful. This is thought to be secondary to hypotension caused by the agent [47]. After patients have stabilized, they should be treated with long-term ACE inhibitor therapy, especially if left ventricular dysfunction is present [48]. There seems to be a class effect with ACE inhibitors, with all having a benefit after infarction. Hyperkalemia, renal failure, and hypotension are the main side effects of these medications.

HMG CoA Reductase Inhibitors (Statins)

Statins work by inhibiting cholesterol formation in the liver. This reduces low-density lipoprotein (LDL) levels and increases high-density lipoprotein (HDL) levels. By decreasing LDL formation, there is a decrease of LDL deposition and decreased oxidation of LDL in tissue. This decrease in oxidized LDL results in lowered inflammatory enzymes and metalloproteinases. This reduction in inflammatory activity leads to increased stability of the fibrinous cap of an atheromatous plaque, thus preventing plaque rupture and ACS. Early (<10 day) high-dose therapy with atorvastatin 80 mg is proven to lower future adverse events [49]. Statin therapy is associated with liver dysfunction and rhabdomyolysis. A periodic check of liver function is warranted with therapy.

References

1. Braunwald E, Antman EM, Beasley JW, et al. ACC/AHA guideline update for the management of patients with unstable angina and non-ST-segment elevation myocardial infarction-2002: summary article: a report of the American College of Cardiology/American Heart Association Task Force on Practice Guidelines (Committee on the Management of Patients With Unstable Angina). Circulation 2002;106: 1893–1900.

2. American Heart Association. 2006 Heart and Stroke Statistical Update. Available at www.americanheart.org.
3. Armstrong PW, Fu Y, Chang WC, et al., for the GUSTO-IIb Investigators. Acute coronary syndromes in the GUSTO-IIb trial: prognostic insights and impact of recurrent ischemia. Circulation 1998;98:1860–1868.
4. Selker HP, Griffith JL, D'Agostino RB. A tool for judging coronary care unit admission appropriateness, valid for both real-time and retrospective use: a time-insensitive predictive instrument (TIPI) for acute cardiac ischemia a multicenter study. Med Care 1991;29:610–627.
5. Jayes RLJ, Beshansky JR, D'Agostino RB, et al. Do patients' coronary risk factor reports predict acute cardiac ischemia in the emergency department? A multicenter study. J Clin Epidemiol 1992;45:621–626.
6. White HD, Barbash GI, Califf RM, et al. Age and outcome with contemporary thrombolytic therapy: Results from the GUSTO-I trial. Global Utilization of Streptokinase and TPA for Occluded coronary arteries trial. Circulation 1996;94:1826–1833.
7. Braunwald E, Mark DB, Jones RH, et al. Unstable angina: diagnosis and management. AHCPR Publication No. 94-0602. Rockville, MD: Agency for Health Care Policy and Research and the National Heart, Lung, and Blood Institute, US Public Health Service, US Department of Health and Human Services; 1994.
8. Braunwald E. Application of current guidelines to the management of unstable angina and non-ST elevation myocardial infarction. Circulation 2003;108:111–128.
9. Stone PH, Thompson B, Anderson HV, et al., for the TIMI III Registry Study Group. Influence of race, sex, and age on management of unstable angina and non-Q-wave myocardial infarction: The TIMI III Registry. JAMA 1996;275:1104–1112.
10. Al-Khatib SM, Granger CB, Huang Y, et al. Sustained ventricular arrhythmias among patients with acute coronary syndromes with no ST-segment elevation: incidence, predictors, and outcomes. Circulation 2002;106:309–312.
11. Granger CB, Goldberg RJ, Dabbous O, et al. Predictors of hospital mortality in the Global Registry of Acute Coronary Events. Arch Intern Med 2003;163:2345–2353.
12. Boersma E, Pieper KS, Steyerberg EW, et al., for the PURSUIT Investigators. Predictors of outcome in patients with acute coronary syndromes without persistent ST-segment elevation. Results from an international trial of 9461 patients. Circulation 2000;101:2557–2567.
13. Antman EM, Cohen M, Bernink PJ, et al. The TIMI risk score for unstable angina/non-ST elevation MI: a method for prognostication and therapeutic decision making. JAMA 2000;284:835–842.
14. de Araujo Goncalves P, Ferreira J, Aguiar C, et al. TIMI, PURSUIT, and GRACE risk scores: sustained prognostic value and interaction with revascularization in NSTE-ACS. Eur Heart J 2005;26:865–872.
15. Antman EM, McCabe CH, Gurfinkel EP, et al. Enoxaparin prevents death and cardiac ischemic events in unstable angina/non-Q-wave myocardial infarction: results of the Thrombolysis In Myocardial Infarction (TIMI) 11B trial. Circulation 1999;100:1593–1601.
16. Cohen M, Demers C, Gurfinkel EP, et al. A comparison of low molecular-weight heparin with unfractionated heparin for unstable coronary artery disease. Efficacy and Safety of Subcutaneous Enoxaparin in Non-Q-Wave Coronary Events Study Group. N Engl J Med 1997;337:447–452.
17. Cannon CP, Weintraub WS, Demopoulos LA, et al. Comparison of early invasive and conservative strategies in patients with unstable coronary syndromes treated with the glycoprotein IIb/IIIa inhibitor tirofiban. N Engl J Med 2001;344:1879–1887.

18. Morrow DA, Antman EM, Snapinn SM, et al. An integrated clinical approach to predicting the benefit of tirofiban in non-ST elevation acute coronary syndromes. Application of the TIMI risk score for UA/NSTEMI in PRISM-PLUS. Eur Heart J 2002;23:223–229.

19. Effects of tissue plasminogen activator and a comparison of early invasive and conservative strategies in unstable angina and non-Q-wave myocardial infarction: results of the TIMI IIIB Trial. Circulation 1994;89:1545–1556.

20. Boden WE, O'Rourke RA, Crawford MH, et al. Outcomes in patients with acute non-Q-wave myocardial infarction randomly assigned to an invasive as compared with a conservative management strategy. N Engl J Med 1998;338:1785–1792.

21. Boden WE, McKay RG. Optimal treatment of acute coronary syndromes—an evolving strategy. N Engl J Med 2001;344:1939–1942.

22. Invasive compared with non-invasive treatment in unstable coronary artery disease: FRISC II prospective randomized multicenter study. Lancet 1999;354:708–715.

23. Karha J, Gibson CM, Murphy SA, et al. Safety of stress testing during the evolution of unstable angina pectoris or non-ST-elevation myocardial infarction. Am J Cardiol 2004;94:1537–1539.

24. Madsen JK, Grande P, Saunamaki K, et al., on behalf of the DANAMI Study Group. Danish multicenter randomized study of invasive versus conservative treatment in patients with inducible ischemia after thrombolysis in acute myocardial infarction (DANAMI). Circulation 1997;96:748–755.

25. The RISC Group. Risk of myocardial infarction and death during treatment with low dose aspirin and intravenous heparin in men with unstable coronary artery disease. Lancet 1990;336:827–830.

26. Lewis HD Jr, Davis JW, Archibald DG, et al. Protective effects of aspirin against acute myocardial infarction and death in men with unstable angina. Results of a Veterans Administration Cooperative Study. N Engl J Med 1983;309:396–403.

27. Collaborative overview of randomised trials of antiplatelet therapy—I: Prevention of death, myocardial infarction, and stroke by prolonged antiplatelet therapy in various categories of patients. Antiplatelet Trialists' Collaboration. BMJ 1994;308:81–106.

28. ISIS-2 (Second International Study of Infarct Survival) Collaborative Group. Randomised trial of intravenous streptokinase, oral aspirin, both, or neither among 17,187 cases of suspected acute myocardial infarction: ISIS-2. Lancet 1988;2:349–360.

29. Topol EJ, Easton D, Harrington RA, et al. Randomized, double-blind, placebo-controlled, international trial of the oral IIb/IIIa antagonist lotrafiban in coronary and cerebrovascular disease. Circulation 2003;108:399–406.

30. Peters RJ, Mehta SR, Fox KA, et al. Effects of aspirin dose when used alone or in combination with clopidogrel in patients with acute coronary syndromes: Observations from the Clopidogrel in Unstable angina to prevent Recurrent Events (CURE) study. Circulation 2003;108:1682–1687.

31. Mehta SR, Yusuf S, Peters RJ, et al. Effects of pretreatment with clopidogrel and aspirin followed by long-term therapy in patients undergoing percutaneous coronary intervention: the PCI-CURE study. Lancet 2001;358:527–533.

32. Pfisterer M, Brunner-La Rocca HP, Buser PT, et al. Late clinical events after clopidogrel discontinuation may limit the benefit of drug-eluting stents. J Am Coll Cardiol 2006;48:2584–2591.

33. Oler A, Whooley MA, Oler J, et al. Adding heparin to aspirin reduces the incidence of myocardial infarction and death in patients with unstable angina: a meta-analysis. JAMA 1996;276:811–815.
34. Becker RC, Ball SP, Eisenberg P, et al. A randomized, multicenter trial of weight-adjusted intravenous heparin dose titration and point-of-care coagulation monitoring in hospitalized patients with active thromboembolic disease. Antithrombotic Therapy Consortium Investigators. Am Heart J 1999;137:59–71.
35. Granger CB, Hirsh J, Califf RM, et al., for the GUSTO-I Investigators. Activated partial thromboplastin time and outcome after thrombolytic therapy for acute myocardial infarction: results from the GUSTO-I Trial. Circulation 1996;93:870–878.
36. Blazing MA, De Lemos JA, Dyke CK, et al. The A-to-Z Trial: Methods and rationale for a single trial investigating combined use of low-molecular-weight heparin with the glycoprotein IIb/IIIa inhibitor tirofiban and defining the efficacy of early aggressive simvastatin therapy. Am Heart J 2001;142:211–217.
37. Goodman SG, Fitchett D, Armstrong PW, et al. Randomized evaluation of the safety and efficacy of enoxaparin versus unfractionated heparin in high-risk patients with non-ST-segment elevation acute coronary syndromes receiving the glycoprotein IIb/IIIa inhibitor eptifibatide. Circulation 2003;107:238–244.
38. SYNERGY Steering Committee. Superior yield of the new strategy of enoxaparin, revascularization and glycoprotein IIb/IIIa inhibitors (SYNERGY): primary results. JAMA 2004;292:45–54.
39. Collet JP, Montalescot G, Lison L, et al. Percutaneous coronary intervention after subcutaneous enoxaparin pretreatment inpatients with unstable angina pectoris. Circulation 2001;103:658–663.
40. The PURSUIT Trial Investigators. Inhibition of platelet glycoprotein IIb/IIIa with eptifibatide in patients with acute coronary syndromes. N Engl J Med 1998;339:436–443.
41. Platelet Receptor Inhibition in Ischemic Syndrome Management in Patients Limited by Unstable Signs and Symptoms (PRISMPLUS) Study Investigators. Inhibition of the platelet glycoprotein IIb/IIIa receptor with tirofiban in unstable angina and non–Qwave myocardial infarction. N Engl J Med 1998;338:1488–1497.
42. The GUSTO IV-ACS Investigators. Effect of glycoprotein IIb/IIIa receptor blocker abciximab on outcome in patients with acute coronary syndromes without early coronary revascularization: the GUSTO IV-ACS randomised trial. Lancet 2001;357:1915–1924.
43. Boersma E, Harrington RA, Moliterno DJ, et al. Platelet glycoprotein IIb/IIIa inhibitors in acute coronary syndromes: a metaanalysis of all major randomised clinical trials. Lancet 2002;359:189–198.
44. COMMIT (Clopidogrel and Metoprolol in Myocardial Infarction Trial) collaborative group. Early intravenous then oral metoprolol in 45,852 patients with acute myocardial infarction: randomised placebo-controlled trial. Lancet 2005;366:1622–1632.
45. Gruppo Italiano per lo Studio della Sopravvivenza nell'Infarto Miocardico. GISSI-3: Effect of lisinopril and transdermal glyceryl trinitrate singly and together on 6-week mortality and ventricular function after acute myocardial infarction. Lancet 1994;343:1115–1122.
46. ISIS-4 Collaborative Group. ISIS-4: Randomized factorial trial assessing early oral captopril, oral mononitrate, and intravenous magnesium sulphate in 58,050 patients with suspected acute myocardial infarction. Lancet 1995;345:669–685.

47. Avanzini F, Ferrario G, Santoro L, et al., for Gruppo Italiano per lo Studio della Sopravvivenza nell'Infarto miocardico-3 Investigators. Risks and benefits of early treatment of acute myocardial infarction with an angiotensin-converting enzyme inhibitor in patients with a history of arterial hypertension: analysis of the GISSI-3 database. Am Heart J 2002;144:1018–1025.
48. Yusuf S, Sleight P, Pogue J, et al., for the Heart Outcomes Prevention Evaluation Study Investigators. Effects of an angiotensin-converting-enzyme inhibitor, ramipril, on cardiovascular events in high-risk patients. N Engl J Med 2000;342:145–153.
49. Cannon CP, Braunwald E, McCabe CH, et al. Intensive versus moderate lipid lowering with statins after acute coronary syndromes. N Engl J Med 2004;350: 1495–1504.

9
Use of Stress Testing for the Risk Stratification of Patients at Low to Intermediate Event Risk According to the PAIN Pathway Algorithm

Seth Uretsky, Randy E. Cohen, and Alan Rozanski

Coronary artery disease is a progressive disease with a wide range of clinical presentations. In some individuals, the development of angina is the first warning sign, but in others, acute coronary syndrome, unheralded myocardial infarction, or sudden death is the initial clinical presentation. The atherosclerotic findings that correspond with these clinical presentations also vary widely. For example, it has been demonstrated that among patients presenting with acute coronary syndromes, approximately 30% of such patients have triple-vessel disease, 30% have double-vessel disease, 30% have single-vessel disease, and approximately 10% are without evidence of significant atherosclerotic narrowing [1–3]. Moreover, various studies have demonstrated that anginal symptoms and inducible myocardial ischemia are not tightly coupled. Patients with typical angina frequently do not manifest inducible ischemia, and conversely, patients with inducible ischemia often do not manifest chest pain (i.e., they manifest "silent ischemia") [4, 5]. For these reasons, the astute clinician learns not to rely solely on clinical evaluation in the workup and follow-up of patients who present with chest pain. Rather, objective measures of cardiac risk, such as the degree of abnormality during cardiac stress testing, is used by clinicians as a decision guide for the clinical management of patients who present with clinical symptoms.

Making a correct diagnosis in the setting of new-onset chest pain is especially important because the a priori risk for significant atherosclerosis is higher in such patients and because progression to very early myocardial revascularization is very important for those having chest pain due to unstable or ruptured atherosclerotic plaque. Accordingly, the St. Luke's-Roosevelt Hospital Center "chest pain pathway" is designed to implement a rapid-response approach to patients presenting to our hospital with acute chest pain. This pathway includes specific indications for the immediate referral to our cardiac catheterization laboratory for those with acute chest pain. These include the immediate referral of patients who present with ST-elevation myocardial infarction or have prolonged chest pain in association with ST changes and/or increase in cardiac enzymes. This pathway has the acronym PAIN, and it is described at length in

Chapter 2. Patients with low to intermediate risk of cardiac events by our pathway include patients with transient chest pain without definitive ST changes or elevations in cardiac enzymes and without signs of new heart failure or hemodynamic instability (see Chapters 12 and 13).

Risk Stratification of Low- to Intermediate-Risk PAIN Pathway Patients

Table 9.1 lists potential methods for evaluating chest pain patients with a low- to intermediate-risk profile. Among these approaches, the performance of stress testing is the most widely used method of risk stratifying such patients. Theoretically, stress testing for our PAIN pathway patients could be performed using either exercise electrocardiography, stress-rest myocardial perfusion single photon computed emission tomography (SPECT) imaging, or stress echocardiography. However, exercise electrocardiography would not be suitable for the evaluation of our patients because this technique does not have sufficient intrinsic sensitivity for excluding angiographically significant disease once coronary artery disease (CAD) likelihood ranges above ~50% (Fig. 9.1). Rather, stress-rest SPECT myocardial perfusion imaging or stress echocardiography are the procedures of choice for the evaluation of our PAIN pathway patients, and both imaging modalities are used at our institution. Unlike exercise electrocardiography, both of these techniques have the ability to size the magnitude of inducible myocardial ischemia, according to a variety of ischemic "extent" and "severity" variables, as listed in Table 9.2. Ischemic "extent" variables, such as the number of stress-induced perfusion abnormalities or stress-induced wall motion abnormalities, roughly indicate the overall area of potentially jeopardized myocardium. Ischemic "severity" variables, such as the regional magnitude of perfusion or wall motion abnormality induced during stress testing, roughly correlate with the severity of angiographic stenosis subtending a given myocardial region. Importantly, Ladenheim et al. demonstrated the extent and severity of ischemia are independent predictors of adverse

TABLE 9.1. Approaches to the risk stratification of PAIN patients.

1. Stress testing
   - Exercise electrocardiography
   - Stress-rest SPECT imaging
        Exercise
        Adenosine/dipyridamole
        Dobutamine
   - Stress echocardiography
        Exercise
        Dobutamine
2. Noninvasive CTA
3. Calcium scanning

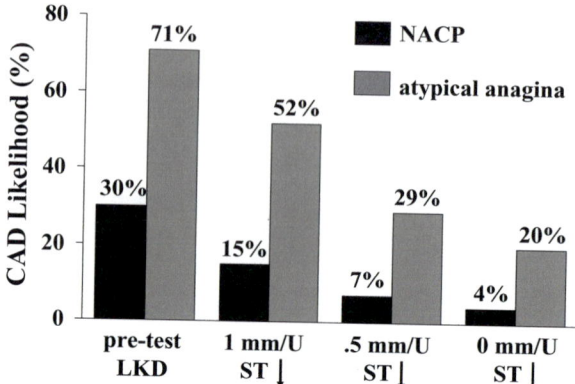

FIGURE 9.1. Shown is the calculated Bayesian likelihood of angiographically significant CAD (vertical axis) for a 55-year-old male without risk factors with 9.7 metabolic equivalents (METS) of exercise, according to whether the patient had nonanginal chest pain (NACP; *black bars*) or atypical angina (*gray bars*). Prior to exercise ECG, the patient with nonanginal chest pain has a low intermediate likelihood of CAD (30%), and the patient with atypical angina has a high intermediate likelihood. Shown are three exercise ST-segment responses (1, 0.5, and 0 mm of upsloping ST-segment depression). Note that for the patient with atypical angina, even a completely normal exercise ECG does not result in a sufficiently low post-test ECG likelihood for excluding the presence of CAD. LKD, likelihood; U, upsloping.

patient outcomes [6]. Moreover, both the extent and severity of ischemia are exponentially related to the future frequency of cardiac events so that those patients having both extensive and severe ischemia are particularly at high risk for future cardiac events (Fig. 9.2) [6].

Patients undergoing cardiac imaging procedures can be divided into four useful clinical groups based on the magnitude of their stress-test findings, including those with: (a) normal stress tests, (b) equivocal stress test findings,

TABLE 9.2. Characterization of the magnitude of ischemia according to "severity" and "extent" of ischemia variables.

	"Severity" of ischemia	"Extent" of ischemia
SPECT imaging		
Number of perfusion defects		++++
Severity of perfusion defects	++++	
Thallium lung uptake	+	+++
Transient ischemic dilatation	++++	++++
Delayed defect reversibility	++++	
Stunned myocardium	++++	
Stress echocardiography		
Number of wall motion abnormalities		++++
Severity of wall motion abnormalities	++++	
Contractile reserve	++++	
Transient ischemic dilatation	++++	++++

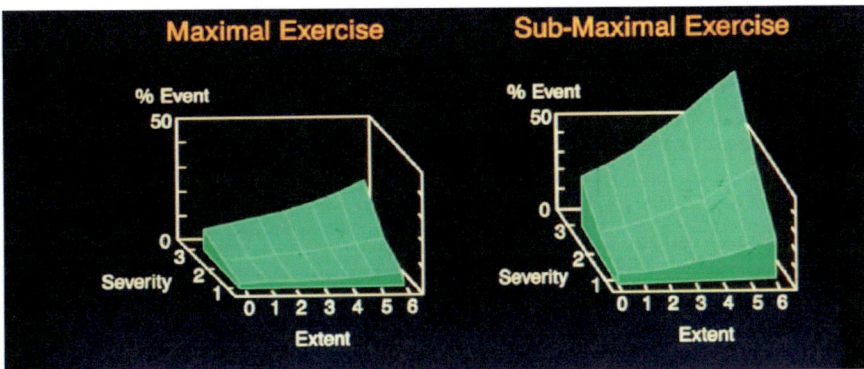

FIGURE **9.2.** Orthogonal axis representing the annualized % event rate (for cardiac death, myocardial infarction, or performance of late coronary bypass surgery) after exercise myocardial perfusion scintigraphy, with results divided according to the extent of perfusion defects (0 to 6 regions) and severity of perfusion defects (from 0 = no defect to 3 = very severe defect). Shown are results for patients who exercised maximally (i.e., to >85% of maximal predicted heart rate) (*left*) and those who did not (*right*). In both groups, event rate was independently and exponentially related to both the extent and severity of perfusion defects, but low achieved heart rate essentially tripled event rate for any magnitude of inducible ischemia. (Reproduced with permission from Ladenheim ML, Pollack BH, Rozanski A, et al. Extent and severity of myocardial hypoperfusion as orthogonal indices of prognosis in patients with suspected coronary artery disease. J Am Coll Cardiol 1986;7:464–471.)

(c) mild ischemia, and (d) moderate to severe ischemia, as shown in Figure 9.3. Patient management is straightforward among patients who do not manifest inducible ischemia. Repeated outcome studies have reliably indicated that such patients have <1%/year annualized cardiac event rate if they have exercised adequately (i.e., to >85% of maximal predicted heart rate). The event rate with a normal pharmacological stress test may be somewhat higher, in the range of

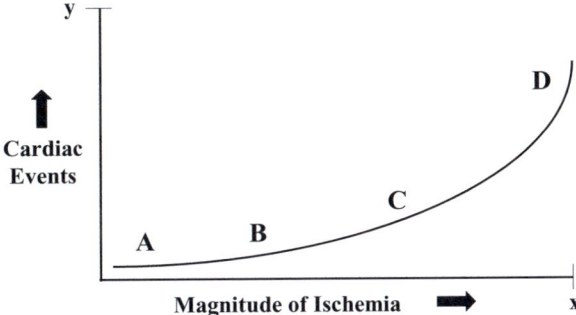

FIGURE **9.3.** Schematic representation of the exponential relationship between the magnitude of inducible ischemia and cardiac events, on which are superimposed the four relevant ranges of test interpretation, as discussed in the text: A, no inducible ischemia; B, an equivocal perfusion defect: C, a mild stress-induced perfusion defect; D, a severe induced defect.

1% to 2%/year, because of a higher a priori risk in such patients, resulting usually from the greater age of such patients and a higher frequency of various comorbidities, such as various chronic inflammatory diseases, which may preclude exercise. Among patients with nonischemic SPECT studies, there exist patient subgroups that may remain at a relatively intermediate risk of cardiac events. These include patients who have diabetes, atrial fibrillation, significant dyspnea, very poor exercise tolerance, and those with substantial discordant findings, such as patients manifesting normal SPECT findings but concomitantly significant ST depression and easily induced chest pain during exercise testing. In the past, there were few available options for evaluating such patients further, but these patients may represent future indications for performing coronary artery calcium (CAC) scanning or computed tomography angiography (CTA), although this has to be tested by prospective study.

Equivocal SPECT studies, such as those involving a very small reversible perfusion, result in diagnostic doubt, but from a prognostic perspective, such studies are very useful because of the exponential relationship between myocardial ischemia and cardiac events (Fig. 9.3). That is, the likelihood of cardiac events in such patients is nearly equivalent to that of a normal stress SPECT study. Thus, patients with equivocal SPECT studies can generally be followed medically.

The clinical management of patients who manifest mild inducible ischemia during stress testing may be somewhat more challenging. This is because the baseline cardiac event rate in this group is in the range of ~2% to 3% per year, which places such patients at intermediate risk for cardiac events. However, in such patients, the assessment of the ancillary information that is available from cardiac stress testing may be very useful for defining high- and low-risk subgroups of patients. These include consideration of exercise duration; the presence, severity, and duration of induced chest pain; and concomitant electrocardiographic and hemodynamic abnormalities induced with stress among patients who undergo exercise testing. For example, patients with mild ischemia but demonstrating excellent exercise duration without induced chest pain or ST-segment depression would generally be considered to be at relatively low risk, and such patients may generally be deserving of conservative medical management. On the other hand, patients with mild ischemia but induced chest pain and/or ST-segment abnormalities at low workloads would be at relatively higher risk and thus generally deserving of the same aggressive management afforded to patients manifesting moderate to severe inducible ischemia. When pharmacological stress testing is employed instead of exercise, these ancillary data are not available.

At the high end of the ischemic spectrum, those who manifest moderate to severe ischemia are at high risk for cardiac events because overall risk increases sharply once moderately severe ischemia is present. Even if such patients have no inducible chest pain or other findings that suggest low risk, such as good exercise duration and the absence of electrocardiographic abnormalities on stress, event risk may not be sufficiently lowered to justify conservative treatment in such patients. It is important to note, however, that virtually all of the outcome data concerning the prognostic significance of patients with both milder and more severe ischemia was obtained from databases that were assembled in the 1980s and early 1990s and thus do not consider the substantial improvements in medical management that have occurred since that time. Currently, this includes the use of beta-blockers, rate lowering calcium channel blockers, antiplatelet agents, angiotensin-converting enzyme inhibitors, and statins. A recent prospective trial randomized 205 patients status post (s/p) acute myocardial infarction (AMI) with large perfusion defects (≥20% of myocardial area) and significant reversible perfusion defects on adenosine SPECT (≥10% of myocardial area), performed soon after AMI, into two treatment arms: intensive medical therapy versus coronary revascularization [7]. Remarkably, both groups showed the same degree of ischemic suppression (Fig. 9.4). Although these data suggest the need for further prospective study, they challenge the notion that postinfarction patients with inducible ischemia necessarily need to be referred for revascularization procedures.

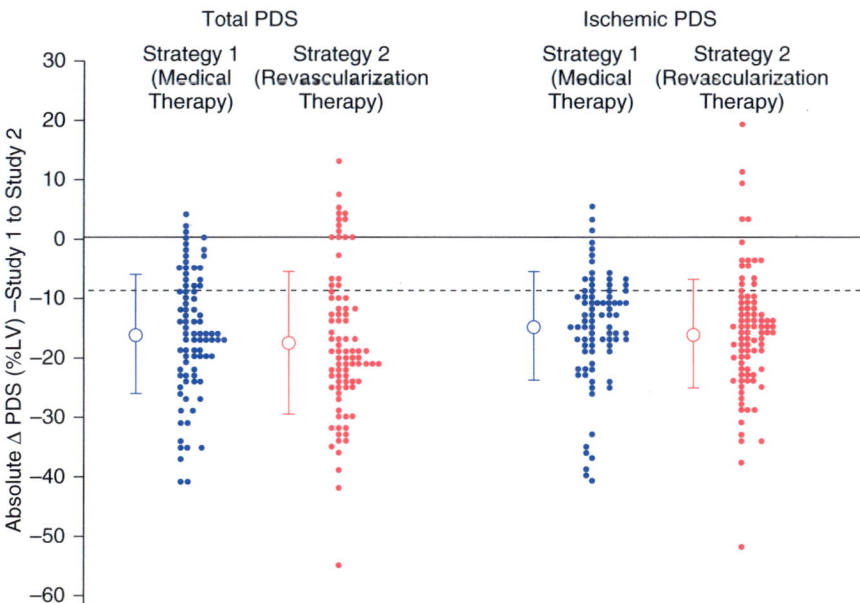

FIGURE 9.4. Reduction in the magnitude of total perfusion defect size (PDS) and ischemic PDS among 205 survivors of acute myocardial infarction undergoing serial adenosine SPECT study after randomization to either aggressive medical therapy, including statin use, or myocardial revascularization. All of these post–myocardial infarction patients had an initial total perfusion defect ≥20% of myocardial area and ischemia defect ≥10% of myocardial area. The magnitude of reduction in perfusion defects and ischemic suppression was comparable for medical therapy versus revascularization. (Reproduced with permission from Mahmarian JJ, Dakik HA, Filipchuk NG. An initial strategy of intensive medical therapy is comparable to that of coronary revascularization for suppression of scintigraphic ischemia in high-risk but stable survivors of acute myocardial infarction. J Am Coll Cardiol 2006;48:2458–2467.)

Selection of Imaging Protocols

In general, patients who have a very low clinical risk profile, such as those who present with transient pain that is deemed to be nonanginal in nature, can undergo either exercise, dobutamine, or vasodilator stress testing. Vasodilator stress testing, using either adenosine or dipyridamole infusion in conjunction with SPECT imaging, may be the procedure of choice for higher risk subsets of patients who are candidates for stress testing, such as patients with medically managed unstable angina or those recovering from uncomplicated myocardial infarction. The safe use of vasodilator stress for imaging patients within days of AMI or unstable angina lies in their ability to cause increased flow in normal coronary vessels without further impairing blood flow in relatively obstructed arteries. Thus, the true induction of ischemia in such patients is uncommon but can occur if vasodilator infusion leads to the development of a vascular steal syndrome in a region of jeopardized blood flow.

Clinical Studies

Many studies have demonstrated the use of both stress-rest myocardial perfusion SPECT and stress echocardiography for the risk stratification of patients with stable chest pain. Accordingly, this literature is not reviewed here. Accumulating data have also demonstrated the efficacy of performing either adenosine or dipyridamole SPECT imaging for the risk stratification of patients with unstable angina and post–myocardial infarction. In early work, Dakik et al. studied 136 patients with unstable angina and negative cardiac enzymes and no new ischemic electrocardiographic changes undergoing SPECT imaging [8]. They found that patients with perfusion defects size (PDS) <15% of the myocardium were much less likely to have a cardiac event than patients with a PDS ≥15%. Similarly, Stratmann et al. studied 128 patients with unstable angina undergoing dipyridamole-sestamibi SPECT imaging and found that patients with normal SPECT images had a significantly lower event rate compared with patients with abnormal SPECT images [9]. With respect to the evaluation of post–myocardial infarction patients, Gibson et al. provided strong early evidence regarding the ability of stress-rest myocardial perfusion scintigraphy to risk stratify patients after myocardial infarction by demonstrating the superiority of myocardial perfusion scintigraphy over catheterization variables for predicting subsequent cardiac events [10]. This initial work was done using submaximal exercise testing, but since then, the focus has shifted to the performance of early pharmacological stress testing, which can be performed safely within 2 days of myocardial infarction using either adenosine or dipyridamole SPECT imaging. In very recent work, Mahmarian et al. enrolled 728 survivors of AMI into the INSPIRE trial, designed to evaluate the prognostic efficacy of adenosine SPECT performed early after myocardial infarction [11]. A low-risk group, which consisted of those patients with a total perfusion defect that was <20% of myocardial area (almost all of which had an left ventricular ejection fraction (LVEF) >35% and reversible perfusion defects that were <10% of myocardial area) had a 1-year event rate of <2%. Cardiac events increased exponentially with the size of total perfusion defects or the size of reversible defects during adenosine infusion (Fig. 9.5).

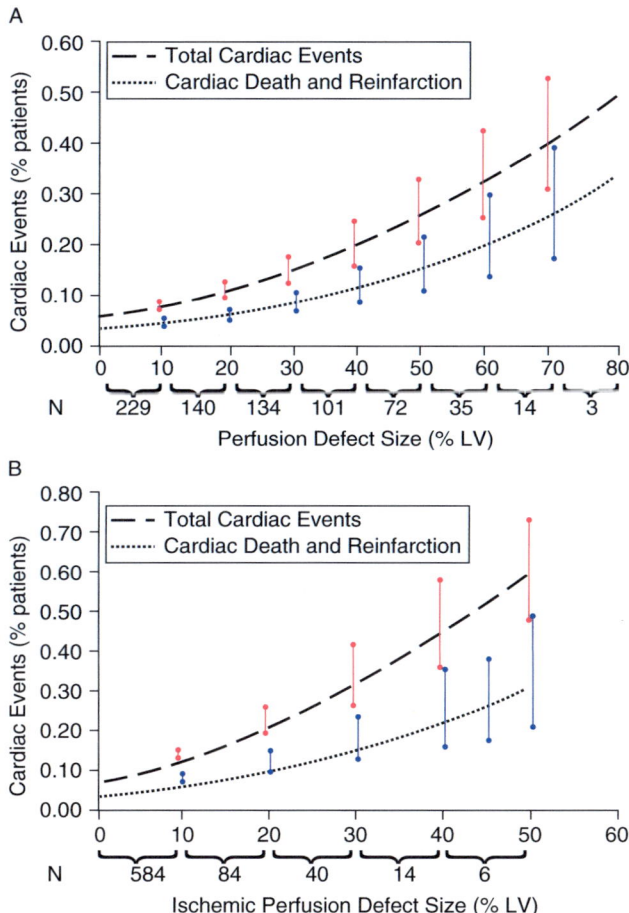

FIGURE 9.5. Predicted 1-year event rates for cardiac death and reinfarction and total cardiac events (also including readmission for acute ischemic syndrome or severe congestive heart failure) among 728 patients undergoing adenosine SPECT after acute myocardial infarction. Cardiac events increased exponentially according to the magnitude of both total perfusion defects and reversible perfusion defects. (Reproduced with permission from Mahmarian JJ, Shaw LJ, Filipchuk NG, et al. A multinational study to establish the value of early adenosine technetium-99 m sestamibi myocardial perfusion imaging in identifying a low-risk group for early hospital discharge after acute myocardial infarction. J Am Coll Cardiol 2006;48:2448–2457.)

Newer Imaging Approaches

The relative role of noninvasive CTA or coronary calcium scanning for the risk stratification of patients who fit into noninvasive evaluation according to our PAIN pathway guidelines remains to be determined by future studies. Various studies have suggested that coronary calcium scanning may be a technique for evaluating patients with chest pain in the emergency room [12, 13]. Similarly, noninvasive CTA is a relatively new technique that has undergone a few generations of improved technology in a matter of only 5 to 7 years. The latest generation of machines, consisting of 64-slice scanners, has shown relatively good correlation with angiographic findings, and importantly, with these latest generation scanners, the number of segments that cannot be evaluated has been reduced to a relatively low percentage. These technological improvements in CTA make it a potential alternative option to the evaluation of patients presenting with chest pain, but its usefulness relative to the potent prognostic information provided by stress testing remains to be determined. Interestingly, noninvasive CT also offers the potential opportunity to look at the morphology of plaque in the vessel wall as well as the lumen [14]. However, the incremental information that may be provided by evaluation of plaque characteristics among patients admitted with acute ischemic syndromes remains to be determined by future study.

Conclusion

For patients identified with a low-risk profile in the PAIN pathway, such as those deemed to have nonanginal chest pain, both SPECT imaging and stress echocardiography may be used to categorize patient risk according to the magnitude of inducible myocardial ischemia. In the subgroup of patients who have a relative contraindication to exercise and dobutamine use, such as patients who are immediately status post myocardial infarction or in recovery from unstable angina, either adenosine or dipyridamole SPECT imaging may be safely used for risk stratification as well. Those with no or only little inducible ischemia are low-risk patients who then can be followed using current approaches to aggressive medical management. Coronary artery calcium scanning, which has recently been used to evaluate patients with acute chest pain in the emergency room, and noninvasive CTA are newer techniques that could complement stress testing in the evaluation of PAIN pathway patients in the future, pending prospective study of their utility.

References

1. Cannon CP, Weintraub WS, Demopoulos LA, et al. Comparison of early invasive and conservative strategies in patients with unstable coronary syndromes treated with the glycoprotein IIb/IIIa inhibitor tirofiban. N Engl J Med 2001;344:1879–1887.

2. Effects of tissue plasminogen activator and a comparison of early invasive and conservative strategies in unstable angina and non-Q-wave myocardial infarction. Results of the TIMI IIIB Trial. Thrombolysis in Myocardial Ischemia. Circulation 1994;89:1545–1556.

3. Boden WE, O'Rourke RA, Crawford MH, et al. Outcomes in patients with acute non-Q-wave myocardial infarction randomly assigned to an invasive as compared with a conservative management strategy. Veterans Affairs Non-Q-Wave Infarction Strategies in Hospital (VANQWISH) Trial Investigators. N Engl J Med 1998;338: 1785–1792.

4. Klein J, Chao SY, Berman DS, Rozanski A. Is "silent" myocardial ischemia really as severe as symptomatic ischemia? The analytic effect of patient selection biases. Circulation 1994;89:1958–1966.

5. Krantz DS, Hedges SM, Gabbay FH, et al. Triggers of angina and ST-segment depression in ambulatory coronary artery disease patients: evidence for an uncoupling of angina and ischemia. Am Heart J 1994;128:703–712.

6. Ladenheim ML, Pollack BH, Rozanski A, et al. Extent and severity of myocardial hypoperfusion as orthogonal indices of prognosis in patients with suspected coronary artery disease. J Am Coll Cardiol 1986;7:464–471.

7. Mahmarian JJ, Dakik HA, Filipchuk NG. An initial strategy of intensive medical therapy is comparable to that of coronary revascularization for suppression of scintigraphic ischemia in high-risk but stable survivors of acute myocardial infarction. J Am Coll Cardiol 2006;48:2458–2467.

8. Dakik HA, Hwang WS, Jatar A, et al. Prognostic value of quantitative stress myocardial perfusion imaging in unstable angina patients with negative cardiac enzymes and no new ischemic ECG changes. J Nucl Cardiol 2005;12:32–36.

9. Stratmann HG, Tamesis BR, Younis LT, et al. Prognostic value of predischarge dipyridamole technetium 99 m sestamibi myocardial tomography in medically treated patients with unstable angina. Am Heart J 1995;130:734–740.

10. Gibson RS, Watson DD, Craddock GB, et al. Prediction of cardiac events after uncomplicated myocardial infarction: a prospective study comparing predischarge exercise thallium-201 scintigraphy and coronary angiography. Circulation 1983;68: 321–336.

11. Mahmarian JJ, Shaw LJ, Filipchuk NG, et al. A multinational study to establish the value of early adenosine technetium-99 m sestamibi myocardial perfusion imaging in identifying a low-risk group for early hospital discharge after acute myocardial infarction. J Am Coll Cardiol 2006;48:2448–2457.

12. Laudon DA, Vukov LF, Breen JF, et al. Use of electron-beam computed tomography in the evaluation of chest pain patients in the emergency department. Ann Emerg Med 1999;33:15–21.

13. McLaughlin VV, Balogh T, Rich S. Utility of electron beam computed tomography to stratify patients presenting to the emergency room with chest pain. Am J Cardiol 1999;84:327–328.

14. Hausleiter J, Meyer T, Hadamitzky M, et al. Prevalence of noncalcified coronary plaques by 64-slice computed tomography in patients with an intermediate risk for significant coronary artery disease. J Am Coll Cardiol 2006;48:312–318.

10

The Role of Echocardiography in Acute Coronary Syndrome

Sandeep Joshi, Eyal Herzog, and Farooq A. Chaudhry

Over the past 25 years, there has been significant progress in the treatment and prevention of acute coronary syndrome (ACS), a myriad of clinical presentations ranging from unstable angina to myocardial infarction, with a strong emphasis on early detection with aggressive management. Echocardiography has emerged globally as a highly effective modality for the detection and identification of regional wall motion abnormalities, which may be typical for ACS, as well as for providing prognostic information for myocardial viability [1, 2]. Echocardiography has gradually evolved into an inexpensive yet highly effective and noninvasive practical tool in assessment of patients with chest pain (Table 10.1) and plays a significant role in the exclusion of other etiologies of chest pain including aortic dissection, pericarditis (with effusion), aortic stenosis, hypertrophic cardiomyopathy, and pulmonary embolism.

Transthoracic echocardiography (TTE) is one of the most useful and widely applicable diagnostic tools available. Developed in the 1960s, echocardiographic images were initially presented in M (motion) mode and supplemented by two-dimensional images, which were promising, yet still compromised imaging quality and information regarding velocities and valvular disorders. The advent of Doppler flow enabled the determination of velocities and blood flow, valvular disease, shunts, and overall function and has revolutionized the identification of cardiac disease.

Transesophageal echocardiography (TEE) was introduced in the 1980s and has also evolved as a useful test with a different role than TTE. Compared with TTE, TEE is an invasive procedure mandating the use of conscious sedation and careful patient monitoring and is contraindicated in certain clinical scenarios such as the presence of esophageal varices and/or the presence of a stricture, which can predispose the patient to esophageal perforation. Even with these limitations, TEE is invaluable for identifying certain cardiac pathology. For instance, TEE provides superior visualization for valvular disorders and areas of the heart not adequately assessed from TTE such as the left atrium, aorta, and the pulmonary veins. It is also routinely used preoperatively when evaluating valvular replacement, aortic dissection, thrombus formation, and endocarditis. It also provides excellent definition of heart structures, allows the

TABLE 10.1. Indication for echocardiography in patients with chest pain.

1. Diagnosis of underlying cardiac disease in patients with chest pain and clinical evidence of valvular, pericardial, or primarily cardiac disease.
2. Evaluation of chest pain in patients with nondiagnostic ECG.
3. Evaluation of chest pain in patients with suspected aortic dissection.
4. Evaluation of Chest pain in patients with severe hemodynamic instability.

visualization of a heart difficult to examine using conventional echocardiography (obese or a thick chest wall), monitoring of heart function during cardiac surgery, and detection of blood clots in the left atrium.

Although not routinely used as the first-line diagnostic option for ACS, it certainly plays a key role in later stages after ACS.

Our goal in this chapter is to examine the role that two-dimensional echocardiography plays in the diagnosis, exclusion, risk stratification, and treatment of ACS and ACS complications as well as the increasing use of echocardiography in the emergency department setting.

The Role of Echocardiography in Myocardial Infarction

Echocardiography plays a pivotal role in the management of acute deterioration of hemodynamics after an acute myocardial infarction [3, 4]. At the molecular level, an ischemic cascade occurs within minutes after ACS (Fig. 10.1). Acute ischemia is followed by the release of lactic acid with subsequent and regional diastolic dysfunction and impairment of contractility, increased filling pressures, EKG changes, and then finally clinical symptoms, angina. This metabolic progression is extremely time dependent, and treatment is critical. The underlying product of ACS or ischemia is a rapid decrease in myocardial contractility secondary to a reduction of sarcomere function. Regional ischemia manifests as abrupt hypokinesia, whereas global ischemia results in complete arrest. During ischemia, the myocardium is mechanically quiescent; however, energy is still required to maintain some degree of cardiac homeostasis. Angina is followed by a prolonged depression of myocardial contractility, often persisting for up to 24 hours or longer.

Several studies have shown that two-dimensional echocardiography can in fact show and identify patients who will experience cardiac events with a greater sensitivity compared with the ECG and is also able to discriminate between unstable angina at high and low risk for adverse cardiac events. In general, it is more sensitive and specific when performed during or immediately after an episode of chest pain. Small studies reported sensitivities and specificities of 86% to 92% and 53% to 90% respectively [5, 6]. Two-dimensional and color flow Doppler may be useful in the setting of an acute myocardial infarction

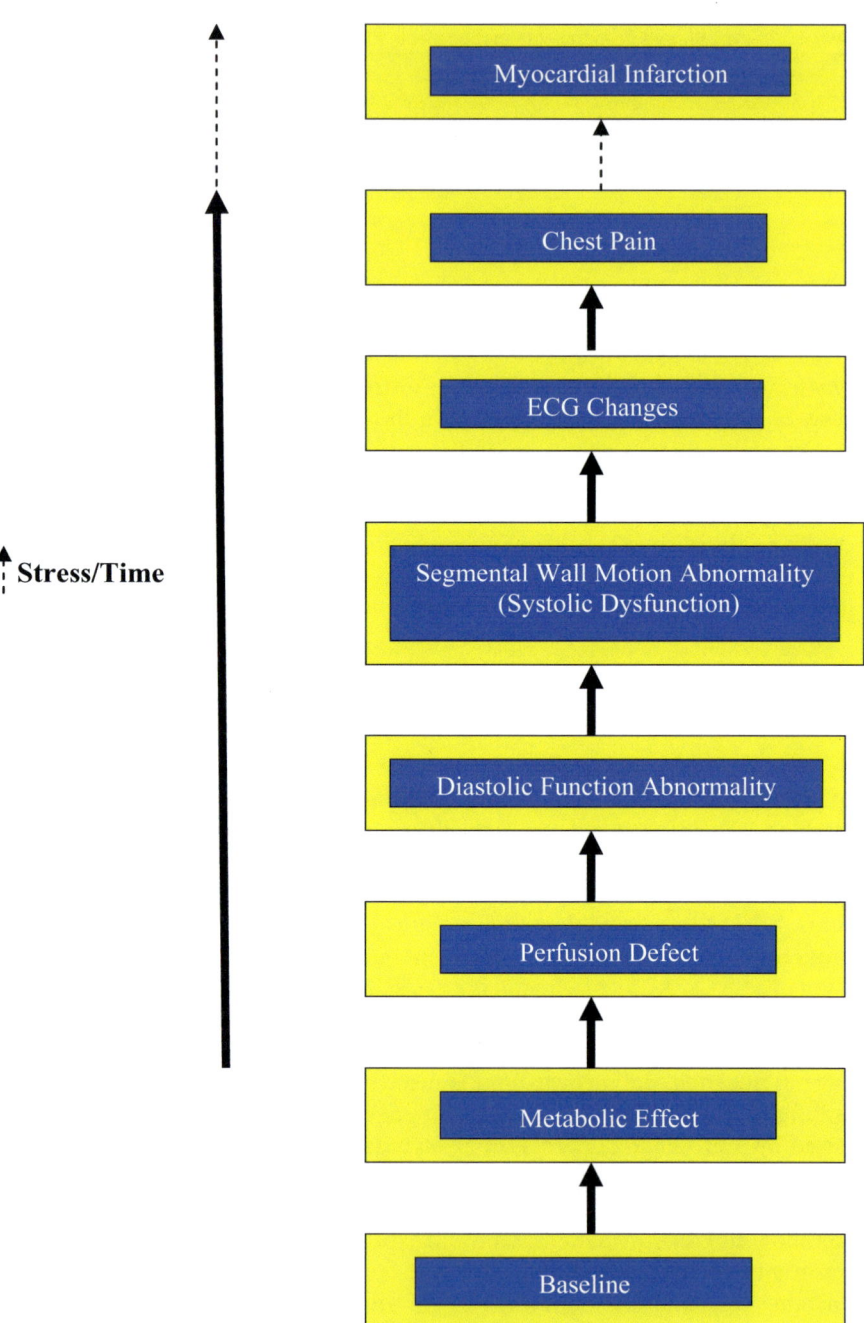

Figure 10.1. Sequence of events in myocardial ischemia.

TABLE 10.2. The role of echocardiography in the detection of complications of ACS.

Acute Phase
1. Rupture of free wall, interventricular septum or papillary muscle.
2. Mitral regurgitation.
3. Left ventricular thrombus.
4. Pericardial effusion/tamponade.
5. Right ventricle infarct.

Chronic Phase
1. Infarct expansion.
2. True ventricular aneurysm.
3. Ventricular pseudoaneurysm.

(AMI), in particular, when assessing infarct size (ejection fraction and ventricular wall motion abnormalities), perfusion and tissue viability, complications such as left ventricular rupture, right ventricular infarction, ruptured ventricular septum or papillary muscle, left ventricular aneurysm, pseudoaneurysm, infarct extension, mural thrombus formation, and pericardial effusion [7, 8] (Table 10.2). Echocardiography also plays a potential role in risk stratification and assessment of prognosis. The availability, ease of use, lack of risk, and wealth of information obtainable from echocardiography make it the ideal noninvasive test of choice in clinical practice.

Echocardiography in Complications of Myocardial Infarction

The topic of this section is discussed in detail in Chapter 11 and is discussed in brief here. Of note, echocardiography is mandatory in the postinfarction patient with a new systolic murmur, pulmonary edema, and sudden cardiac decompensation.

Left Ventricle Rupture

Left ventricular rupture is often a life-threatening situation mandating immediate and accurate diagnosis because of pooling of blood within the pericardial space and possibly acute cardiac tamponade; although in certain instances rupture may be contained by adhesions and/or thrombus. Echocardiography can occasionally identify the site of rupture and can also guide treatment. Clues to the diagnosis may include a localized or diffuse pericardial effusion with or without a regional wall motion abnormality. Containment of the rupture leads to the formation of a pseudoaneurysm. Echocardiographic features include a narrow neck at the rupture site, thrombus filling the aneurysm, and a clearly defined transition from healthy myocardial tissue to aneurysm tissue at an acute angle. Although the prognosis is poor, surgical repair is the mainstay of therapy and is mandated as the risk of impending rupture exists.

Ventricular Septal Rupture

Ventricular septal rupture occurs in the days after an AMI and is one of the etiologies of a new systolic murmur on cardiac auscultation. This entity entails a focal area of necrosis with eventual rupture of the interventricular septum. Two-dimensional echocardiography can identify the site of rupture by localizing a site of impaired wall motion, which may be subtle due to the fact that this complication has been observed to occur secondary to small infarcts. In addition, via color Doppler the identification of a left-to-right shunt with an interrupted septum can help delineate an infarct-related rupture. Right ventricular infarction may be associated with posterior septal wall ruptures. Moore et al. [8] examined the role of echocardiography in the identification and location of site of infarct in patients after septal rupture. The data showed that (1) mortality is higher when ventricular septal rupture complicates inferior myocardial infarction (MI) versus when it complicates anterior MI, and (2) the prediction of outcome is highly accurate, and combined right ventricular and septal dysfunction has a substantial impact on prognosis.

Right Ventricular Infarction

Usually occurring in patients with concomitant inferior left ventricular infarction and rarely occurring in the isolated form, right ventricular infarction should be suspected in patients with inferior left ventricular infarction with unexplained, persistent hypotension, clear lung fields, and elevated jugular venous pressure. Echocardiography is the diagnostic procedure of choice. The ECG, although not as sensitive compared with TTE, reveals ST-segment elevations in the right precordial leads, particularly leads RV_4–RV_6. Echocardiography provides better assessment of the extent and severity compared with other imaging modalities and reveals right ventricular dilatation, hypokinesis, and/or akinesis. In addition, echocardiography can evaluate complications of right ventricular infarction. Functional tricuspid regurgitation is common; rarer complications are papillary muscle rupture and hypoxemia from shunting through a patent foramen ovale secondary to raised right atrial pressure. Right ventricular dilatation, segmental wall motion abnormality of the right ventricular free wall, decreased descent of the right ventricular base, paradoxical septal motion, tricuspid regurgitation, dilated inferior vena cava, right-to-left interatrial septal bowing, right-to-left shunting across a patent foramen ovale, and pulmonary regurgitant jet pressure half-time of less than 150 milliseconds are all echocardiographic findings associated with right ventricular infarction [9].

Treatment is often fluid administration with the addition of inotropic support in the form of dobutamine.

Papillary Muscle Rupture

This is the most serious cause of mitral regurgitation in the setting of AMI. Rupture of the head of the papillary muscle results in severe mitral regurgitation; rupture of the entire trunk is inevitably fatal. Rupture of the head of the papillary muscle has the highest incidence at 3 to 5 days after myocardial infarction (75%), whereas the incidence is 25% on days 1 to 2 or days 6 to 10 after a myocardial infarction. Partial or complete rupture is associated with a high mortality rate and may be recognized on two-dimensional echocardiography as a flail leaflet with an attached papillary head that may prolapse into the left atrium during cardiac systole. A TEE is usually the procedure of choice unless the diagnosis can be made via a TTE.

Aneurysm Formation and Left Ventricular Thrombus

True left ventricular aneurysms are defined as a "dyskinetic" region with a deformed diastolic and systolic left ventricle contour abnormality. The underlying premise is a dilatation of an area of scarred myocardial tissue. Echocardiography is quite sensitive for the diagnosis but occasional false negatives may occur, especially when the aneurysm involves a small part of the apex or the basal anterolateral wall. A true aneurysm is lined by a thin myocardium, harbors a ratio of the diameter of the junction between the aneurysm and the remainder of the left ventricle to the maximum aneurysm diameter >0.5, and most commonly occurs in the apex but inferobasal aneurysms may be seen as well.

A pseudoaneurysm consists of a wall composed of pericardium (no myocardial fibers), a narrow neck, and a ratio of the diameter at the "neck" to the maximum diameter of the aneurysm of <0.5 and typically partially filled with thrombus, and often flow into and out of the pseudoaneurysm. Overall, aneurysm formation is a poor prognostic sign associated with decompensated heart failure, various arrhythmias, and thrombus formation.

Left ventricular thrombi often form in regions of stasis such as the apex but may also occur in the lateral and inferior aneurysms. Certain echocardiographic characteristics such as pedunculated and mobile thrombi are associated with higher risk of embolization [10]. Thrombi most commonly develop in the presence of a large infarction. Echocardiography has high sensitivity (95%) and high specificity (85%) for identification of a left ventricular thrombus. Characteristically, a thrombus is identified as an area of increased homogenicity with a margin distinct from the underlying wall, which may present as akinetic or dyskinetic. False positives may occur; false chordae or false tendon spanning the left ventricle apex as well as coarse trabeculations associated with left ventricular hypertrophy and near-field artifacts (commonly present with low-frequency transducers) may mimic the echocardiographic findings. High-frequency transducers can differentiate true thrombus from these artifacts, and color Doppler flow or intravenous contrast agents may outline the contours of the thrombus, creating a filling defect and improving the detection of the thrombus. TEE may not visualize the apex as well as TTE.

Pericardial Effusion

Echocardiography is quite sensitive for the detection and diagnosis of pericardial effusion, a nonspecific response after a transmural infarction. Patients may be asymptomatic or manifest the signs and symptoms of pericarditis. Although the presence of pericardial effusion is often associated with a low mortality rate, cardiac tamponade can occur and progress to an adverse outcome. Two-dimensional echocardiography can identify and localize the site for percutaneous drainage and may be used to monitor the procedure, if necessary (Fig. 10.2).

Mitral Regurgitation

Mechanisms of acute mitral regurgitation (Fig. 10.3) after an AMI may be secondary to left ventricular cavity and mitral annulus dilatation, papillary muscle dysfunction and/or rupture. Papillary muscle rupture mandates urgent mitral valve repair and/or replacement. TEE is the diagnostic test of choice and may guide decision making for surgical intervention.

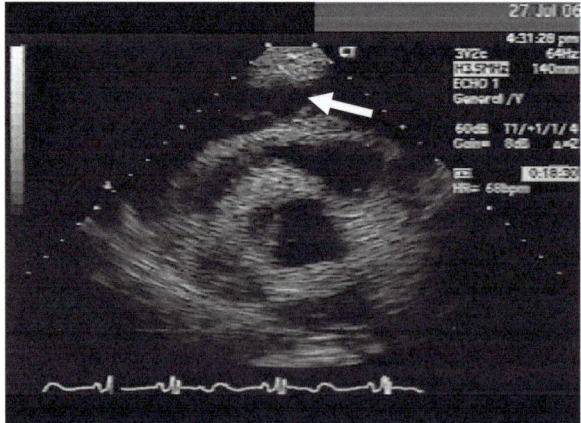

FIGURE 10.2. Acute aortic dissection with large pericardial effusion (*arrow*).

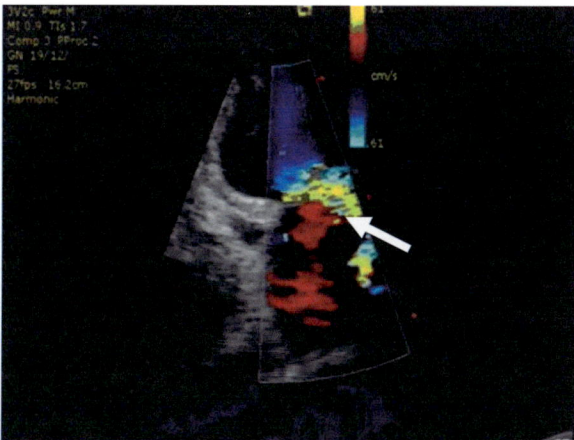

Figure 10.3. Mitral regurgitation (*arrow*).

The Role of Echocardiography in the Cardiac Care Unit

In the setting of an AMI in the cardiac care unit, echocardiography is of great value in that it aids in identifying the location and extent of myocardium at risk and may serve as a reliable gauge for the effects of reperfusion therapy in that it may identify successful reperfusion and normalization of wall motion. In terms of long-term benefits after an AMI, echocardiography can evaluate overall global function and cardiac remodeling. Prior to interventional or reperfusion therapy, echocardiography provides a noninvasive means of overall assessment of function, valvular disease, and right heart function. Both TTE and TEE may be employed for the patient in the cardiac care unit setting. TEE is of tremendous value as the cardiac care unit is a monitored setting, ideal for administering conscious sedation of the patient. It also is beneficial for ventilated patients, postoperative patients, and patients too hemodynamically unstable; hence, TEE may be performed for evaluating complications after an ACS such as valvular disorders, pericardial effusion, and aneurysm formation in hemodynamically unstable patients [11–12]. Furthermore, echocardiography plays a pivotal role in the detection of cardiac remodeling, a marker of worse outcome; hence, patients with extensive regional wall motion abnormalities should have follow-up echocardiography, which may demonstrate remodeling. Data from Cerisano et al. [13] revealed that a correlation exists between serial changes in left ventricular volumes with changes in filling patterns and that a simple, early measurement of left ventricular diastolic function can predict late left ventricular dilatation. Repeated echocardiographic measurements are of great value as they reflect left ventricular remodeling characterized by alterations in left ventricular size, shape, and wall thickness [14]. Cardiac remodeling correlates with increased wall motion stress, further dilation, and eventually deterioration of left ventricular function. Early remodeling and left ventricular aneurysm have been shown to be compatible with a poor outcome. Three-dimensional echo-cardiography is more accurate than two-dimensional echocardiography in left ventricular size and shape and may play an important role in the detection of remodeling, however as this is a novel technique, further investigative work is required to corroborate this data. Also, there are several new techniques that are used to evaluate left ventricular function and ischemia such as tissue Doppler imaging, strain rate imaging, as well as tissue characterization. Many cardiac care units are fully equipped with an echocardiogram machine. This greatly facilitates patient management both routinely and in the emergent setting and overall results in a lower mortality rate and a higher rate of discharge from the unit setting. One caveat that lies herein is that an experienced sonographer and interpreting physician are required to perform and interpret these studies, which, as mentioned earlier, may be entail both TTE and TEE.

Echocardiography in the Emergency Department

In the setting of chest pain with a nondiagnostic ECG, echocardiography can provide valuable assessment and evaluation of regional and global wall motion abnormalities and can therefore serve as a useful guide for clinical decision making. A segmental wall motion abnormality indicates an acute ischemic event, ischemia ,or a chronic infarct. The presence of a new wall motion abnormality may warrant immediate reperfusion or interventional therapy. Normal wall motion during acute chest pain makes the diagnosis of ACS unlikely, whereas normal wall motion after chest pain has resolved may prove to be less diagnostic as often wall motion abnormalities may be present only in the presence of chest pain. Both of these scenarios depict the potential usefulness of echocardiography in patient management in the emergency department setting. The challenge herein lies in the diagnosis of low-risk patients without sacrificing the care of higher-risk patients, especially when considering reperfusion therapy. Several studies have demonstrated the role and efficacy of echocardiography in AMI. From these data, it appears that echocardiography is more sensitive than other diagnostic modalities, for the diagnosis of infarction. Echocardiography provides incremental information that may be prognostic for the identification of patients at risk for cardiac events.

Many emergency departments have now a designated "chest pain center" where patients who fit the ECG, biochemical, and clinical profiles of ACS are treated promptly, whereas those patients with chest pain with ambiguous ECG and/or biochemical markers undergo echocardiographic stress testing. Many centers have found this to be of tremendous value for risk-stratification purposes. Moreover, it can provide valuable insight into patient decision making in terms of immediate interventional treatment, conservative management, and cardiac care unit admission versus telemetry unit admission as well as discharge home. Trippi et al. [15] demonstrated the aggressive use of stress echocardiography in the emergency department setting. The study evaluated 163 chest pain patients with no ECG evidence of ischemia or infarction and with normal cardiac enzyme markers. Average length of stay was 5.4 hours, dramatically decreased from patients who are eventually admitted to the hospital. Dobutamine stress echocardiography had a negative predictive value of 98.5% based on clinical follow-up. The study proved to be quite interesting because of the aggressive approach to achieve patient discharge, the use of tele-echocardiography, and the presence of nursing supervision in lieu of a cardiologist being on-site as well as the choice of pharmacological stress. Several other studies have shown similar results, and although carrying certain limitations such as the availability of a nursing staff to supervise stress testing on a 24-hour basis and the availability of an experienced interpreting physician on a 24-hour basis, this treatment strategy can immensely lower unnecessary testing and procedures and reduce hospital admissions thereby saving the health care industry billions of dollars annually.

In summary, echocardiography in the emergency department may facilitate the early diagnosis and treatment of myocardial infarction in those patients with a high clinical suspicion of myocardial infarction but a nondiagnostic ECG. It may also diagnose unstable angina if performed during pain. Aggressive use of rest and stress echocardiography can reduce hospital admissions, but some false negatives will occur and small subendocardial infarctions may not be otherwise detected. What remains a critical logistic factor is the necessity for an experienced staff available on a 24-hour basis.

There are handheld, battery-powered echocardiography devices that are used quite frequently in emergency rooms. Data from these devices reveal that they are sensitive and more accurate than physical diagnosis; however, the limitations remain in that they can result in significant errors; Doppler functions on these devices are substantially inferior to two-dimensional imaging. Weston et al. [16] examined the role of handheld echocardiography in the diagnosis of ACS among 150 patients presenting to the emergency department with chest pain and suggested a possible role for handheld echo devices among patients with a low likelihood of myocardial schema or infarction and symptoms suggestive of ACS. The widespread use of these devices and the optimal setting yet remains to be seen, as adequate training in the interpretation of images remains a critical factor and may be subject to extreme variability.

Conclusion

In conclusion, the role of echocardiography in ACS is a critical factor in the detection and treatment of patients with ACS [4]. Echocardiography is a powerful technique that can provide invaluable information in the acutely ill cardiac patient. It can help in the early diagnosis of conditions causing acute chest pain such as AMI and aortic dissection and can help diagnose the causes of underlying hemodynamic instability and can also help determine the patient management strategy. After an AMI, it can provide information regarding the size of risk area; status of other regions of the myocardium; effect of reperfusion therapy on regional myocardial function; presence or absence of mechanical complications; and patients at risk for immediate or late cardiac events. It is likely that in the future with concomitant advances in technology and widespread use, this technique will find routine use in every emergent setting. However, in the workup of ACS, a thorough history and physical examination in conjunction with the brilliance of echocardiography is the key to diagnosis and patient management.

References

1. Greaves SC. Role of echocardiography in acute coronary syndromes. Heart 2002;88: 419–425.
2. Loh IK, Charuzi I, Beeder C, et al. Early diagnosis of non-transmural myocardial infarction by two-dimensional echocardiography. Am Heart J 1982;104:963–968.
3. Chirillo F, Cavarzerani A, Ius P, et al. Role of transthoracic, transesophageal, and transgastric two-dimensional and color Doppler echocardiography in the evaluation of mechanical complications of acute myocardial infarction. Am J Cardiol 1995; 76(11):833–836.
4. Assmann PE, Roelandt JR. Two-dimensional and Doppler echocardiography in acute myocardial infarction and its complications. Ultrasound Med Biol 1987;13(9): 507–517.
5. Feinberg MS, Schwammenthal E, Shlizerman L, et al. Prognostic significance of mild mitral regurgitation by color Doppler echocardiography in acute myocardial infarction. Am J Cardiol 2000;86:903–907.
6. DiPasquale P, Cannizzaro S, Scalzo S, et al. Sensitivity, specificity and predictive value of the echocardiography and troponin-T test combination in patients with non-ST elevation acute coronary syndromes. Int J Cardiovasc Imaging 2004;20: 37–46.
7. Kishon Y, Iqbal A, Oh JK, et al. Evolution of echocardiographic modalities in detection of post myocardial infarction ventricular septal defect and papillary muscle rupture: study of 62 patients. Am Heart J 1993;126(3 Pt 1):667–675.
8. Moore CA, Nygaard TW, Kaiser DL, et al. Postinfarction ventricular septal rupture: the importance of location of infarction and right ventricular function in determining survival. Circulation 1986;74(1):43–55.
9. Goldberger JJ, Himelman RB, Wolfe CL, et al. Right ventricular infarction: recognition and assessment of its hemodynamic significance by two-dimensional echocardiography. J Am Soc Echocardiogr 1991;4:140–146.
10. Jugdutt BI, Sivaram CA. Prospective two-dimensional echocardiographic evaluation of LV thrombus and embolization after acute myocardial infraction. J Am Coll Cardiol 1989;13:554–564.
11. Sabia P, Afrookteh A, Touchstone DA, et al. Value of regional wall motion abnormality in the emergency room diagnosis acute myocardial infarction. A prospective study using two-dimensional echocardiography. Circulation 1991;84:85–92.
12. Kang DH, Kang SH, Song JM, et al. Efficacy of myocardial contrast echocardiography in the diagnosis and risk stratification of acute coronary syndrome. Am J Cardiol 2005;96:1498–1502.

13. Cerisano G, Bolognese L, Carrabba N, et al. Doppler derived mitral deceleration time. An early predictor of LV remodeling after reperfused anterior acute myocardial infarction. Circulation 1991;99:230–236.

14. Korup E, Kober L, Torp-Pedersen C, and the TRACE study group. Prognostic usefulness of repeated echocardiographic evaluation after acute myocardial infarction. Am J Cardiol 1999;83:1559–1562.

15. Trippi JA, Lee KS, Kopp G, et al. Dobutamine stress tele-echocardiography for evaluation of emergency department patients with chest pain. J Am Coll Cardiol 1997;30: 627–632.

16. Weston BS, Alexander JH, Patel MR, et al. Hand-held echocardiographic examination of patients with symptoms of acute coronary syndromes in the emergency department: The 30-day outcome associated with normal left ventricular wall motion. Am Heart J 2004;148:1096–1101.

11
Mechanical Complications of Acute Myocardial Infarction

Gregory Janis, Atul Kukar, Eyal Herzog, and Farooq A. Chaudhry

Mechanical complications of acute myocardial infarction (AMI) result in some of the deadliest outcomes. It is difficult to assess the true incidence of these complications as both clinical and autopsy series differ considerably, though they are thought to be responsible for about 15% of all AMI deaths [1]. In general, patients at increased risk include elderly women, first AMI, and hypertension. Mechanical complications can be subdivided into two basic categories: the acute phase and the chronic phase. The acute phase usually involves rupture of damaged myocardium. This can take the form of rupture of the ventricular free wall, the interventricular septum, or a papillary muscle. The chronic phase usually involves formation of a ventricular aneurysm. This results in either a true aneurysm or a pseudoaneurysm. The following chapter will discuss how to detect, diagnose, and treat each of these entities.

The initial assessment of all patients who are considered to have a mechanical complication of AMI includes:

- Complete history and physical
  - Pay particular attention to:
    - New or change in a murmur
    - New or change in hemodynamic stability
    - Signs of acute heart failure: jugular venous distention (JVD), rales, S3
- Labs
  - Complete blood count, chemistries, cardiac markers (troponin, B-natriuretic peptide (BNP)), coagulation profile, type and screen
- ECG
  - Nonspecific for mechanical complications of AMI
- Echocardiography
  - Stat for any occurrence of change in hemodynamics or new/changing murmur
  - Most important part of pathway for mechanical complications of AMI

Ventricular Free Wall Rupture

Free wall rupture is one of the most devastating mechanical complications of AMI. It is often fatal as many patients are unable to tolerate the hemodynamic compromise long enough to make it to the operating room. This devastating complication occurs in about 1% of all patients with AMI [1]. Early recanalization, with either thrombolysis or primary percutaneous coronary intervention (PCI), has reduced its incidence dramatically. Albeit controversial due to conflicting data, nonsteroidal anti-inflammatory agents (NSAIDs) as well as steroids may increase the risk of rupture, believed secondary to impaired healing and scar formation. Also, late thrombolysis, greater than 6 hours after AMI, may increase the risk of rupture due to thinning out of the myocardium.

Although it can occur on either the left or right side of the myocardium and in either the atrium or ventricle, it most commonly occurs in the left ventricle. The anterior and lateral walls are at highest risk, being supplied by the distal left anterior descending artery (LAD). Unlike other complications of AMI, the left circumflex (LCX) is a common culprit in free wall rupture [2]. Although its occurrence has been reported between day 1 and up to as long as 3 weeks after an AMI, it usually occurs between day 1 and day 4 after the inciting event. Of note, it is less likely to occur in patients with prior coronary artery disease as these patients often have collateral circulation, which limits infarct size.

The only form of treatment for cardiac rupture is open heart surgical repair. Mortality is very high but some patients may have a temporary respite due to containment of the rupture by pericardial adhesions or by thrombosis at the rupture site. Temporary hemodynamic support with vasopressors and/or an intraaortic balloon pump (IABP) is usually required. Often, patients do not survive long enough and die from hemopericardium and subsequent tamponade.

Key Points in the Diagnosis and Management of Free Wall Rupture

- History
  - Usually occurs within 1 week (median 4 days) of an AMI
  - Has been reported between 1 day and 3 weeks after infarction
  - If acute, can lead to immediate death
  - If subacute, the patient can feel nauseated, with dyspnea and a pericardial type of discomfort [1]
- Physical exam
  - Acute hemodynamic compromise: severe hypotension, tachypnea
  - Signs of failure: JVD, rales, S_3
  - May see signs of acute tamponade: JVD, pulsus paradoxus, muffled heart sounds
- ECG
  - Generally nonspecific but may see signs of anterior or lateral wall infarct

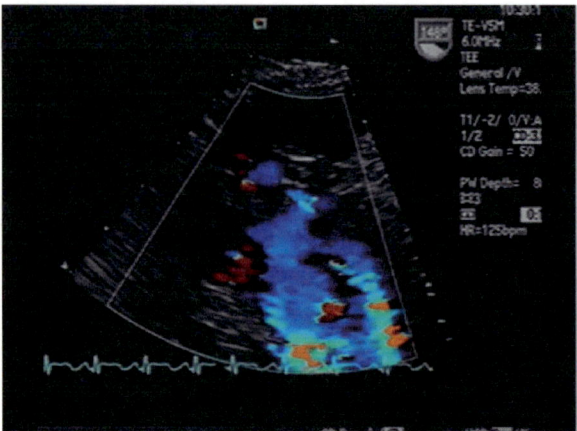

Figure 11.1. Transesophageal echo of ventricular free wall rupture, showing flow across the ventricular free wall.

- May see signs of pericarditis with evidence of progressive or recurrent ST elevation in the absence of recurrent ischemia [3]
- Echocardiography (Fig. 11.1)
  - Diffuse or localized pericardial effusion and a discrete segmental wall motion abnormality [4]
  - Rarely flow from the ventricle into the pericardial space can be demonstrated on Doppler techniques
- Treatment
  - Cardiothoracic (CT) surgery to repair mechanical defect
  - Hemodynamic support with pressors ± IABP

Interventricular Septum Rupture

In addition to rupture of a free wall, the interventricular septum may also rupture after an AMI. Its risk increases with age, hypertension, anterior wall infarction, and a lack of collaterals. It occurs most frequently in elderly women with no previous myocardial infarction. Fifty percent of patients have only single-vessel coronary artery disease, and about 55% are due to inferior wall AMIs and 45% due to anterior wall AMIs [2]. It is often detected with a change in hemodynamics and the presence of a harsh, loud holosystolic murmur heard over the left lower sternal border, often with a thrill. This specific finding is often difficult to distinguish from mitral regurgitation secondary to ischemia or even papillary muscle rupture. In these conditions, as with any hint of a mechanical complication, echocardiogram becomes an essential part of the evaluation. Traditionally, it is also possible to diagnose this rupture with an oxygen saturation run (oxygen measurements in the superior and inferior vena cava, right atrium, right ventricle, and pulmonary artery) via a right heart catheterization. There will be high right ventricular and pulmonary artery PaO_2 levels when compared with the right atrium and superior vena cava due to shunting of oxygenated blood from the left to right ventricle.

Septal rupture, without surgical intervention, can carry a mortality rate as high as 100%. Even with surgical intervention, it still carries a high mortality rate of up to 80% [5]. Of note, a septal rupture carries a higher mortality when in the setting of an inferior wall AMI with right ventricular involvement versus in the setting of an anterior wall AMI. This is predominately due to the fact that in the former, the right ventricle will not be able to handle the excess blood flowing into it from the left ventricle.

It is necessary to treat hemodynamically unstable patients immediately with either open surgical repair using a patch graft or transcutaneously with an umbrella device. If the patient is able to tolerate the defect, some surgeons prefer to wait a few weeks in order to allow the muscular septum to undergo healing and fibrosis, which makes the surgical repair easier.

Key Points in the Diagnosis and Management of Interventricular Septal Rupture

- History
  - Change in symptoms within the first week of AMI (median 3 to 6 days)
  - Acute shortness of breath (SOB), weakness, nausea, and occasional chest heaviness
- Physical exam
  - Acute hemodynamic instability: severe hypotension, tachypnea
  - A harsh, loud, holosystolic murmur over the left lower sternal border
  - Often evidence of a thrill
  - Signs of failure: JVD, rales, and so forth
- ECG
  - If normal, suggests a small ventricular septal defect (VSD) [4]
  - Left ventricular hypertrophy (LVH) with right ventricular hypertrophy (RVH) with large biphasic QRS complexes in limb and precordial leads suggests a large defect with variable degrees of pulmonary hypertension (HTN) [4]
- Echocardiography (Fig. 11.2)
  - Echocardiographic evaluation begins with color flow imaging, which will show systolic turbulent flow on the right ventricular side, owing to the higher pressures normally found in the left ventricle.
  - Further evaluation with Doppler ultrasound will show a high-velocity left-to-right systolic jet recorded with continuous-wave Doppler ultrasound
  - Also, the defect is always located in the region of thinned myocardium with a wall motion abnormality
- Cardiac catheterization
  - Right heart cath will show a "step-up" in O_2 saturation in blood from the right ventricle (RV) and pulmonary artery (PA) compared with those from

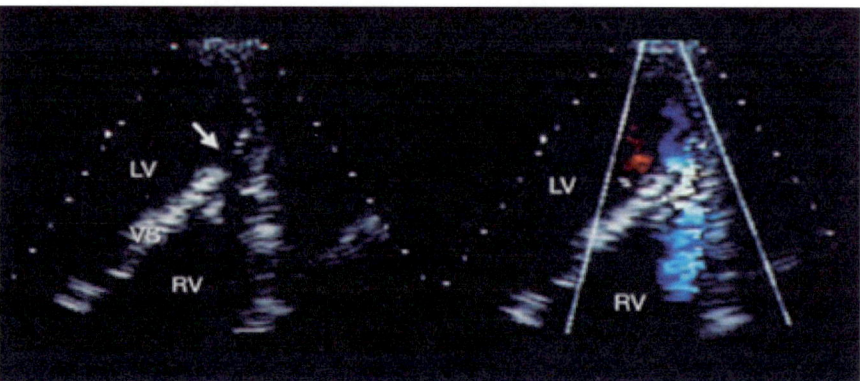

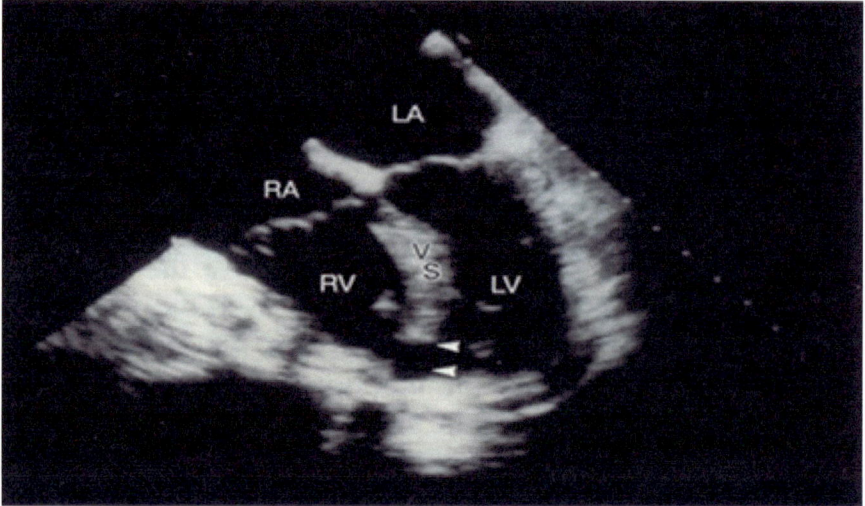

Figure 11.2. Two-dimensional echo of ventricular septum rupture. Evidence of the defect through the ventricular septum with Doppler flow from the left ventricular cavity to the right ventricular cavity. LV, left ventricle; RV, right ventricle; RA, right atrium; LA, left atrium; VS, ventricular septum. (Permission for pictures by Mayo foundation for Medical Education and Research. All rights reserved.)

the right atrium (RA). This test is often performed in a hemodynamically stable patient if echocardiogram is inconclusive and the coronary anatomy requires definition prior to surgical intervention [1]

- Treatment
  - Urgent CT surgical consult
  - IABP insertion and use of inotropes
  - Vasodilator therapy should be initiated if blood pressure permits
  - Straight to the operating room if evidence of hemodynamic compromise
  - Most surgeons prefer to wait a few weeks if the patient is stable

Papillary Muscle Rupture

Another dreaded complication of an AMI is rupture of the papillary muscle, which supports the mitral or tricuspid valve. In comparison with wall rupture, papillary muscle rupture is more often associated with smaller infarcts. The mitral valve papillary muscles are more often affected and carry more profound hemodynamic compromise. The condition is often diagnosed with the same clinical and physical exam findings as seen with interventricular septal rupture, mainly a new holosystolic murmur and worsening heart failure. However, a thrill is often absent and pulmonary edema is often present with a full tear of the mitral valve papillary muscle.

The posteromedial papillary muscle has a single source of blood supply, mainly coming from the posterior lateral branch, which comes off the dominant coronary artery, more often the right coronary artery (RCA). Occasionally, this papillary muscle is supplied by an obtuse marginal branch of the LCX. The anterolateral leaflet has dual blood supply by both a diagonal branch off the LAD and an obtuse marginal from the LCX. Thus, the posteromedial leaflet is more susceptible to tear/rupture because of its single blood supply and is typically injured in inferior wall AMIs. It occurs 6 to 10 times more frequently than in the anterolateral leaflet, which is damaged in anterolateral myocardial infarctions.

A full tear of the papillary muscle is usually incompatible with life because of the acute massive amount of regurgitation, which overcomes the ability of the heart to compensate with the pressure overload. Usually, the muscle undergoes various degrees of tear rather than full rupture, which allows the valve to maintain a certain degree of integrity, making it possible to survive long enough to undergo surgical repair.

The definitive treatment of choice is open heart surgery, involving either a new valve (mechanical or bioprosthetic) or, if possible, valve repair. Even with the ability to repair this devastating complication, the mortality rate is still about 17% if surgery is performed within 24 hours [2]. As with interventricular septal rupture, many surgeons prefer to wait in order to allow the muscle to undergo fibrosis and to make suturing easier. Although IABP can be used as a bridge to surgery, hemodynamic instability often dictates the urgency to operate.

Key Points in the Diagnosis and Management of Papillary Muscle Rupture

- History
  - Change in symptoms within 1 to 4 days of AMI
  - Usually flash pulmonary edema (septal rupture may not have this)
- Physical exam
  - Acute hemodynamic instability: severe hypotension, tachypnea

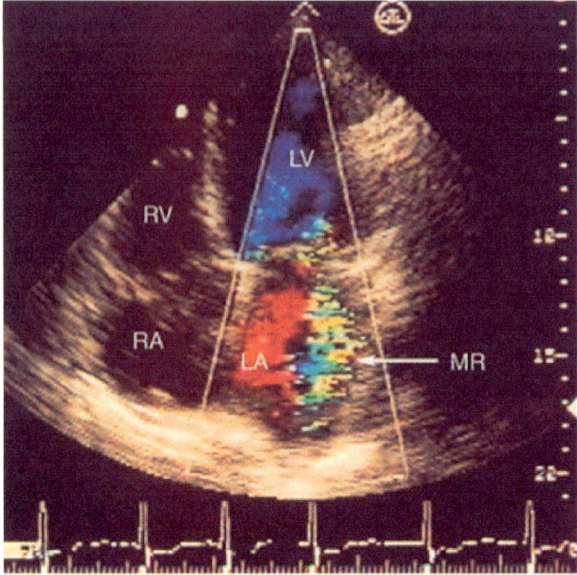

FIGURE 11.3. Two-dimensional echo of severe mitral regurgitation from papillary muscle rupture. Doppler flow in the apical four-chamber view showing severe mitral regurgitation. LV, left ventricle; RV, right ventricle; RA, right atrium; LA, left atrium; MR, mitral regurgitation. (Reprinted from Otto CM. Texbook of Clinical Echocardiography 3rd ed, 2004; p. 214, with permission from Elsevier.)

- A harsh, loud holosystolic murmur; may not be pansystolic but will end with a sudden drop-off in intensity because of high end-diastolic pressure [5]
- Less often evidence of a thrill (compared with septal rupture)
- Signs of failure: JVD, rales, S$_3$
- ECG
  - Anterolateral papillary muscle infarction may see ST depression in inferior leads [3]
  - Posteromedial papillary muscle infarction may show ST-segment depression in lead I or aVL
- Echocardiography (Fig. 11.3)
  - Presence and severity of regurgitation evaluated using two-dimensional imaging with Doppler techniques
  - Will see a flail valve leaflet with an attached mass (the papillary muscle head) that prolapses into the left atrium during systole [4]
- Cardiac catheterization
  - Right heart catheterization may show tall c-v waves in both the pulmonary capillary and pulmonary arterial tracings, distinguishing it from a ventricular septal rupture [1]
- Treatment
  - Emergent valve replacement for those hemodynamically unstable

- IABP insertion and use of inotropes
- Vasodilator therapy should be initiated if blood pressure permits
- If stable, can wait for ruptured muscle to undergo fibrosis so that it may be more amenable to primary repair

Aneurysm

AMI can also be complicated with the formation of aneurysms. This can be divided into either true or pseudoaneurysms. In its true form, the aneurysm contains all the layers of the myocardium and has a wide neck. A cardiac pseudoaneurysm has a small neck with a wall rupture that is contained by the pericardium. It is more dangerous in reference to its risk for embolism as well as rupture (Fig. 11.4) and requires surgical intervention.

There are many variations in clinical studies on aneurysms, making it difficult to pool them together for long-term therapy options, and there are no controlled trials with new therapy options. In general, small to moderate true aneurysms have an excellent survival rate of up to 90% at 5 years. They can be managed with afterload reduction, antiplatelet therapy, and anticoagulation in the setting of severe left ventricular dysfunction or thrombus. A large aneurysm is traditionally treated in the same manner, with closer follow-up for dilatation. Surgery can be considered in the setting of heart failure, angina, recurrent emboli despite anticoagulation therapy, and malignant ventricular arrhythmias.

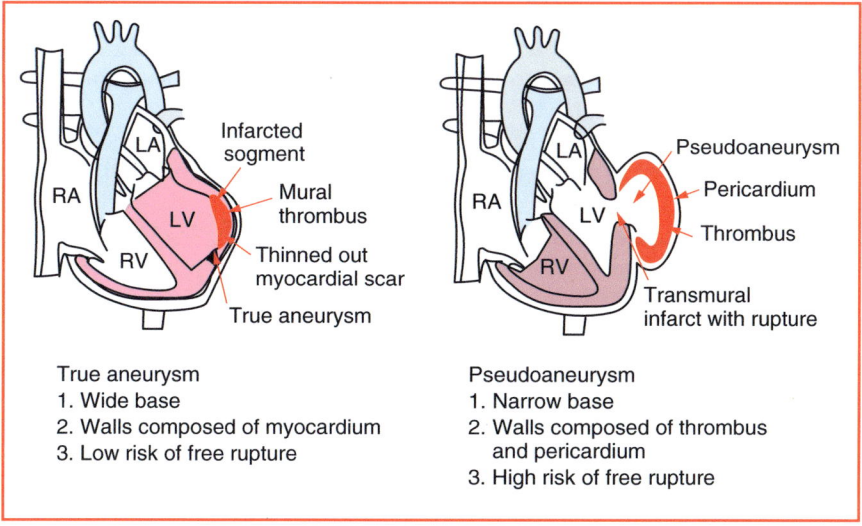

FIGURE 11.4. Diagram of true aneurysm vs. pseudoaneurysm. LV, left ventricle; RV, right ventricle; RA, right atrium; LA, left atrium. (Adapted from Elsevier Saunders for Medical Education and Research, Brawnwield's Heart Disease: 7th ed., 2005)

Even though rare in the era of primary PCI and improved preventive measures, it is of vital importance that we train and learn about these complications, as we must know them the first time we see them in order to try to overcome the extremely high mortality from mechanical complications of AMI.

Key Points in the Diagnosis and Management of Cardiac Aneurysms

- History
  - 50% with moderate or large aneurysms have symptoms of heart failure with or without angina [1]
- Physical exam
  - True aneurysm
    - Occasionally as a palpable paradoxic (systolic) outward bulge at the site of the aneurysm [5]
  - Pseudoaneurysm
    - An apical systolic murmur may be heard when flow goes in and out of the pseudoaneurysm
- ECG
  - Abnormal Q waves in precordial leads correlate with asynergy of the anterior segment of the left ventricle [3]
  - Persistent ST elevation with T-wave inversion lasting more than a month indicates a large degree of left ventricular asynergy and myocardial scarring [4]
  - These findings are more prevalent in true aneurysms
- Echocardiography (Figs. 11.5 and 11.6)
  - True aneurysm
    - A smooth transition exists from normal myocardium to the infarcted, thinned myocardium with an obtuse angle between the aneurysm and the body of the left ventricle [4]
    - Ratio of the diameter of the junction between the aneurysm and the remainder of the left ventricle to the maximum aneurysm diameter is >0.5
    - Most common in the apex but inferobasal aneurysms may be seen
    - A dyskinetic region with hinge points and diastolic contour abnormality may be seen [4]
  - Pseudoaneurysm
    - Abrupt transition from normal myocardium to the aneurysm with the wall composed of pericardium (no myocardial fibers) [4]
    - Has an acute angle between the normal myocardium and the aneurysm [4]
    - Has a narrow neck. The ratio of the diameter at the "neck" to the maximum diameter of the aneurysm is <0.5 [4].
    - Typically partially filled with thrombus
    - Often has flow in and out of the pseudoaneurysm

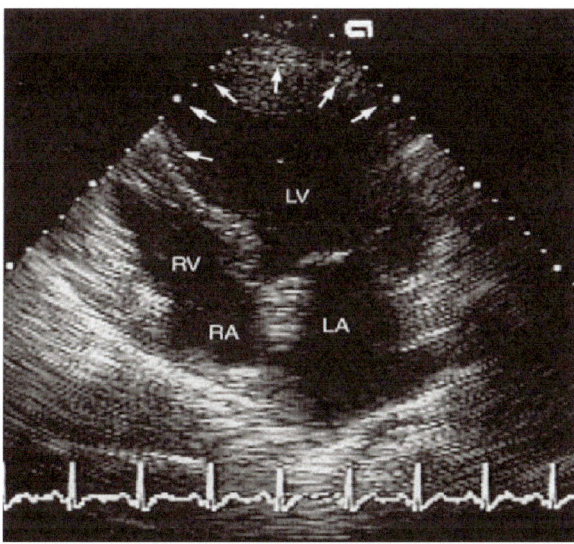

FIGURE 11.5. Two-dimensional echo of a true aneurysm. Apical four-chamber view with evidence of a true aneurysm. LV, left ventricle; RV, right ventricle; RA, right atrium; LA, left atrium. (Reprinted from Otto CM. Textbook of Clinical Echocardiography 3rd ed., 2004; p. 218, with permission from Elsevier.)

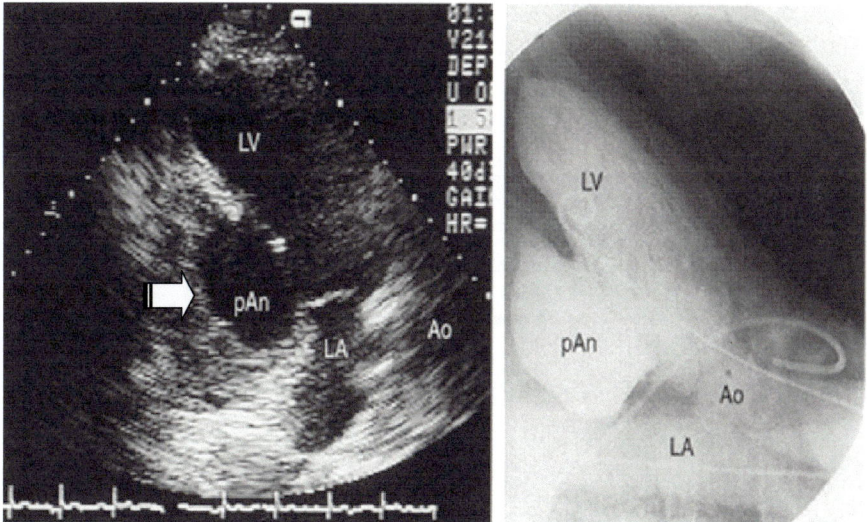

FIGURE 11.6. Two-dimensional echo of a pseudoaneurysm. On the left is an apical three-chamber view with evidence of a pseudoaneurysm in the posterior wall. On the right is a left ventriculography during cardiac catheterization showing the same. LV, left ventricle; pAn, pseudoaneurysm; LA, left atrium; Ao, aorta. (Reprinted from Otto CM. Textbook of Clinical Echocardiography 3rd ed., 2004; p. 218, with permission from Elsevier.)

- Treatment
  - True aneurysm
    - Anticoagulation for evidence of a thrombus
    - Generally do not rupture
    - May perform aneurysmectomy for symptomatic aneurysms
  - Pseudoaneurysm
    - Anticoagulation for thrombus within the aneurysm
    - Tend to rupture more than true aneurysms
    - Nonemergent surgical evaluation for aneurysmectomy

References

1. Antman EM. ST elevation myocardial infarction: management. In: Zipes D, Libby P, Bonow R, Braunwald E, eds. Braunwald's heart disease: a textbook of cardiovascular medicine, 7th ed. Philadelphia: Elsevier Saunders; 2005:1167–1226.
2. Mayo Clinic Cardiology Board Review. Mayo Foundation for Education and Research. Rochester, 2006.
3. Surawicz B, Knilans T. Chou's electrocardiography in clinical practice, 5th ed. Philadelphia: Elsevier Health Sciences; 2001.
4. Otto CM. Textbook of clinical echocardiography in clinical practice, 5th ed. Philadelphia: Elsevier Health Sciences, 2001.
5. Orient JM. Sapira's art and sciences of bedside diagnosis, 3rd ed. Philadelphia: Lippincott Williams & Wilkins; 2005.
6. Oh J. The echo manual, 3rd ed. Philadelphia: Lippincott Williams & Wilkins; 2006.

12
Diagnosis and Treatment of Congestive Heart Failure

David M. Wild, Emad Aziz, Eyal Herzog, and Marrick Kukin

Patients presenting to the emergency department with acute heart failure (AHF) pose a major health care problem [1]. Acute heart failure accounts for more than 1 million hospitalizations per year in the United States with an in-hospital mortality rate of 4.1% and a mean length of stay of 6.5 days. Whether due to inadequate in-hospital treatment, refractory disease, noncompliance with diet or medications, or comorbidities, there is a hospital readmission rate of 20% within 30 days and 50% during the next 6- to 12-month interval. Additionally, there is a 10% mortality rate at 30 days, which increases to 20% to 40% at 12 months [2].

Heart failure can occur in the setting of acute coronary syndrome (ACS) and acute myocardial infarction (AMI). Other chapters in this book focus on the primary care of these conditions (i.e., angioplasty/revascularization) and treatment of mechanical complications associated with AMI and heart failure. In this chapter, we will focus on the medical diagnosis and therapy of acute decompensated heart failure—both in the setting of ACS and in chronic heart failure patients with acute heart failure decompensation.

The American College of Cardiology and the American Heart Association (ACC/AHA) have recently published revised guidelines for the management of chronic heart failure in adults [2]. The European Society of Cardiology has also developed guidelines for chronic heart failure [3]. Both sets of guidelines focus on outpatient management of chronic heart failure; treatment options for acutely decompensated heart failure (ADHF) and new-onset heart failure are not addressed. To address this deficiency, we have developed a unified pathway for the management of patients presenting with AHF to the emergency department. This pathway is simple yet comprehensive and covers the entire spectrum of patient care, from the time of emergency department presentation through their admission and the discharge plan (Fig. 12.1).

This pathway does not describe new treatments for heart failure. Rather, it is an attempt to incorporate, in a user-friendly format, the keys to initial diagnosis and management of heart failure. This is followed by a comprehensive guideline to therapy with a goal of shortening length of stay (LOS) without compromising medical stabilization, optimal diuresis, and implementation of

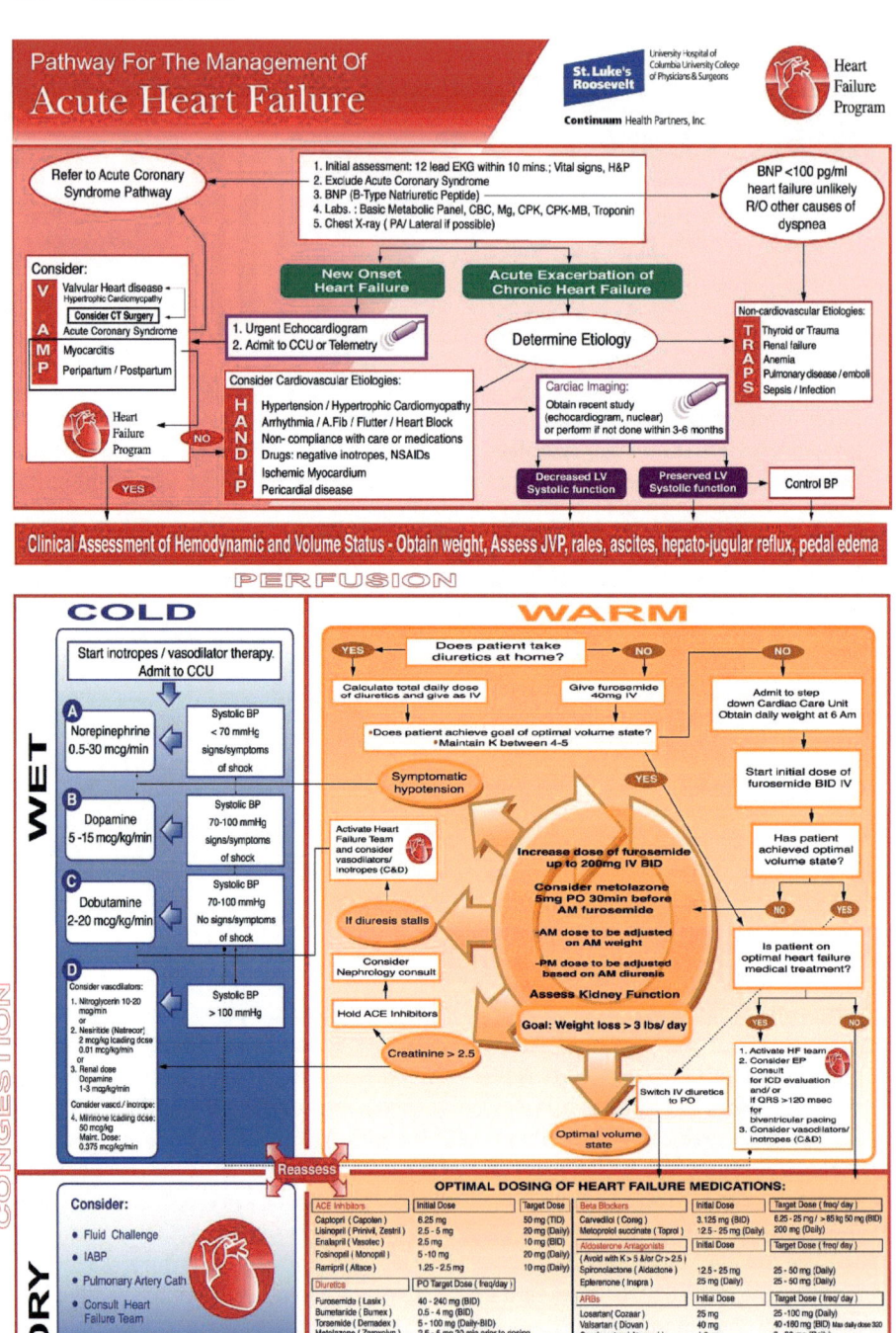

Figure 12.1. Pathway for the evaluation and management of acute heart failure.

outpatient therapies based on the proven results of clinical trials. The use of aggressive loop diuretics with daily weight monitoring is empirically derived from our clinical experience, whereas the usage and dosing of the other medications are derived from clinical trials [2] and published Advanced Cardiac Life Support (ACLS) guidelines [4].

The ESCAPE trial [5] evaluated the use of the pulmonary artery catheter in patients admitted with decompensated heart failure. The results demonstrated that outcomes are not improved by invasive hemodynamic monitoring for the patients that would generally be eligible for the pathway described herein. A careful history and physical exam (H&P) combined with clinical judgment and incorporation of clinically proven therapies are the guiding principles in the development of this pathway.

Diagnosis

The first step in the management of the patient with heart failure is a rapid but thorough evaluation of the patient in the emergency department. This includes a 12-lead ECG within 10 minutes, vital signs, H&P, labs, and chest x-ray. The primary goal is to exclude ACS, which would lead to different, more aggressive therapy. In addition, one can obtain a brain natriuretic peptide (BNP) level to exclude noncardiovascular causes of dyspnea [6] when the diagnosis of heart failure may be in doubt (Fig. 12.2).

The development of assays for the natriuretic peptides (NPs), BNP and N-terminal pro-BNP (NT-proBNP), have become increasingly important for evaluation of dyspneic patients and, depending on the results of clinical trials, may prove useful to guide treatment of congestive heart failure.

BNP is synthesized and secreted mainly by the ventricular myocardium; it is derived from the precursor pre–pro-BNP. Pro-BNP gene expression must be upregulated before it can be released into the blood, thus the concentration of BNP does not fluctuate as quickly as does atrial NP. Under conditions of sustained ventricular expansion and pressure overload, pro-BNP is released into the blood, where it is cleaved into BNP, the active hormone, and N-terminal BNP (NT-BNP), an inactive metabolite. BNP has a biologic half-life of approximately 20 minutes, making it a valuable tool for the diagnosis of congestive

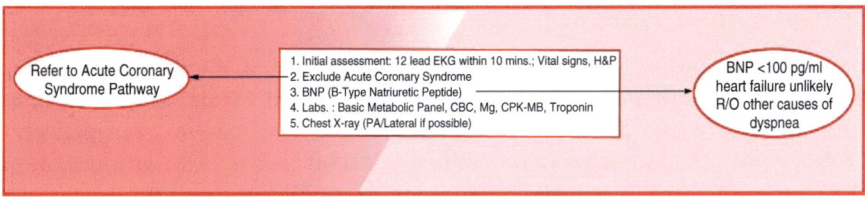

FIGURE 12.2. Initial evaluation of patients presenting to the emergency department with suspected AHF.

heart failure (CHF) and potentially useful for optimizing the treatment of ADHF patients [7].

The Breathing Not Properly study used BNP levels to evaluate the causes of dyspnea in 1,586 patients. BNP levels were found to be more accurate predictors of CHF than any history, physical findings, or laboratory value [8]. A BNP value of 100 pg/mL had a sensitivity of 90% and a specificity of 76% for differentiating CHF from other causes of dyspnea, and a cutoff level of 50 pg/mL had a negative predictive value of 96%. BNP levels, had they been available to clinicians, would have reduced the rate of indecision from 43% to 11%. Incorporating BNP into the clinical evaluation of dyspneic patients was found to increase the absolute diagnostic accuracy by 10% [9].

Differentiating cardiac from pulmonary causes of dyspnea is a great challenge. Morrison et al. studied 321 patients who presented to the emergency department with dyspnea [10]. BNP distinguished heart failure (HF) (mean BNP, 759 ± 798 pg/mL) from pulmonary disease (61 ± 10 pg/mL) and other clinical presentations with high specificity and sensitivity. Moreover, when patients who had a history of heart failure but whose dyspnea was caused by chronic obstructive pulmonary disease (COPD; mean BNP, 47 ± 23 pg/mL) were compared with patients who had a history of COPD but whose dyspnea was caused by heart failure (731 ± 764 pg/mL), a BNP value of 94 pg/mL yielded a sensitivity and specificity of 86% and 98%, respectively, and differentiated heart failure from lung disease with an accuracy of 91%. BNP has therefore emerged as a strong diagnostic and prognostic indicator of left ventricular (LV) dysfunction and heart failure.

Elevations of BNP have been shown to be a powerful marker for prognosis and risk stratification in the setting of HF. Furthermore, changes in plasma BNP levels are significantly related to changes in limitation of physical activities and thus a powerful predicator of the functional status deterioration. Maisel et al. followed 325 patients for 6 months after an index visit to the emergency department [11]. Higher BNP levels were associated with a progressively worse prognosis. The relative risk of 6-month CHF admission or death in patients with BNP levels >230 pg/dL was 24 times the risk of levels less than this. BNP levels might not only be helpful in assessing whether or not a dyspneic patient has HF, but also it may assist in making subsequent triage and management decisions [11].

BNP as a Prognostic Tool

In a prospective study at St. Luke's Roosevelt Hospital, 87 patients admitted with HF were evaluated according to our HF pathway. Median BNP on admission was 623 pg/mL (25th to 75th percentile, 286 to 877 pg/mL, respectively). Twenty-two (25%) patients were readmitted (21%) or died (3%) within 30 days. Patients with admission BNP values >75th percentile (877 pg/mL) had greater risk of rehospitalization compared with values <877 pg/mL (66% vs. 2%, respectively; $P < 0.001$) with a negative predictive value of 87%, (95% CI, 0.62 to 0.96).

BNP values >75th percentile were associated with a 4.1 hazard ratio (HR) of early readmission or death (95% CI, 2.38 to 7.32; $P < 0.0001$), regardless of other comorbid diseases. We concluded that admission BNP levels were the strongest predictor of early readmissions (within 30 days) or death due to HF, irrespective of other substantial comorbidities and advanced age.

New-Onset HF Versus Acute Exacerbation of Chronic HF

The next diagnostic step would be to differentiate between new-onset heart failure and acute exacerbations of chronic heart failure. This early recognition emphasizes that new-onset heart failure is an urgent situation, which may require cardiothoracic surgery involvement for acute valvular problems (i.e., flail mitral leaflet) or chronic valvular problems with acutely decompensated heart failure (i.e., critical aortic stenosis) (Fig. 12.3). If the heart failure is believed to be new onset, the patient should have an urgent echocardiogram to rule out valvular disease and one should consider other etiologies including acute coronary syndromes, myocarditis, and peripartum/postpartum cardiomyopathy (Fig. 12.3). If the heart failure is believed to be an exacerbation of chronic heart failure, it is necessary to determine the etiology of the decompensation by considering causes with the reminder acronym, HANDIP:

- H, Hypertension
- A, Arrhythmias: atrial fibrillation, atrial flutter, heart block
- N, Noncompliance with care (i.e., diet, fluid excess) or medications
- D, Drugs: negative inotropes (i.e., calcium channel blockers), nonsteroidal anti-inflammatory drugs (NSAIDs), alcohol, illicit drug use
- I, Ischemic myocardium
- P, Pericardial disease

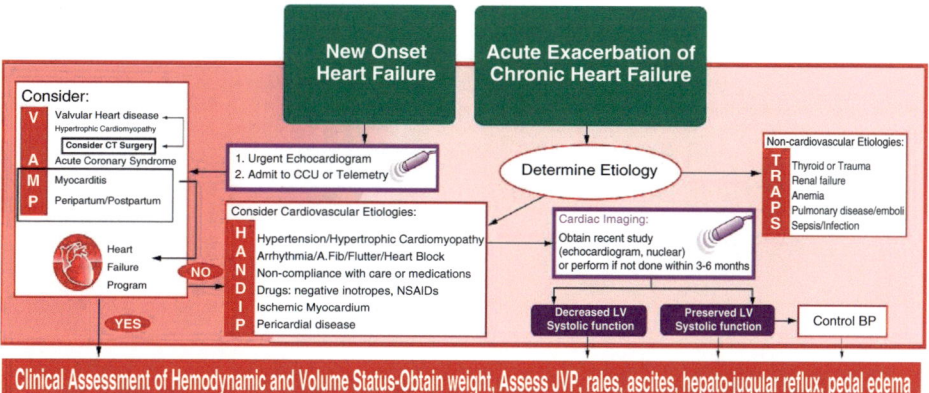

FIGURE 12.3. Differential diagnosis between new-onset heart failure and acute exacerbation of chronic heart failure with timing of imaging and consideration of precipitating pathophysiology.

In addition, noncardiovascular causes of heart failure should be considered using the acronym TRAPS as a guide:

- T, Thyroid or trauma
- R, Renal failure
- A, Anemia
- P, Pulmonary disease, pulmonary emboli
- S, Sepsis, infection

For newly diagnosed heart failure, is routine cardiac catheterization indicated? In the absence of angina, diagnostic electrocardiogram of ischemia, or multiple coronary risk factors, the answer is not clear. Certainly, when there is an index of suspicion, all reversible causes of heart failure, such as ischemia, must be considered. However, in a young patient with no coronary risk factors, the risks of cardiac catheterization must be carefully weighed against the low probability of finding coronary artery disease. When in doubt, we would err on the side of performing a cardiac catheterization. However, in the absence of anginal symptoms or multiple risk factors, the majority of these procedures document clean coronaries. A second procedure often debated is endomyocardial biopsy [2]. This is not recommended in the practice guidelines (level of evidence = C).

Bedside Assessment

Cardiac imaging is used to determine whether LV function is decreased or preserved as this distinction affects therapy. Once the etiology has been established, the next phase of management is rapid clinical assessment of hemodynamics based on perfusion and congestion [12, 13]. This assessment is based on bedside examination: whether the clinical symptoms indicate the adequacy of filling pressure/perfusion (warm or cold) and the volume status of the patient based on history and physical exam (wet or dry) (Fig. 12.4). The sizing of the

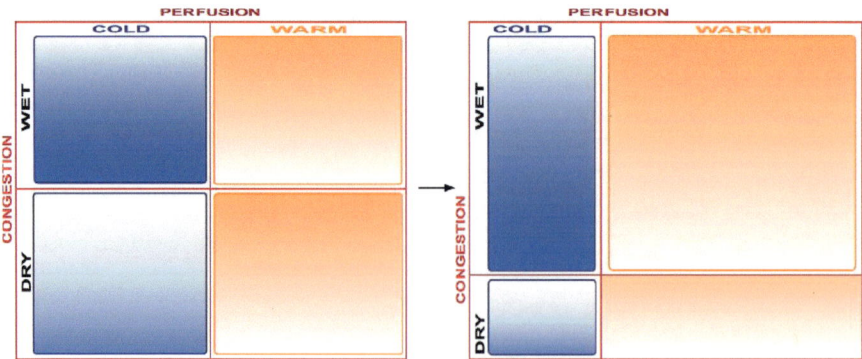

FIGURE 12.4. Depiction of perfusion and congestion concept with consideration of disproportionate group size of each quadrant.

four quadrants (warm-wet, warm-dry, cold-wet, cold-dry) is not equal, reflecting the actual proportionate distribution of these patient admissions into the hospital based on their clinical presentation [13]. Thus, the group of warm-wet patients is visually the largest part of the pathway emphasizing their relative frequency compared with all HF admissions (Fig. 12.4).

Therapy

The determination of volume status will have implications in the pharmacological management of the patient. Most patients admitted with symptomatic heart failure will have warm-wet physiology, and the key in their management will be aggressive loop diuretic management (Fig. 12.5). This recognition and early

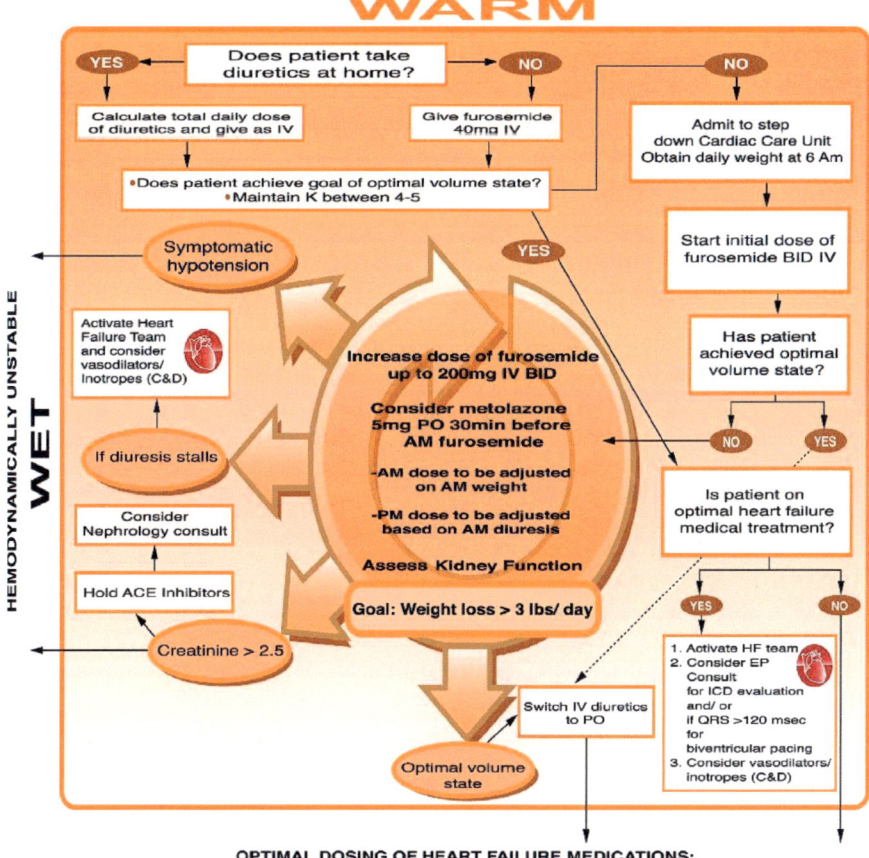

FIGURE **12.5.** The "loop" concept of aggressive usage of loop diuretics to rapidly and safely diurese patients, shorten LOS, and transition to oral therapy upon successful completion of diuresis.

aggressive treatment is the key to decreasing the length of in-hospital stay. Three major decisions regarding pharmacological treatment need to be addressed based on the hemodynamic assessment: What regimen of diuretic should be used? If the patient is on chronic therapy with beta-blockers, should it be discontinued or reduced? Does the patient require inotropes? In Figure 12.5, the algorithm shows the optimal method of deciding appropriate diuretic doses. If the patient has been taking oral diuretics as an outpatient, that total daily dose should be given intravenously as a bolus infusion. If the patient has not been taking diuretics, the patient should be given an intravenous loop diuretic (i.e., furosemide 40 mg).

Once an optimal volume state is achieved, then the patient can be changed to oral therapy and begun on a chronic heart failure regimen. If the patient does not initially achieve a euvolemic state, then the patient should be admitted to a monitored setting and have the diuretic dose doubled and given twice daily. If this still does not work, the dose of diuretic can be increased and consideration given to adding other diuretics, such as metolazone. If there is difficulty in achieving a euvolemic state or if the patient develops symptomatic hypotension or a significant increase in serum creatinine, which together can signify a low-flow state, the patient should be started on appropriate inotropic therapy (Fig. 12.6). Guidelines of management of hemodynamically unstable patients are based on the ACLS guidelines, incorporating vasodilators and inotropic infusions [4]. In these circumstances, it is appropriate to activate the heart failure team (if there is one present at the institution).

Beta-Blockers

The next question is what to do if the patient is chronically being treated with beta-blockers. The use of beta-blockers in chronic heart failure has been well established in multiple randomized trials [14–16]. However, the majority of heart failure patients we encounter in the hospital are in decompensated heart failure. It is in these patients where there is ambiguity as to the role of beta-blockers. There are no clear guidelines as to whether to stop or reduce the dose of the beta-blocker.

There are two major questions yet to be answered regarding beta-blockers and acutely decompensated heart failure: (1) In patients currently taking beta-blockers, should the beta-blocker be held completely or have the dose reduced when these patients are admitted with fluid overloaded states? (2) In these patients who are admitted with acute exacerbations of heart failure who have not been on chronic beta-blocker therapy, when is it safe to start a beta-blocker?

The theoretical concern with continuing beta-blockers in decompensated heart failure is that administration of a beta-blocker may exacerbate the fluid overload state because of its negative inotropic effects. However, there are no data to suggest that this is true. On the other hand, it may be desirable to continue beta-blockers because doing so may help avoid the long process of having to uptitrate the medications and may decrease the delay of ultimately reaching

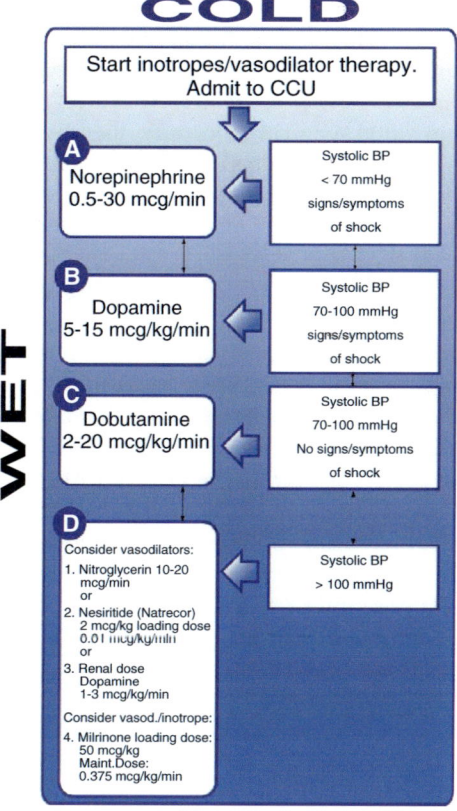

FIGURE 12.6. Management of hemodynamically unstable heart failure patients adapted from ACLS guidelines.

target doses. In addition, there are data suggesting that patients with systolic dysfunction have poorer outcomes after stopping beta-blocker therapy [17, 18]. Recently, two studies have examined the safety of continuing beta-blocker therapy in patients admitted with acutely decompensated heart failure [19, 20]. These studies examined two large databases of heart failure patients admitted with fluid overload: the OPTIME-CHF and ESCAPE databases. However, these studies have shown that continuing beta-blockers during the hospitalization is not associated with an increase in adverse outcomes and even suggest that there may be improved outcomes in patients in whom the beta-blockers are continued. These studies were observational and nonrandomized and therefore cannot be used as definitive evidence.

In view of these recent developments and lack of randomized studies examining beta-blocker therapy in this group of patients, we recommend the following: In patients who are "warm and wet" upon hospitalization with no evidence of poor perfusion or low-flow state, such as prerenal azotemia, and not requiring intubation or bilevel position airway pressure for respiratory distress, the beta-blocker should be continued at the same dose as outpatient. However, if there is difficulty after 24 to 48 hours in achieving a euvolemic state, then the dose should be reduced to 50% or stopped entirely. In the very small population of "cold and wet" patients requiring inotropic therapy for low-flow state, the beta-blocker should be discontinued altogether until there is significant improvement in the fluid status. Thought should be given to the choice of inotropic therapy because of differential effects of the various inotropes depending on which beta-blocker the patient was on chronically. Data suggest that patients on carvedilol do not respond as well to dobutamine as to milrinone, a phosphodiesterase inhibitor [21–23].

In patients admitted with decompensated heart failure who are not already taking beta-blockers, there is controversy regarding the appropriate time to initiate therapy. Heart Failure Society of America guidelines recommend that beta-blockers should not be initiated during a hospitalization for an exacerbation of heart failure [24]. However, in the IMPACT-HF trial published in 2004, they conclude that predischarge initiation of beta-blockers improves the probability of use of beta-blockers at subsequent visits without increasing side effects or LOS [25]. We recommend starting therapy with an approved beta-blocker at the lowest dose once patients are believed to be euvolemic. Outpatient uptitration as tolerated to target doses as established in mortality trials should follow.

Oral Medications

Once patients are stabilized and are believed to be euvolemic, attention should be given to placing the patient on an optimal medical regimen [26] (Fig. 12.7). Albeit representative, not all medications in some categories are included in the chart due to space constraints. Early ambulation of these patients during their hospital stay and exercise regiments are encouraged. In addition, for appropriate patients, a heart failure and/or an electrophysiology (EPS) consult should be considered because current therapy for heart failure now encompasses electrical devices and close collaboration with electrophysiologists.

ACE Inhibitors	Initial Dose	Target Dose	Beta Blockers	Initial Dose	Target Dose (freq/ day)
Captopril (Capoten)	6.25 mg	50 mg (TID)	Carvedilol (Coreg)	3.125 mg (BID)	6.25 - 25 mg / > 85 kg 50 mg (BID)
Lisinopril (Prinivil, Zestril)	2.5 - 5 mg	20 mg (Daily)	Metoprolol succinate (Toprol)	12.5 - 25 mg (Daily)	200 mg (Daily)
Enalapril (Vasotec)	2.5 mg	10 mg (BID)	Aldosterone Antagonists	Initial Dose	Target Dose (freq/ day)
Fosinopril (Monopril)	5 -10 mg	20 mg (Daily)	(Avoid with K > 5 &/or Cr > 2.5)		
Ramipril (Altace)	1.25 - 2.5 mg	10 mg (Daily)	Spironolactone (Aldactone)	12.5 - 25 mg	25 - 50 mg (Daily)
Diuretics	PO Target Dose (freq/day)		Eplerenone (Inspra)	25 mg (Daily)	25 - 50 mg (Daily)
Furosemide (Lasix)	40 - 240 mg (BID)		ARBs	Initial Dose	Target Dose (freq/ day)
Bumetanide (Bumex)	0.5 - 4 mg (BID)		Losartan(Cozaar)	25 mg	25 -100 mg (Daily)
Torsemide (Demadex)	5 - 100 mg (Daily-BID)		Valsartan (Diovan)	40 mg	40 -160 mg (BID) Max daily dose 320
Metolazone (Zaroxolyn)	2.5 - 5 mg 30 min prior to dosing		Candesartan (Atacand)	4-8 mg	8 - 32 mg (Daily)
Lanoxin (Digoxin)	0.125 - 0.25 mg (Daily) - Consider age/ Cr.		Consider for African Americans: Hydralazine/ ISDN 37.5/ 20 - 75/40mg (TID)		

Figure 12.7. Initiation and target dosages of oral heart failure medications.

Incorporated into the pathway is the timing and consideration of biventricular pacemakers (BIVPMs) in patients with wide QRS complexes and the consideration of implantable cardioverter-defibrillators (ICDs) based on MADIT-2 [27], SCD-HEFT [28], and COMPANION [29] criteria (Fig. 12.5).

This acute heart failure pathway flows as the patient progresses toward the warm/dry group, which is a segue to outpatient management of heart failure. The ACC/AHA [2] and European guidelines [3] detail the major trials and dosing of the appropriate heart failure medications. The key point in this algorithm is that upon discharge, all HF patients should be on, at a minimum, starting doses of angiotensin-converting enzyme (ACE) inhibitors and beta-blockers, unless contraindicated. Angiotensin receptor blockers (ARBs) should be used instead of ACE inhibitors when ACE inhibitors cannot be given, (i.e. ACE inhibitor–induced cough). In certain instances, it may be appropriate to combine an ACE inhibitor and ARB [30]. Data from RALES [31] and EPHESUS [32] would support the addition of aldosterone antagonists with the precaution of monitoring potassium and creatinine levels on therapy [33].

With the recent publication of the results of A-HeFT [34], consideration should be given to the addition of hydralazine/isosorbide dinitrate in African Americans. Most U.S. physicians use digoxin for patients with New York Heart Association (NYHA) class III/IV heart failure with an age/creatinine nomogram. Dosages of oral diuretics should be adjusted to maintain the euvolemic state achieved during the hospitalization, along with adherence to a 2-g sodium diet and daily weight monitoring. A motivated patient with a home scale can be taught to self-adjust diuretics based on his or her morning weight.

References

1. Fonarow GC, Weber JE. Rapid clinical assessment of hemodynamic profiles and targeted treatment of patients with acutely decompensated heart failure. Clin Cardiol 2004;27(Suppl V):V-1–V-9.
2. Hunt SA, Baker DW, Chin MH, et al. ACC/AHA guidelines for the evaluation and management of chronic heart failure in the adult: a report of American College of Cardiology/American Heart Association Task Force on Practice Guidelines (Committee to Revise the 1995 Guidelines for the Evaluation and Management of Heart Failure). J Am Coll Cardiol 2001;38:2101–2113.
3. Remme WJ, Swedberg K. Comprehensive guidelines for the diagnosis and treatment of chronic heart failure. Task force for the diagnosis and treatment of chronic heart failure of the European Society of Cardiology. Eur J Heart Fail 2002;4:11–22.
4. Mary FH, Richard OC, John MF. AHA 2000 handbook of emergency cardiovascular care for healthcare providers American Heart Association; Dallas, 2000.
5. Shah MR, Stevenson LW. Evaluation Study of Congestive Heart Failure and Pulmonary Artery Catheterization Effectiveness (ESCAPE). American Heart Association Scientific Sessions, New Orleans, LA, November 9, 2004.
6. Maisel SA, Krishnaswamy P, Nowak, RM, et al. Rapid measurement of b-type natriuretic peptide in the emergency diagnosis of heart failure. N Engl J Med 2002;347: 161–167.

7. Bhalla V, Willis S, Maisel AS. B-type natriuretic peptide: the level and the drug partner in the diagnosis and management of congestive heart failure. Congest Heart Fail 2005;3:161.

8. Maisel AS, Krishnaswamy P, Nowak RM, et al. Breathing Not Properly Multinational Study Investigators. Rapid measurement of B-type natriuretic peptide in the emergency diagnosis of heart failure. N Engl J Med 2002;347:161–167.

9. McCullough PA, Nowak RM, McCord J, et al. B-type natriuretic peptide and clinical judgment in emergency diagnosis of heart failure: analysis from Breathing Not Properly (BNP) Multinational Study. Circulation 2002;106:416–422.

10. Morrison LK, Harrison A, Krishnaswamy P, et al. Utility of a rapid B-natriuretic peptide assay in differentiating congestive heart failure from lung disease in patients presenting with dyspnea. J Am Coll Cardiol 2002;39:202–209.

11. Maisel AS. The diagnosis of acute congestive heart failure: role of BNP measurements. Heart Fail Rev 2003;8:327–334.

12. Stevenson LW. Tailored therapy of hemodynamic goals for advanced heart failure. Eur J Heart Fail 1999;1:252–257.

13. Nohria A, Tsang SW, Fang JC, et al. Clinical assessment identifies hemodynamic profiles that predict outcomes in patients admitted with heart failure. J Am Coll Cardiol 2003;41:1797–1804.

14. Packer M, Coats AJ, Fowler MB, et al. Effect of carvedilol on survival in severe chronic heart failure. N Engl J Med 2001;344:1651–1658.

15. MERIT-HF study group. Metoprolol CR/XL Randomised Intervention trial in congestive heart failure (MERIT-HF). Lancet 1999;353:2001–2007.

16. Packer M, Bristow MR, Cohn JN, et al. The effect of carvedilol on morbidity and mortality in patients with chronic heart failure. U.S. Carvedilol Heart Failure Study Group. N Engl J Med 1996;334:1349–1355.

17. Morimoto S, Shimizu K, Yamada K, et al. Can beta-blocker therapy be withdrawn from patients with dilated cardiomyopathy? Am Heart J 1999;138:456–459.

18. Waagstein F, Caidahl K, Wallentin I, et al. Long term beta blockade in dilated cardiomyopathy. Effects of short- and long- term metoprolol treatment followed by withdrawal and readministration of metoprolol. Circulation 1989;80:551–563.

19. Gattis WA, O'Connor CM, Leimberger JD, et al. Clinical outcomes in patients on beta-blocker therapy admitted with worsening chronic heart failure. Am J Cardiol 2003;91:169–174.

20. Butler J, Young JB, Abraham WT, et al. Beta-blocker use and outcomes among hospitalized heart failure patients. J Am Coll Cardiol 2006;47:2462–2469.

21. Lowes BD, Tsvetkova T, Eichhorn EJ, et al. Milrinone versus dobutamine in heart failure subjects treated chronically with with carvedilol. Int J Cardiol 2001;81:141–149.

22. Metra M, Nodari S, D'Aloia A, et al. Beta-blocker therapy influences the hemodynamic response to inotropic agents in patients with heart failure: a randomized comparison of dobutamine and enoximone before and after chronic treatment with metoprolol or carvedilol. J Am Coll Cardiol 2002;40:1248–1258.

23. Bollano E, Tang MS, Hjalmarson A, et al. Different responses to dobutamine in the presence of carvedilol or metoprolol in patients with chronic heart failure. Heart 2003;89:621–624.

24. Heart Failure Society of America Guideline Committee. HFSA guidelines for the management of patients with heart failure caused by left ventricukar systolic dysfunction: pharmacologic approaches. J Card Fail 1999;5:357–382.

25. Gattis WA, O'Connor CM, Gallup DS, et al., and IMPACT-HF Investigators and Coordinators. Predischarge initiation of carvedilol in patients hospitalized for decompensated heart failure: results of the Initiation Management Predischarge: Process for Assessment of Carvedilol therapy in Heart Failure (IMPACT-HF) Trial. J Am Coll Cardiol 2004;43:1534–1541.

26. Bukharovich IF, Kukin ML. Optimal medical therapy for heart failure. Prog Cardiovasc Dis 2006;48:372–385.

27. Moss AJ, Zareba W, Hall WJ, et al. Prohylactic implantation of a defibrillator in patients with myocardial infraction and reduced ejection fraction. N Engl J Med 2002;346:877–883.

28. Bardy GH, Lee KL, Mark DB, et al. Amiodarone or an implantable cardioverter-defibrillator for congestive heart failure. N Engl J Med 2005;352:225–237.

29. Bristow MR, Saxon LA, Boehmer J, et al. Cardiac-resynchronization therapy with or without an implantable defibrillator in advance chronic heart failure. N Engl J Med 2004;350:2140–2150.

30. McMurray JJV, Östergren J, Sweedberg K, et al. Effects of candesartan in patients with chronic heart failure and reduced left-ventricular systolic function taking angiotensin-converting-enzyme inhibitors; the CHARM-Added trial. Lancet 2003; 362:767–771.

31. Pitt B, Zannad F, Renne WJ, et al. The effect of spironolactone on morbidity and mortality in patients with severe heart failure. N Engl J Med 1999;341:709–717.

32. Pitt B, Willem R, Zannad F, et al. Eplerenone, a selective aldosterone blocker, in patients with ventricular dysfunction after myocardial infarction. N Engl J Med 2003;348:1309–1321.

33. Juurklink D, Mamdani MM, Lee DS, et al. Rates of hyperkalemia after publication of the Randomized Aldactone Evaluation Study. N Engl J Med 2004;351:543–551.

34. Taylor AL, Ziesche S, Yancy C, et al. Combination of isosorbride dinitrate and hydralazine in blacks with heart failure. N Engl J Med 2004;351:2049–2057.

13
Diagnosis and Treatment of Cardiogenic Shock

Angela Palazzo, Sripal Bangalore, Jacqueline E. Tamis-Holland, and Amy Chorzempa

Cardiogenic shock is the leading cause of death in patients hospitalized with acute myocardial infarction [1, 2]. Cardiogenic shock is characterized by a state of inadequate tissue perfusion due to cardiac dysfunction and is classically manifested by systemic hypotension and end-organ hypoperfusion in the setting of adequate or elevated left ventricular filling pressures. The hemodynamic definition includes sustained hypotension (systolic blood pressure <90 mm Hg or a decrease >30 mm Hg or more in mean arterial pressure from baseline for at least 30 minutes) and a reduced cardiac index ($<2.2\,L\,min^{-1}\,m^{-2}$) [3]. In the SHould we emergently revascularize Occluded Coronaries for cardiogenic shocK (SHOCK) Trial [4], tissue hypoperfusion was defined as cold peripheries (extremities colder than core), oliguria (<30 mL/h), or both. Subjects requiring pharmacological or mechanical circulatory support to maintain blood pressure are also included in this category.

In the setting of an acute myocardial infarction, hypotension, tachycardia, peripheral vasoconstriction, decreased urine output, and altered mentation are all manifestations of the syndrome, which can range from "preshock" to fully developed pump failure.

It is important to recognize the preshock syndrome because early investigation of its etiology and early intervention may reduce the development of frank cardiogenic shock. In this state, systolic blood pressure may be normal to borderline without pressors, but this "stability" occurs at the expense of an elevated peripheral resistance and elevated heart rate that support a borderline stroke volume. The signs of peripheral hypoperfusion may be obvious or subtle. This is also known as nonhypotensive cardiogenic shock and is associated with ineffective tissue perfusion and a severely depressed cardiac index. The preshock syndrome is associated with a high in-hospital mortality (43%), which is lower than that in patients with classic cardiogenic shock (66%) [5]. This syndrome predominately occurs in the setting of a large anterior wall myocardial infarction (MI). Recognition of this "preshock state" is important to avoid potentially cardiodepressant medications and to identify patients who might benefit from aggressive revascularization strategies.

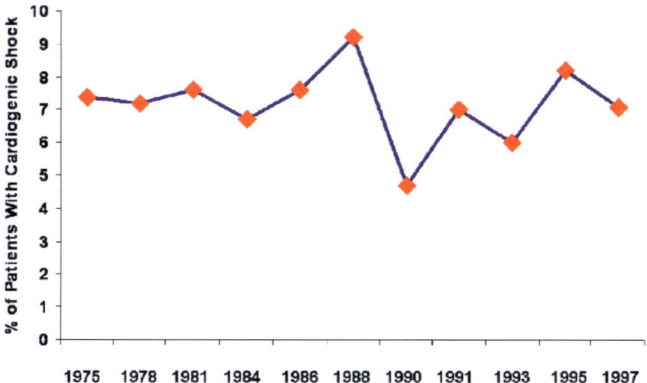

FIGURE 13.1. Temporal trends in the incidence of cardiogenic shock in patients with myocardial infarction. (Adapted from Goldberg RJ, Samad NA, Yarzebski J, et al. Temporal trends in cardiogenic shock complicating acute myocardial infarction. N Engl J Med 1999;340(15):1162–1168.)

Incidence

Cardiogenic shock occurs in 7.2% of patients with ST-segment elevation MI (STEMI) [6] and in 2% to 3% of patients with non–ST-segment elevation MI (NSTEMI) [7, 8]. The incidence of cardiogenic shock has not changed significantly over time despite the introduction of pharmacological reperfusion therapy and percutaneous coronary intervention (PCI). Studies evaluating temporal trends in cardiogenic shock from 1975 until 2001 have reported similar rates of shock over this time period, averaging 7% to 9% of patients with acute myocardial infarction (Fig. 13.1) [1, 9].

Risk Factors

Certain clinical variables have been identified that increase the likelihood for developing cardiogenic shock after myocardial infarction. These include older age, diabetes, a history of prior infarction or known preexisting systolic dysfunction. Anterior wall infarction, a large myocardial infarction as evidenced by higher cardiac enzyme levels, and multivessel disease increase the risk of cardiogenic shock [2, 4, 10, 11].

The risk of cardiogenic shock is greater with a higher number of such risk factors. In one study [2], the probability of developing cardiogenic shock was 17.9% for patients with three risk factors and 54.4% among patients with five risk factors.

Etiology

Cardiogenic shock complicating acute MI can be the result of pump failure or mechanical complications. It is important to recognize the etiology of cardio-

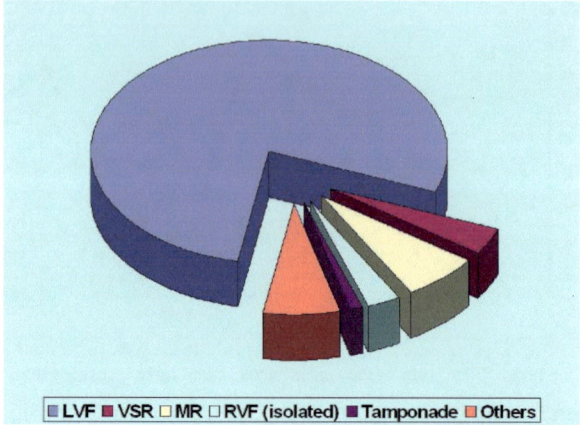

FIGURE 13.2. Etiology of cardiogenic shock. LVF, left ventricular failure; MR, mitral regurgitation; RVF, right ventricular failure; VSR, ventricular septal rupture. (Adapted from Menon V, Hochman JS. Management of cardiogenic shock complicating acute myocardial infarction. Heart 2002;88(5):531–537.)

genic shock because the management will differ with each cause. In the SHOCK Trial registry [4, 10], 74.5% of patients had predominant left ventricular failure and 3.4% had isolated right ventricular shock. Mechanical complications leading to cardiogenic shock occurred in 12% of patients including acute mitral regurgitation (8.3%), ventricular septal rupture (4.6%), and tamponade or free wall rupture (1.7%) (Fig. 13.2).

Left Ventricular Failure

Predominant left ventricular (LV) pump failure in the setting of a large MI is the most common etiology of cardiogenic shock. It has been documented that at least 40% of the total LV mass is infarcted in patients with death due to cardiogenic shock [12, 13]. Cardiogenic shock can also result from smaller infarctions in patients with preexisting LV dysfunction, severe multivessel disease, and widespread ischemia. Delayed shock may result from infarction extension or reinfarction.

Pathophysiology of Left Ventricular Shock

In data from the SHOCK Registry [14], 74.1% of patients presented with early shock (<24 hours) and 46.6% presented with shock very early (<6 hours). Early shock is more indicative of widespread necrosis, whereas shock that develops later may be secondary to expansion or extension of the infarct. The classic explanation of the mechanisms of LV shock shows how both jeopardized myocardium as well as more distant myocardium is affected by hypotension and increased LV end-diastolic pressure. These effects are magnified when there is flow-limiting stenosis in remote, nonculprit vessels. Compensating mechanisms such as tachycardia and increased metabolic demand in both ischemic and nonischemic regions lead to further global dysfunction (Fig. 13.3) [15].

Right Ventricular Shock

Right ventricular (RV) infarction leading to cardiogenic shock can be seen in the presence of an acute inferior wall MI with RV involvement. The typical findings of significant right ventricular infarction are hypotension, clear lung fields, and jugular venous distension. Although these may also be seen in cardiac tamponade or acute RV failure secondary to pulmonary emboli, in the presence of an acute inferior wall MI they are diagnostic of RV infarct. Often, these patients will have an exaggerated hypotensive response to vasodilating agents. Pulmonary congestion may be seen when extensive LV infarction/scar is also present, and rarely, severe right ventricular dysfunction can cause RV distension and septal shift resulting in LV compromise with clinical evidence of pulmonary congestion [16].

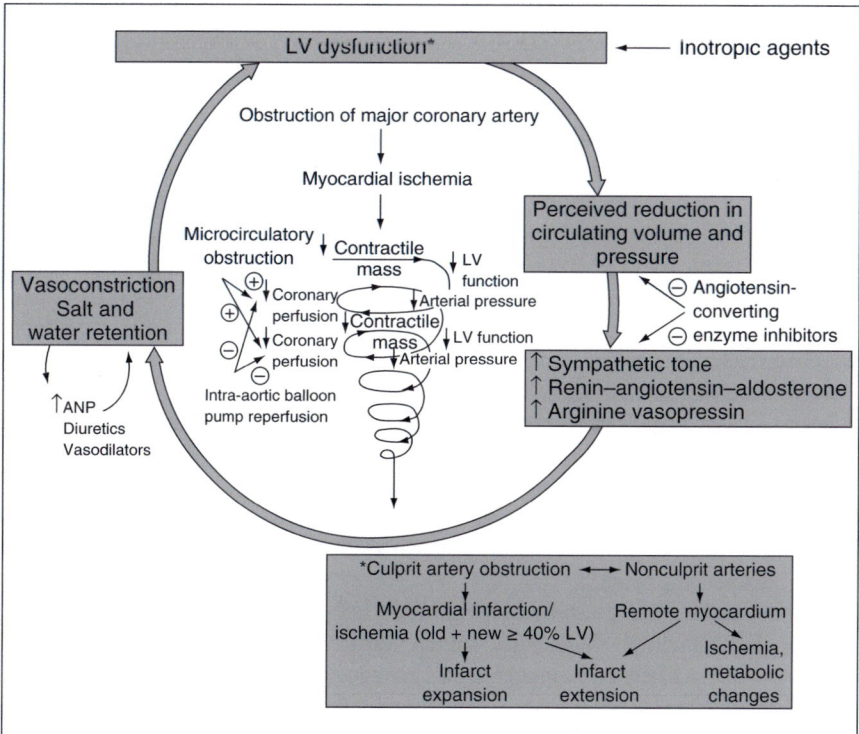

FIGURE 13.3. Pathophysiology of left ventricular shock. (Adapted from Califf RA, Bengtson JR. Cardiogenic shock. In: Braunwald E, Califf RM, eds. Atlas of Heart Disease-Acute Myocardial Infarction and other Acute Ischemic Syndromes. 2nd ed. Philadelphia: Current Medicine; 2001: pp. 149–178.)

Mechanical Complications Leading to Cardiogenic Shock

Mechanical complications of acute MI resulting in cardiogenic shock include acute mitral regurgitation caused by papillary muscle dysfunction or rupture, rupture of the interventricular septum, or rupture of the free wall with resultant contained tamponade. Free wall rupture with tamponade is usually characterized by hypotension, tachycardia, clear lungs, and jugular venous distension, and can easily be differentiated from RV infarct by echocardiogram. Free wall rupture that is not contained usually results in immediate death. Acute papillary muscle rupture or rupture of the interventricular septum are both characterized by hypotension in the setting of pulmonary vascular congestion and a new murmur. They can be differentiated from each other by echocardiogram. (See chapters 11 and 12 for details.)

Diagnosis

Cardiogenic shock is a catastrophic event with an extremely high mortality. Early diagnosis is essential to provide rapid and potentially lifesaving therapies. Once the diagnosis of MI has been established, the presence of cardiogenic shock or impending shock can be rapidly assessed by physical examination. The combination of a large MI and tachycardia, with or without hypotension, should alert the physician to the possibility of cardiogenic shock or preshock. Tachycardia may be masked by the use of beta-blockers, increased vagal tone, or inappropriate chronotropic reserve. Frank hypotension should immediately be investigated, but the absence of hypotension does not exclude the diagnosis of shock [5]. Evidence of increased vasoconstriction such as cyanosis or cool extremities and signs of hypoperfusion such as decreased urine output or an altered sensorium must raise suspicion.

On physical examination, the quality of the peripheral pulses may be altered or absent. Jugular venous distention may be present. Pulmonary rales are usually appreciated, but in isolated RV failure or early tamponade they may be absent. A precordial heave resulting from left ventricular dyskinesis or an RV heave from right ventricular volume overload secondary to a ventricular septal rupture may be palpable. The heart sounds may be distant, and a third or fourth heart sound is sometimes present. A new pansystolic murmur may be heard with or without a palpable thrill if acute mitral regurgitation or ventricular septal rupture is present.

Electrocardiography can be helpful in the initial evaluation of the etiology of cardiogenic shock. Patients with pump failure as the cause for cardiogenic shock are more likely to have extensive electrocardiographic changes supporting an anterior wall infarction or multivessel infarction or ischemia. An inferior-posterior infarct is more frequently noted in patients with acute severe mitral regurgitation and papillary muscle rupture/dysfunction. Low-voltage QRS complexes with electrical alternans supports possible tamponade, whereas

RV infarct is suspected when there are significant (>1 mm) ST-segment elevations in the RV precordial leads.

Echocardiography

Echocardiography is the most rapid and specific examination in the investigation of the etiology of cardiogenic shock. Its ease of performance and universal availability mandate its early use. Both RV and LV functions are readily assessed by echocardiography, and pulmonary artery pressure can be estimated. In early free wall rupture, infarct thinning and pericardial effusion may be seen. When frank cardiac tamponade is present, the echocardiogram will demonstrate a moderate to large pericardial effusion with right atrial and/or right ventricular diastolic collapse and respiratory variation in the mitral inflow velocities. Pseudoaneurysms, as is seen in cases of contained free wall rupture, may be distinguished from true aneurysms by echocardiography as well.

When mechanical complications of myocardial infarction are suspected, transesophageal echocardiography (TEE) is invaluable. Mitral valvular abnormalities and acute mitral regurgitation are readily distinguished from ventricular septal rupture by TEE. Papillary muscle rupture, chordal tear, or a flail mitral leaflet can be diagnosed by TEE. Echocardiographic analysis of a patient with ventricular septal defect may demonstrate color flow across the ventricular septum. This is usually noted in the setting of septal wall thinning and akinesis.

Cardiac Catheterization

Cardiac catheterization is important for invasive hemodynamic monitoring, to diagnose and treat coronary artery disease, and to exclude or quantify mechanical complications.

Right heart catheterization (RHC) provides objective hemodynamic data that can help to support or discount the diagnosis of cardiogenic shock. The hemodynamic profile of cardiogenic shock from LV pump failure includes a pulmonary capillary occlusion pressure greater than 15 mm Hg and a cardiac index less than $2.2 \, L \, min^{-1} \, m^{-2}$ in the setting of hypotension or decreased tissue perfusion. When ventricular septal rupture is being considered, oxygen saturations should be measured in the RA and the RV to detect a "step-up" in oxygen saturation and to quantify a left-to-right shunt. A large "V" wave on the pulmonary capillary wedge (PCW) tracings can support the diagnosis of severe mitral regurgitation, although it is neither a specific nor sensitive finding. The hemodynamic profile of right ventricular infarction includes high right-sided filling pressures in the presence of normal or low pulmonary wedge pressures. Kussmaul's sign, which is an elevation of RA pressure during inspiration, may be identified. Cardiac tamponade is characterized by pulsus paradoxus, which is a fall in arterial pressure greater than 15 mm Hg on inspiration. Elevation and equalization of diastolic filling pressures and a steep X and absent Y descent on RA pressure tracings may also be seen.

Left heart catheterization is used to assess the presence and degree of coronary artery disease and to determine the feasibility of PCI or coronary bypass surgery. In the SHOCK Trial [17], left main stenosis was present in 21% of patients, three-vessel disease in 65% of patients, and two-vessel disease in approximately 23%. It is important to note that the extent of ventricular dysfunction and hemodynamic instability should correlate with the extent and severity of coronary artery disease. When the amount of coronary disease does not support a large ischemic/infarct burden, then LV shock is unlikely unless there is a preexisting cardiomyopathy or a mechanical complication [16].

In patients with cardiogenic shock, left ventriculography assesses the left ventricular ejection fraction and defines wall motion abnormalities. Ventriculography will also identify patients with mechanical complications such as mitral regurgitation and ventricular septal rupture.

Therapeutic Options (Figure 13.4)

The initial approach to the patient with cardiogenic shock is stabilization. It is critical to maintain adequate oxygenation, and mechanical ventilation is often required. Supplemental oxygen in nonintubated patients should be administered to maintain an arterial oxygen saturation of greater than 90%. Correction of acidosis and other metabolic abnormalities is important to reduce arrhythmias and optimize the effect of pharmacological therapies. Relief of pain and anxiety is important to reduce excessive sympathetic activity and decrease oxygen demand. This may be accomplished with morphine sulfate, anxiolytics, or fentanyl. Beta-blockers, angiotensin-converting enzyme inhibitors, and nitrates should be avoided in the patient with cardiogenic shock and preshock because exacerbation of hypotension is likely to occur [18, 19]. In patients with RV infarct and hypotension, fluid resuscitation should be initiated. If hypotension does not readily respond to initial fluids, inotropic support should be started.

As with all patients presenting with acute infarction, antiplatelet therapy should be given. Aspirin should be administered with an initial dose of 162 to 325 mg and continued daily. Clopidogrel should be started unless early coronary bypass surgery is a high probability. Treatment with glycoprotein IIb/IIIa inhibitors should be initiated if thrombolytics are not given, especially if PCI is anticipated. Antithrombin therapy with weight-adjusted unfractionated heparin is a class I indication in cardiogenic shock [20].

In patients with adequate intravascular volume but with persistent hypotension and hypoperfusion, inotropic and vasopressor therapy should be promptly initiated. Dobutamine acts on β_1-adrenergic receptors to increase cardiac contractility. It may exacerbate hypotension in some patients and should not be used as a sole agent when SBP is <80 mm Hg unless blood pressure can be sup-

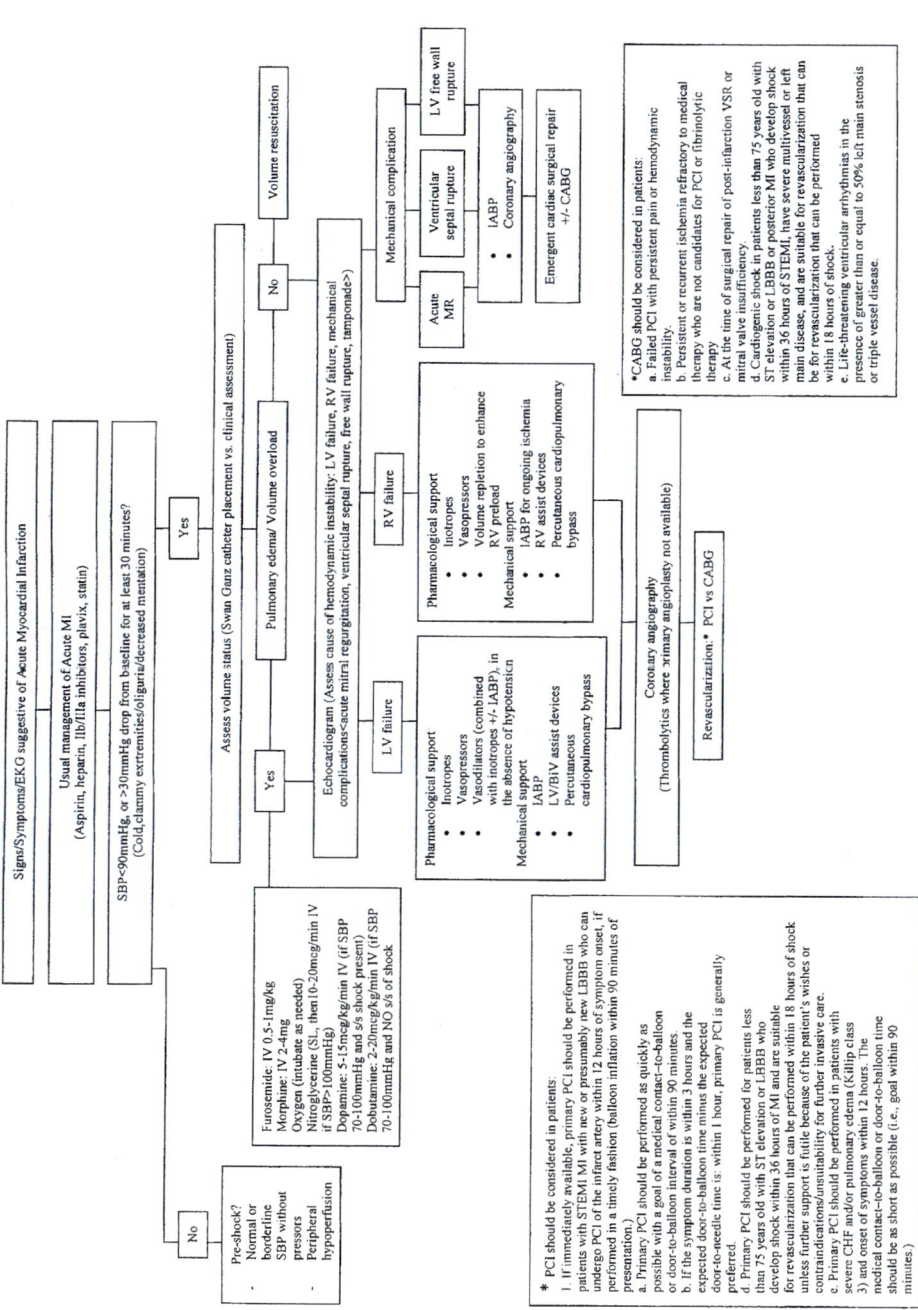

FIGURE 13.4. Algorithm for evaluation and management of patients in cardiogenic shock.

ported with intraaortic balloon pump (IABP) counterpulsation. Vasopressors such as dopamine are indicated when systolic blood pressure (SBP) is <80 mm Hg. Dopamine acts as both an inotropic agent via its action on β_1-adrenergic receptors and also as a vasoconstrictor by its release of norepinephrine. Combination therapy with both dopamine and dobutamine may be effective in some patients. In patients with profound hypotension, other vasopressor agents such as norepinephrine or epinephrine may be used, but tachycardia and increased peripheral resistance may increase myocardial oxygen consumption and worsen ischemia.

Phosphodiesterase inhibitors such as milrinone or amrinone may improve cardiac contractility without tachyarrhythmias, but vasodilation can worsen hypotension therefore limiting their usefulness. Likewise, nitroglycerin is an effective venodilator that reduces preload and pulmonary congestion and is a potent coronary artery vasodilator; however, the use of this agent is contraindicated in cardiogenic shock unless blood pressure is supported.

The combination of pharmacological therapy with mechanical support devices is an effective approach to the initial stabilization of cardiogenic shock. IABP is the most readily available device. These catheters are placed percutaneously in the descending aorta just distal to the aortic arch. The balloon catheter inflates in diastole thereby improving diastolic blood flow to the coronary arteries and cerebral circulation. The balloon deflates in systole, resulting in decreased peripheral resistance. Through this design, intraaortic balloon counterpulsation reduces afterload, increases coronary and cerebral perfusion, and decreases cardiac work. It is an important adjunct to definitive revascularization therapy. In the SHOCK registry, in-hospital mortality was lower among those patients in whom IABP therapy was initiated than among those in whom IABP therapy was not used [21].

In selected patients, LV or biventricular assist devices can be used as a bridge to revascularization, transplantation, or recovery. Small studies [22–24] of LV assist devices (LVAD) support in the setting of cardiogenic shock after acute myocardial infarction have reported favorable mortality rates of 24% to 44% with this approach, although the definitive role of such devices is still to be determined. In select patients with irreversible cardiogenic shock in spite of aggressive treatment with revascularization, mechanical assistance and pharmacological therapy, the use of artificial hearts [25] and emergent transplantation can be considered.

Reperfusion, Revascularization, and Repair

In patients with STEMI and cardiogenic shock due to LV failure, an early revascularization strategy with either PCI or coronary artery bypass grafting (CABG) has been shown to result in decreased mortality over time with the greatest benefit in patients less than 75 years of age. In the SHOCK study, early revascularization resulted in a 13% absolute decrease in mortality at 1 year [4]. According to the American College of Cardiology/American Heart Association

(ACC/AHA) guidelines, early revascularization with either PCI or CABG is recommended as a class I therapy for the treatment of an acute STEMI in patients less than 75 years old with cardiogenic shock, if performed within 36 hours of infarction and within 18 hours of the development of shock. Early revascularization should be considered on a case-by-case basis for patients aged 75 years and older who have good functional status [20]. For patients requiring transfer for angiography, IABP placement at the local hospital with the use of a fibrinolytic agent if the delay is expected to be greater than 2 hours [16] is a reasonable strategy. Fibrinolytic therapy may also be of value in patients who are unsuitable for an invasive strategy [20].

The mode of revascularization performed should be decided on a case-by-case basis and dictated by coronary anatomy as well as clinical variables. In a post hoc analysis of the SHOCK trial data, there was no difference in survival at 30 days or at 1 year in the PCI versus CABG groups [26]. Therefore, CABG should be considered for extensive coronary disease and left main disease if it can be performed by an experienced team in a timely manner.

In patients with a mechanical basis for cardiogenic shock after acute MI, emergent referral for cardiac surgery may be lifesaving. In a small cohort of patients in the SHOCK study who had free wall rupture, survival with surgery or pericardiocentesis was 39.3%, which was similar to other shock patients [27]. Similarly, patients with cardiogenic shock and ventricular septal rupture had increased survival with surgery [28].

Prognosis

In-hospital mortality rates remain about 50% in patients with cardiogenic shock complicating acute infarction, even with emergency revascularization [21]. The prognosis of patients with shock is influenced by the time to onset of shock and by the presence of mechanical complications. Patients with early shock (<24 hours) had a slightly higher mortality compared to patients with late shock (>24 hours) [14], and patients with LV shock have a lower in-hospital mortality than patients with mechanical complications [29]. It is still a devastating complication of acute myocardial infarction in spite of primary intervention. Further research may focus on the role of mechanical assist devices to support circulation and the use of metabolic therapies to limit injury in patients at high risk.

References

1. Goldberg RJ, Samad NA, Yarzebski J, et al. Temporal trends in cardiogenic shock complicating acute myocardial infarction. N Engl J Med 1999;340(15):1162–1168.
2. Hands ME, Rutherford JD, Muller JE, et al. The in-hospital development of cardiogenic shock after myocardial infarction: incidence, predictors of occurrence, outcome and prognostic factors. The MILIS Study Group. J Am Coll Cardiol 1989; 14(1):40–46; discussion 47–48.

3. Forrester JS, Diamond G, Chatterjee K, et al. Medical therapy of acute myocardial infarction by application of hemodynamic subsets (first of two parts). N Engl J Med 1976;295(24):1356–1362.

4. Hochman JS, Sleeper LA, Webb JG, et al. Early revascularization in acute myocardial infarction complicated by cardiogenic shock. SHOCK Investigators. Should We Emergently Revascularize Occluded Coronaries for Cardiogenic Shock. N Engl J Med 1999;341(9):625–634.

5. Menon V, Slater JN, White HD, et al. Acute myocardial infarction complicated by systemic hypoperfusion without hypotension: report of the SHOCK trial registry. Am J Med 2000;108(5):374–380.

6. Holmes DR Jr, Bates ER, Kleiman NS, et al. Contemporary reperfusion therapy for cardiogenic shock: the GUSTO-I trial experience. The GUSTO-I Investigators. Global Utilization of Streptokinase and Tissue Plasminogen Activator for Occluded Coronary Arteries. J Am Coll Cardiol 1995;26(3):668–674.

7. Hasdai D, Harrington RA, Hochman JS, et al. Platelet glycoprotein IIb/IIIa blockade and outcome of cardiogenic shock complicating acute coronary syndromes without persistent ST-segment elevation. J Am Coll Cardiol 2000;36(3):685–692.

8. Holmes DR Jr, Berger PB, Hochman JS, et al. Cardiogenic shock in patients with acute ischemic syndromes with and without ST-segment elevation. Circulation 1999;100(20):2067–2073.

9. Babaev A, Frederick PD, Pasta DJ, et al. Trends in management and outcomes of patients with acute myocardial infarction complicated by cardiogenic shock. JAMA 2005;294(4):448–454.

10. Hochman JS, Buller CE, Sleeper LA, et al. Cardiogenic shock complicating acute myocardial infarction–etiologies, management and outcome: a report from the SHOCK Trial Registry. SHould we emergently revascularize Occluded Coronaries for cardiogenic shocK? J Am Coll Cardiol 2000;36(3 Suppl A):1063–1070.

11. Leor J, Goldbourt U, Reicher-Reiss H, et al. Cardiogenic shock complicating acute myocardial infarction in patients without heart failure on admission: incidence, risk factors, and outcome. SPRINT Study Group. Am J Med 1993;94(3):265–273.

12. Alonso DR, Scheidt S, Post M, et al. Pathophysiology of cardiogenic shock. Quantification of myocardial necrosis, clinical, pathologic and electrocardiographic correlations. Circulation 1973;48(3):588–596.

13. Page DL, Caulfield JB, Kastor JA, et al. Myocardial changes associated with cardiogenic shock. N Engl J Med 1971;285(3):133–137.

14. Webb JG, Sleeper LA, Buller CE, et al. Implications of the timing of onset of cardiogenic shock after acute myocardial infarction: a report from the SHOCK Trial Registry. SHould we emergently revascularize Occluded Coronaries for cardiogenic shocK? J Am Coll Cardiol 2000;36(3 Suppl A):1084–1090.

15. Hochman J, Palazzo A, Holmes DR. Cardiogenic shock complicating acute myocardial infarction. In: Braunwald E, Califf RM, eds. Atlas of heart disease acute myocardial infarction and other acute ischemic syndromes. 2nd ed. Philadelphia: Current Medicine; 2001: pp. 149–178.

16. Menon V, Hochman JS. Management of cardiogenic shock complicating acute myocardial infarction. Heart 2002;88(5):531–537.

17. Sanborn TA, Sleeper LA, Webb JG, et al. Correlates of one-year survival in patients with cardiogenic shock complicating acute myocardial infarction: angiographic findings from the SHOCK trial. J Am Coll Cardiol 2003;42(8):1373–1379.

18. Gunnar RM, Bourdillon PD, Dixon DW, et al. ACC/AHA guidelines for the early management of patients with acute myocardial infarction. A report of the American College of Cardiology/American Heart Association Task Force on Assessment of Diagnostic and Therapeutic Cardiovascular Procedures (subcommittee to develop guidelines for the early management of patients with acute myocardial infarction). Circulation 1990;82(2):664–707.
19. Pfisterer M, Cox JL, Granger CB, et al. Atenolol use and clinical outcomes after thrombolysis for acute myocardial infarction: the GUSTO-I experience. Global Utilization of Streptokinase and TPA (alteplase) for Occluded Coronary Arteries. J Am Coll Cardiol 1998;32(3):634–640.
20. Antman EM, Anbe DT, Armstrong PW, et al. ACC/AHA guidelines for the management of patients with ST-elevation myocardial infarction: Executive summary; a report of the American College of Cardiology/American Heart Association Task Force on Practice Guidelines (Committee to Revise the 1999 Guidelines for the Management of Patients with Acute Myocardial Infarction). Circulation 2004;110(9): 588–636.
21. Sanborn TA, Sleeper LA, Bates ER, et al. Impact of thrombolysis, intra-aortic balloon pump counterpulsation, and their combination in cardiogenic shock complicating acute myocardial infarction: a report from the SHOCK Trial Registry. SHould we emergently revascularize Occluded Coronaries for cardiogenic shocK? J Am Coll Cardiol 2000;36(3 Suppl A):1123–1129.
22. Chen JM, DeRose JJ, Slater JP, et al. Improved survival rates support left ventricular assist device implantation early after myocardial infarction. J Am Coll Cardiol 1999; 33(7):1903–1908.
23. Leshnower BG, Gleason TG, O'Hara ML, et al. Safety and efficacy of left ventricular assist device support in postmyocardial infarction cardiogenic shock. Ann Thorac Surg 2006;81(4):1365–1370; discussion 1370–1361.
24. Park SJ, Nguyen DQ, Bank AJ, et al. Left ventricular assist device bridge therapy for acute myocardial infarction. Ann Thorac Surg 2000;69(4):1146–1151.
25. Arusoglu L, Reiss N, Morshuis M, et al. [Implantation of CardioWest total artificial heart in irreversible acute myocardial infarction shock-new hope for patients with infaust prognosis.] Z Kardiol 2003;92(11):916–924.
26. White HD, Assmann SF, Sanborn TA, et al. Comparison of percutaneous coronary intervention and coronary artery bypass grafting after acute myocardial infarction complicated by cardiogenic shock: results from the Should We Emergently Revascularize Occluded Coronaries for Cardiogenic Shock (SHOCK) trial. Circulation 2005;112(13):1992–2001.
27. Slater J, Brown RJ, Antonelli TA, et al. Cardiogenic shock due to cardiac free-wall rupture or tamponade after acute myocardial infarction: a report from the SHOCK Trial Registry. Should we emergently revascularize occluded coronaries for cardiogenic shock? J Am Coll Cardiol 2000;36(3 Suppl A):1117–1122.
28. Menon V, Webb JG, Hillis LD, et al. Outcome and profile of ventricular septal rupture with cardiogenic shock after myocardial infarction: a report from the SHOCK Trial Registry. SHould we emergently revascularize Occluded Coronaries in cardiogenic shocK? J Am Coll Cardiol 2000;36(3 Suppl A):1110–1116.
29. Wong SC, Sanborn T, Sleeper LA, et al. Angiographic findings and clinical correlates in patients with cardiogenic shock complicating acute myocardial infarction: a report from the SHOCK Trial Registry. SHould we emergently revascularize Occluded Coronaries for cardiogenic shocK? J Am Coll Cardiol 2000;36(3 Suppl A):1077–1083.

14
Management of Pericardial Disease Complicating Acute Coronary Syndrome

Seth Uretsky, Dan L. Musat, Mark V. Sherrid, and Eyal Herzog

Anatomy and Physiology of the Pericardium

Anatomy

The pericardium is a sac containing the heart and proximal parts of the great vessels [1, 2]. It consists of two layers:

- The *visceral* pericardium is a single-layer serous membrane that reflects back near the origins/insertions of the great vessels and becomes continuous with and forming the inner layer of the parietal pericardium.
- The *parietal* pericardium is an acellular tough, fibrous coat composed mainly of collagen and elastin fibers, about 2 mm thick, and surrounds most of the heart.

The space between the two serous layers is named *pericardial space* and normally contains up to about 50 mL of plasma ultrafiltrate. The left atrium is largely an extrapericardial chamber, explaining why the effusions generally are not seen behind this structure [2, 3]. The parietal pericardium is anchored by ligamentous attachments to the diaphragm inferiorly and to the sternum anteriorly. These ligamentous attachments ensure that the heart occupies a relatively fixed central position within the thoracic cavity regardless of phase of respiration and body position. Pericardium receives its arterial supply from branches of internal thoracic and musculophrenic arteries as well as directly from descending aorta. The veins are tributaries of the azygos system [2]. Pericardium is innervated by branches from vagus, phrenic nerves, and the sympathetic trunks [2]. Of importance is the fact that phrenic nerves descend on the lateral sides, between the fibrous pericardium and mediastinal pleura.

Physiology

The normal pericardium serves four primary functions [2]: fixing the heart within the mediastinum; limiting cardiac distension during sudden increases in intracardiac volume; limiting the spread of infection from the adjacent lungs; and providing lubrication in between the two layers.

Pericardial Disease Complicating Acute Coronary Syndrome

Pericardial Chest Pain: Differential Diagnosis

Chest pain can arise from cardiovascular structures (heart, pericardium, aorta) or noncardiovascular structures (skin, chest wall, intrathoracic structures, or subdiaphragmatic organs). It is often difficult to accurately determine the source of chest pain in distressed patient as all structures are supplied by sensory fibers from the same spinal segments and may cause similar pain syndromes [4].

It is crucial to differentiate pericarditis from myocardial infarction as outlined in Table 14.1. This can be very challenging, but there are some clinical

TABLE **14.1.** Differentiation of acute pericarditis from acute ischemia.

	Acute pericarditis	Acute ischemia
Characteristics of pain		
Onset	More often sudden	Usually gradual, crescendo
Main location	Substernal or left precordial	Same as pericarditis or confined to zones of radiation
Radiation	Most common to the back or same as ischemic	Shoulders, arms, neck, jaw
Quality	Sharp, stabbing	Heavy pressure or burning
Duration	Persistent; may wax and wane	Intermittent; <30 minutes each recurrence, longer for unstable angina
Inspiration	Worse	No effect unless associated with peri-infarction pericarditis
Body movements	Increased	No effect
Posture	Worse on recumbency; improved on sitting, leaning forward	No change upon sitting
Nitrates	No effect	Usually relief
Physical examination		
Friction rub	Most cases	Only if with infarction pericarditis
S1	Intact	Often dull, not distinct, after first day
S4	Absent unless preexisting	Nearly always present
Pulmonary congestion	Absent	May be present
Murmurs	Absent unless preexisting	May be present
ECG findings		
J point–ST segments	Diffuse elevation; saddle-shaped or concave, without reciprocal depressions; except aVR and V_1	Localized deviation; convex (dome-shaped), with reciprocal changes in typical distribution
PR segment depressions	Frequent, with PR elevation in aVR	Rare
T waves	Inverted after ST-segment return to baseline	Hyperacute or inverted while the ST still elevated
Arrhythmias/conduction abnormalities	None	Frequent

Source: Adapted from Spodick DH. Acute pericarditis: current concepts and practices. JAMA 2003;289:1150–1153.

hints that can lead the physician to one diagnosis or the other. An algorithm for patients with acute coronary syndrome (ACS) who present to the emergency department with suspicion of pericardial involvement is seen in Figure 14.1. Acute viral pericarditis is often preceded by a viral syndrome with upper respiratory infection symptoms, malaise, and fever in the days/week before pain started.

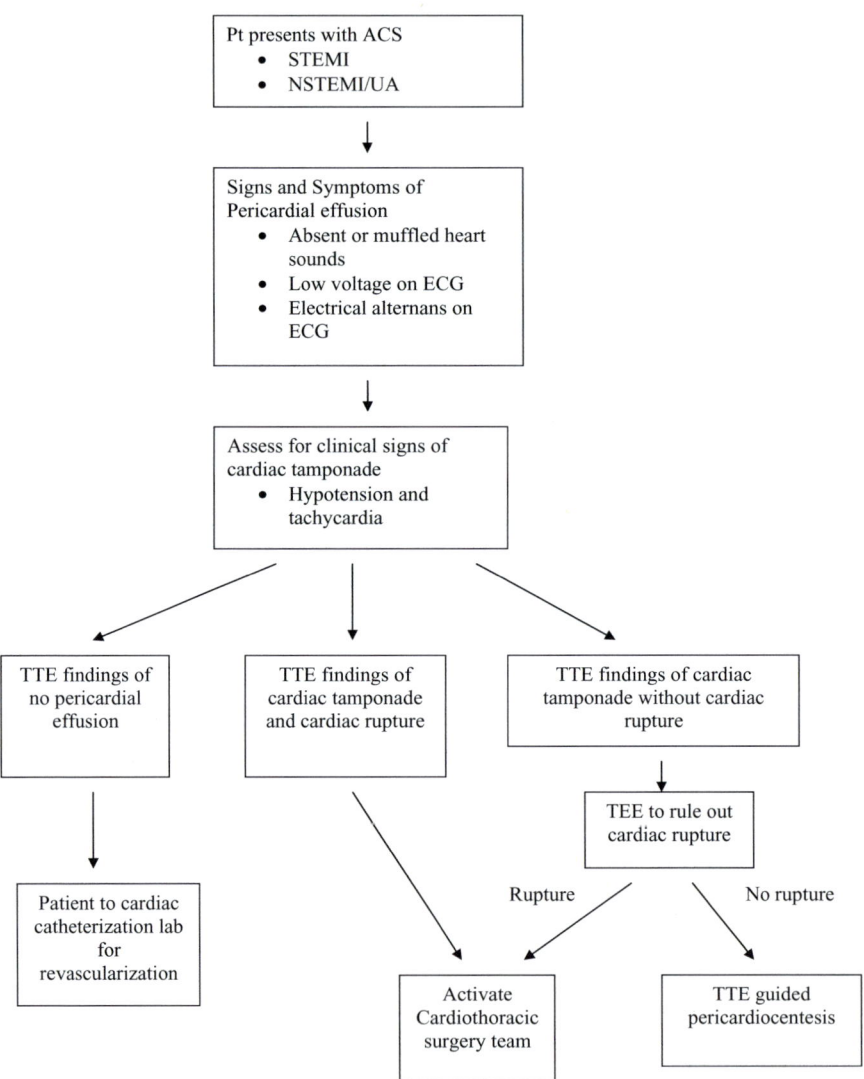

FIGURE 14.1. Algorithm for patients with ACS presenting to the emergency department with suspicion of pericardial involvement.

Pericarditis pain can be characterized as [4]:

- Sharp, precordial, and knife-like
- Pleuritic, worse on inspiration
- Radiating to the shoulders, upper back, and neck
- Increased when lying down
- Relieved by sitting up or leaning forward

On physical examination, the presence of a friction rub may be suggestive of acute pericarditis but cannot exclude an acute myocardial infarction (AMI) as a series showed that 8% to 23% of patients admitted with AMI had a rub due to AMI-associated pericarditis [5, 6].

Electrocardiogram (ECG) features of pericarditis include [7] diffuse concave ST elevations and PR segment depression.

Echocardiography is an important tool in differentiating pericardial disease from AMI and can dramatically change decisions for further treatment. Echocardiographic findings that suggest pericarditis are pericardial effusion. If segmental wall motion abnormalities are seen on echocardiography, myocardial ischemia should be suspected.

Serologic markers of myocardial damage are usually negative in acute pericarditis and are not helpful in diagnosis.

Pericardial Involvement in AMI

Pericardial involvement in AMI is usually secondary to inflammation. Very rarely, constrictive pericarditis had been reported as a cause for myocardial ischemia, angina, and AMI [8]. In patients presenting with AMI, there can be three major types of pericardial complications: (1) early infarct-associated pericarditis (often termed *infarction pericarditis*); (2) pericardial effusion due to free wall rupture (with or without tamponade); and (3) post–myocardial infarction (Dressler's syndrome).

Infarction Pericarditis

The incidence of infarction pericarditis is decreasing in recent years with the use of thrombolytics and percutaneous coronary intervention in the treatment of AMI [6, 9–11]. Pericardial pain and pericardial friction rub define early postinfarction pericarditis and usually develop on day 2 or 3 after a transmural AMI [12] and are usually short lived, lasting only few days [13]. Clinical features that predispose to early infarction pericarditis include [5, 6, 9–11, 14] male sex, smoking, transmural myocardial infarction, anterior wall involvement, large infarcts, delayed presentation to the hospital, low ejection fraction, and congestive heart failure.

On short- and long-term follow-up, these findings did not translate into a significant increased mortality in this subset of patients [5, 6, 13]. In some studies, a trend was noticed for both in-hospital and 1-year mortality, but infarction pericarditis was not found to be an independent prognostic factor [9–11, 15]. This finding made some authors to conclude that clinical course is benign and the prognosis of the patient is not altered by development of this complication [12]. The preferred form of therapy for early postinfarction pericarditis is aspirin [16]. Corticosteroids and nonsteroidal anti-inflammatory drugs (NSAIDs) should be carefully considered because of the reported complications caused by these agents [12, 13].

It is usually not necessary to stop anticoagulation therapy in patients who develop infarction pericarditis. Wall et al. showed that cardiac tamponade did not occur clinically in any of 40 patients who developed pericarditis among 810 patients admitted for AMI [9]. However, the 2004 guidelines of the American College of Cardiology (ACC) and the American Heart Association (AHA) recommended that anticoagulation should be immediately discontinued if a pericardial effusion develops or increases [16]. On the other hand, Gregoratos states that a stable small pericardial effusion is not an absolute contraindication for anticoagulation [12].

Pericardial Effusion Due to Free Wall Rupture

Free wall rupture (FWR) is a mechanical complication of ST-elevation myocardial infarction (STEMI) and is most often fatal. The rupture often occurs in the watershed zone between infarcted and noninfarcted tissue and is thought to be mediated by inflammatory factors. The incidence of FWR has decreased with the use of thrombolytics and percutaneous coronary intervention. However, the delayed use of thrombolytics has been implicated in an increased incidence of FWR [17]:

- FWR is the second most common cause of in-hospital mortality after left ventricular failure in AMI.
- Overall incidence of cardiac rupture ranges from 0.8% to 6.2%.
- It accounts for 15% to 30% of fatalities from AMI.

FWR tends to occur 3 to 5 days after AMI at the anterior or lateral wall of the left ventricle at the midpapillary level. Clinical features that predispose to FWR include [17, 18]: increased age, female gender, lower body weight, peri-infarct hypertension, and infarct expansion.

FWR should be suspected in patients with shock or severe chest pain suggestive of infarct expansion. The most common clinical features of acute FWR are asystole, pulseless electrical activity, and severe chest pain.

Approximately one third of patients with FWR present with the subacute form. Clinical signs of cardiac tamponade can be appreciated prior to hemodynamic collapse. The most common features of subacute FWR are [19, 20] recurrent chest pain, syncope, hypotension, shock, nausea, arrhythmia, restlessness, transient bradycardia, and transient pulseless electrical activity.

Diagnosis of FWR

Echocardiography is considered the diagnostic tool of choice for FWR [21, 22]. Transthoracic echocardiography (TTE) can readily identify pericardial effusion and intrapericardial clot secondary to FWR. TTE is useful in determining the site of rupture and the flow of blood into the pericardial space. Transesophageal echocardiography can be used if the TTE images are not satisfactory.

Treatment

Medical Therapy. Medical therapy should only be used to stabilize the patient prior to mechanical repair of the FWR [23]. Intravenous delivery of fluids and inotropes can help stabilize the patient prior to repair. All anticoagulants should be stopped.

Percutaneous Therapy. Pericardiocentesis can be used as a temporizing measure to relieve cardiac tamponade [24], although this is not the definitive therapy.

Mechanical Closure. Survival without mechanical closure of FWR is rare. There are several techniques that can be used to repair the rupture including [25] infarcterectomy and prosthetic patch; and use of Dacron, Teflon, pericardial patch without infarcterectomy.

Thrombolytics and FWR

Hemopericardium after use of thrombolytics necessitates prompt echocardiographic evaluation for cardiac rupture. However, not all cases of hemopericardium associated with the use of thrombolytic therapy are secondary to cardiac rupture. Renkin et al. reported 4 of 392 patients, who developed hemopericardium within 24 hours of thrombolytic therapy without cardiac rupture [26].

Cardiac Tamponade

Pathophysiology

The pericardial sac is a nondistensible sac; therefore, acute accumulations of even small amounts of fluid in the pericardial sac can result in high pressures in the intrapericardial space. This increase in intrapericardial pressure impinges on the cardiac chambers, impairing their ability to fill during diastole, thus affecting cardiac output [27]. We have developed a flowchart presenting the hemodynamic changes present in cardiac tamponade as seen in Figure 14.2.

Signs and Symptoms

The following changes are the physiologic basis for the hallmark clinical signs and symptoms of cardiac tamponade: tachycardia; and hypotension.

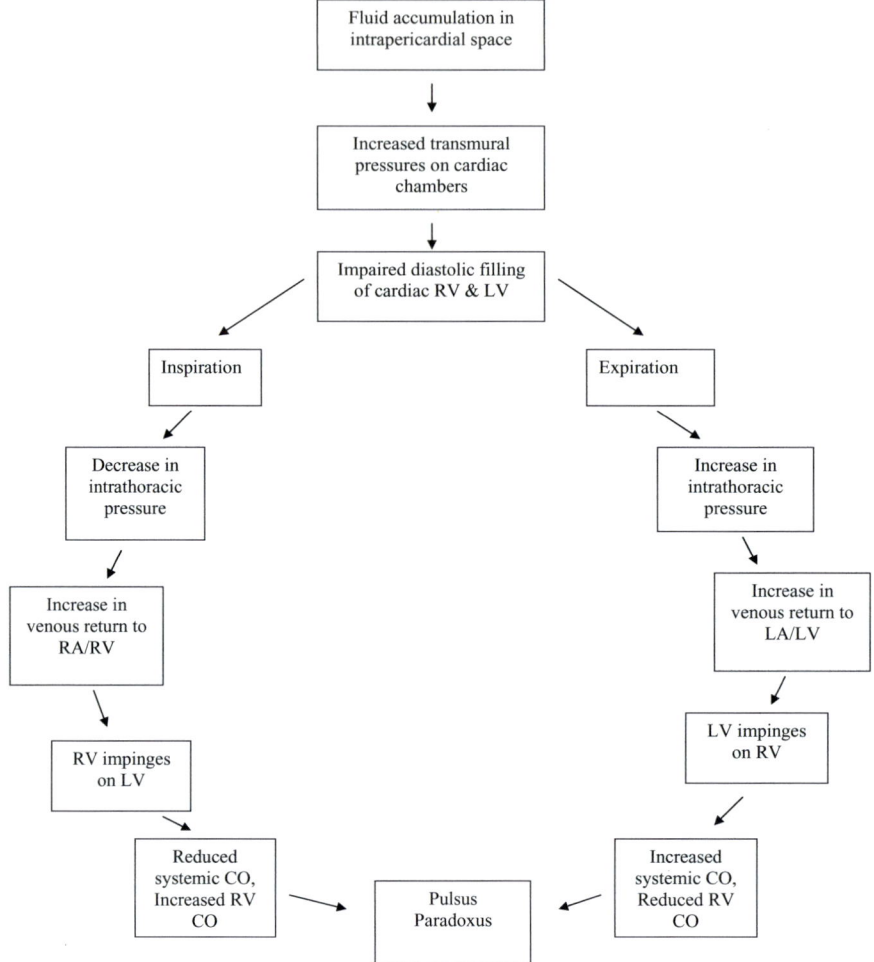

FIGURE 14.2. Hemodynamic changes present in cardiac tamponade.

If the patient has large pericardial effusion, further signs of tamponade may be seen: muffled or absent heart sounds; low voltage and/or electrical alternans on ECG; rounded flask-like cardiac silhouette on chest x-ray film.

The gold standard for evaluating and assessing hemodynamic derangements due to cardiac tamponade is echocardiography. Echocardiography allows accurate quantification of effusion size. Two-dimensional echocardiographic signs used to assess for the substrate of tamponade include [27] exaggerated diastolic collapse RA and diastolic RV collapse.

Doppler signs used to assess for the substrate of tamponade include [27] exaggerated changes in mitral and tricuspid valve inflow during inspiration and expiration, and loss of forward flow from the inferior vena cava during diastole.

Treatment

Cardiac tamponade occurring in the context of STEMI must be considered FWR and is usually an indication for immediate surgery. Treatment of cardiac tamponade is removal of the pericardial effusion, which will immediately reverse the hemodynamic derangements. In the emergent setting, pericardiocentesis is the procedure of choice. Using echocardiography to guide the pericardiocentesis decreases the morbidity and mortality associated with this procedure. If echocardiography is not available, then a subxiphoid approach is preferred.

Post–Myocardial Infarction Syndrome

The post–myocardial infarction syndrome (Dressler's syndrome) is a late complication, mainly of transmural myocardial infarction, which develops typically during the second or third week after AMI but may be seen as early as 24 hours and as late as several months after the MI [12, 28, 29]. The incidence of Dressler's syndrome dropped from 1% to 5% in the prethrombolytic/early intervention era to almost zero, with only few case reports now. It is hypothesized that smaller infarct size and shortened time of exposure of the myocardial antigens with early revascularization contribute to these findings [28–31]. Another factor that may contribute to low incidence now is the widespread use of aspirin and adjunctive therapies, angiotensin-converting enzyme (ACE) inhibitors, statins, and beta-blockers that have immunomodulatory properties [29].

It is thought that immunologic factors play an important role in pathogenesis of Dressler's syndrome. Myocardial injury may release cardiac antigens that stimulate antibody formation. The immune complexes then are deposited onto the pericardium, pleura, and lungs, eliciting an inflammatory response [29]. An alternative hypothesis for this syndrome includes the release of blood in the pericardial space due to a prolonged and exaggerated early postinfarction pericarditis [12, 29].

Clinically, post–myocardial infarction syndrome is manifested by fever, leukocytosis, malaise, chest pain, presence of a pericardial and possibly pleuropericardial friction rub, sometimes pericardial effusion (occasionally large and rarely cardiac tamponade and may require pericardiocentesis), and pulmonary infiltrates [12].

Symptoms of Dressler's syndrome generally resolve after the administration of aspirin, NSAIDs, or corticosteroids. Anecdotally, it has been reported that colchicine may be helpful in this scenario [32]. This complication of myocardial infarction does not seem to have negative prognostic implications.

References

1. Gabella G. The pericardium. In: Gray H, Williams PL, Bannister LH, eds. Gray's anatomy: the anatomical basis of medicine and surgery. New York: Churchill-Livingstone; 1995:1471–1472.
2. Chiles CD, Stauffer GA. Pericardial disease: clinical features and treatment. In: Marschall SR, Magnus EO, eds. Netter's cardiology. 1st ed. Icon Learning Systems; 2004;334–345.
3. Hoit B, Faulx MD. Diseases of the pericardium. In: Fuster V, Alexander RW, eds. Hurst's the heart. 11th ed. New York: McGraw-Hill Professional; 2004:1977–1998.
4. Wilke A, Noll B, Maisch B. Angina pectoris in extracoronary diseases. Herz 1999; 24:132–139.
5. Dubois C, Smeets JP, Demoulin JC, et al. Frequency and clinical significance of pericardial friction rubs in the acute phase of myocardial infarction. Eur Heart J 1985;6:766–768.
6. Aydinalp A, Wishniak A, van den Akker-Berman L, et al. Pericarditis and pericardial effusion in acute ST-elevation myocardial infarction in the thrombolytic era. Isr Med Assoc J 2002;4:181–183.
7. Teh BS, Walsh J, Bell AJ, et al. Electrical current paths in acute pericarditis. J Electrocardiol 1993;26:291–300.
8. Topaz O, Nair R, Mackall JA. Observations of angina and myocardial infarction in constrictive pericarditis. Int J Cardiol 1993;39:121–129.
9. Wall TC, Califf RM, Harrelson-Woodlief L, et al. Usefulness of a pericardial friction rub after thrombolytic therapy during acute myocardial infarction in predicting amount of myocardial damage. The TAMI Study Group. Am J Cardiol 1990;66: 1418–1421.
10. Correale E, Maggioni AP, Romano S, et al. Comparison of frequency, diagnostic and prognostic significance of pericardial involvement in acute myocardial infarction treated with and without thrombolytics. Gruppo Italiano per lo Studio della Sopravvivenza nell'Infarto Miocardico (GISSI). Am J Cardiol 1993;71:1377–1381.
11. Tofler GH, Muller JE, Stone PH, et al. Pericarditis in acute myocardial infarction: characterization and clinical significance. Am Heart J 1989;117:86–92.
12. Gregoratos G. Pericardial involvement in acute myocardial infarction. Cardiol Clin 1990;8:601–608.
13. Toole JC, Silverman ME. Pericarditis of acute myocardial infarction. Chest 1975; 67:647–653.
14. Martinez Sande JL, Amaro Cendon A, Jacquet Herter M, et al. [Pericarditis in the acute phase of myocardial infarction: incidence and clinical significance.] Rev Port Cardiol 1992;11:733–737.
15. Correale E, Maggioni AP, Romano S, et al. Pericardial involvement in acute myocardial infarction in the post-thrombolytic era: clinical meaning and value. Clin Cardiol 1997;20:327–331.
16. Antman E, Anbe, DT, Armstrong, PW, et al. ACC/AHA guidelines for the management of patients with ST-elevation myocardial infarction—executive summary: a report of the American College of Cardiology/American Heart Association Task Force on Practice Guidelines (Writing Committee to Revise the 1999 Guidelines for the Management of Patients With Acute Myocardial Infarction). Circulation 2004; 110:e82–292.

17. Birnbaum Y, Chamoun AJ, Anzuini A, et al. Ventricular free wall rupture following acute myocardial infarction. Coron Artery Dis 2003;14:463–470.
18. Lopez-Sendon J, Gonzalez A, Lopez de Sa E, et al. Diagnosis of subacute ventricular wall rupture after acute myocardial infarction: sensitivity and specificity of clinical, hemodynamic and echocardiographic criteria. J Am Coll Cardiol 1992;19:1145–1153.
19. Figueras J, Curos A, Cortadellas J, et al. Reliability of electromechanical dissociation in the diagnosis of left ventricular free wall rupture in acute myocardial infarction. Am Heart J 1996;131:861–864.
20. Lavie CJ, Gersh BJ. Mechanical and electrical complications of acute myocardial infarction. Mayo Clin Proc 1990;65:709–730.
21. Lindower P, Embrey R, Vandenberg B. Echocardiographic diagnosis of mechanical complications in acute myocardial infarction. Clin Intensive Care 1993;4:276–283.
22. Buda AJ. The role of echocardiography in the evaluation of mechanical complications of acute myocardial infarction. Circulation 1991;84:I109–121.
23. Figueras J, Cortadellas J, Evangelista A, et al. Medical management of selected patients with left ventricular free wall rupture during acute myocardial infarction. J Am Coll Cardiol 1997;29:512–518.
24. Purcaro A, Costantini C, Ciampani N, et al. Diagnostic criteria and management of subacute ventricular free wall rupture complicating acute myocardial infarction. Am J Cardiol 1997;80:397–405.
25. Komiya T, Ishii O, Yamazaki K, et al. [Surgical treatment for subacute left ventricular free wall rupture complicating acute myocardial infarction—pericardial patch gluing method.] Nippon Kyobu Geka Gakkai Zasshi 1996;44:806–810.
26. Renkin J, de Bruyne B, Benit E, et al. Cardiac tamponade early after thrombolysis for acute myocardial infarction: a rare but not reported hemorrhagic complication. J Am Coll Cardiol 1991;17:280–285.
27. Feigenbaum H, Ryan T. Feigenbaum's echocardiography. Sixth ed. Philadelphia: Lippincott Williams & WIlkins; 2005.
28. Shahar A, Hod H, Barabash GM, et al. Disappearance of a syndrome: Dressler's syndrome in the era of thrombolysis. Cardiology 1994;85:255–258.
29. Bendjelid K, Pugin J. Is Dressler syndrome dead? Chest 2004;126:1680–1682.
30. Reinecke H, Wichter T, Weyand M. Left ventricular pseudoaneurysm in a patient with Dressler's syndrome after myocardial infarction. Heart 1998;80:98–100.
31. Welin LVA, Wilhelmsson C. Characteristics, prevalence, and prognosis of postmyocardial infarction syndrome. Br Heart J 1983;50:140–145.
32. Madsen SM, Jacobsen TJ. Colchicine treatment of recurrent steroid-dependent pericarditis in a patient with post-myocardial-infarction syndrome (Dressler's syndrome). Ugeskr Laeger 1992;154:3427–3428.

15
Surgical Intervention in Acute Coronary Syndrome

Sandhya K. Balaram and Daniel G. Swistel

Surgical management of patients with acute coronary syndrome (ACS) has advanced significantly over the past ten years. Much of the improvement in outcomes can be attributed to the of early coronary angiography followed by immediate percutaneous. Coronary angiography is used to assess anatomy, myocardium at risk, and previous damage. Percutaneous interventions, anticoagulants, and aortic counterpulsation restore flow to threatened myocardium for patients with ACS.

Cardiac muscle in ACS may be infarcted, stunned, or hibernating. Immediate evaluation of contractile dysfunction is determined by estimation of ejection fraction with a left ventriculogram. The use of intraoperative transesophageal echocardiography (TEE) gives further information into wall motion, valve function, and potentially recoverable myocardium. In the subacute period, methods to determine cardiac muscle viability includes radionuclide imaging, positron emission tomography, dobutamine stress echocardiography, stress-thallium studies, and magnetic resonance imaging [1].

Much of the initial patient stabilization is performed prior to the arrival of the surgical team. This includes administration of nitroglycerin, heparin, glycoprotein IIb/IIIa inhibitors, aspirin, and invasive monitoring prior to transfer to the cardiac catheterization laboratory.

There is often only a short period of time to determine the best treatment for the unstable cardiac patient. A survey of the patient's comorbidities must be performed rapidly and accurately. Preoperative risk assessment is important in helping make decisions regarding therapy. Table 15.1 includes most of the variables required to complete a risk assessment. There are multiple risk-stratification scores available to determine a patient's risk and facilitate optimal outcome [2–4]. In addition, elevated troponin levels are a tool that can be used as a powerful predictor of surgical outcome in ACS and correlate with increasing length of stay and in-hospital mortality [5].

TABLE 15.1. Preoperative risk assessment of patient with ACS.

1. Age
2. Ejection fraction
3. Sex
4. Emergency status
5. Hemodynamic instability
6. Concomitant valvular disease
7. Renal function
8. History of cerebrovascular accident
9. Peripheral vascular disease
10. Chronic obstructive pulmonary disease
11. Diabetes mellitus
12. Reoperative status

Surgical Revascularization in ACS

In a patient with ACS, immediate therapy is often focused on thrombolytics or percutaneous interventions (PCI). There have been no randomized trials comparing coronary artery bypass grafting (CABG) with PCI during acute myocardial infarction (AMI). Given the immediacy of angiography with time to reperfusion, PCI with stents is most often utilized in the acute setting. However, there is a definite role for CABG in certain specific settings that require urgent or emergent surgical revascularization. The current American College of Cardiology class I indications for CABG in the presence of ACS are well-defined [6].

CABG is recommended for patients with ACS non–ST-segment elevation myocardial infarction (NSTEMI) (Fig. 15.1) and

1. Left main lesions;
2. Left main equivalent (significant proximal LAD >70% and significant proximal circumflex >70%); and
3. PCI is not optimal or possible and patients have ongoing ischemia not responsive to maximal nonsurgical therapy.

CABG is recommended for patients with ACS ST-segment elevation myocardial infarction (STEMI) (Fig. 15.2) and:

1. Failed PCI with persistent pain or hemodynamic instability with suitable coronary anatomy;
2. Persistent, refractory ischemia not amenable to PCI;
3. Concurrent postinfarct ventricular septal defect or mitral valve insufficiency;
4. Mitral regurgitation;
5. Cardiogenic shock for patients <75 years old with ST-segment elevation or left bundle branch block (LBBB) or posterior AMI who develop shock within 36 hours of AMI and are suitable for revascularization; and
6. Life-threatening ventricular arrhythmias with >50% left main and/or three vessel disease.

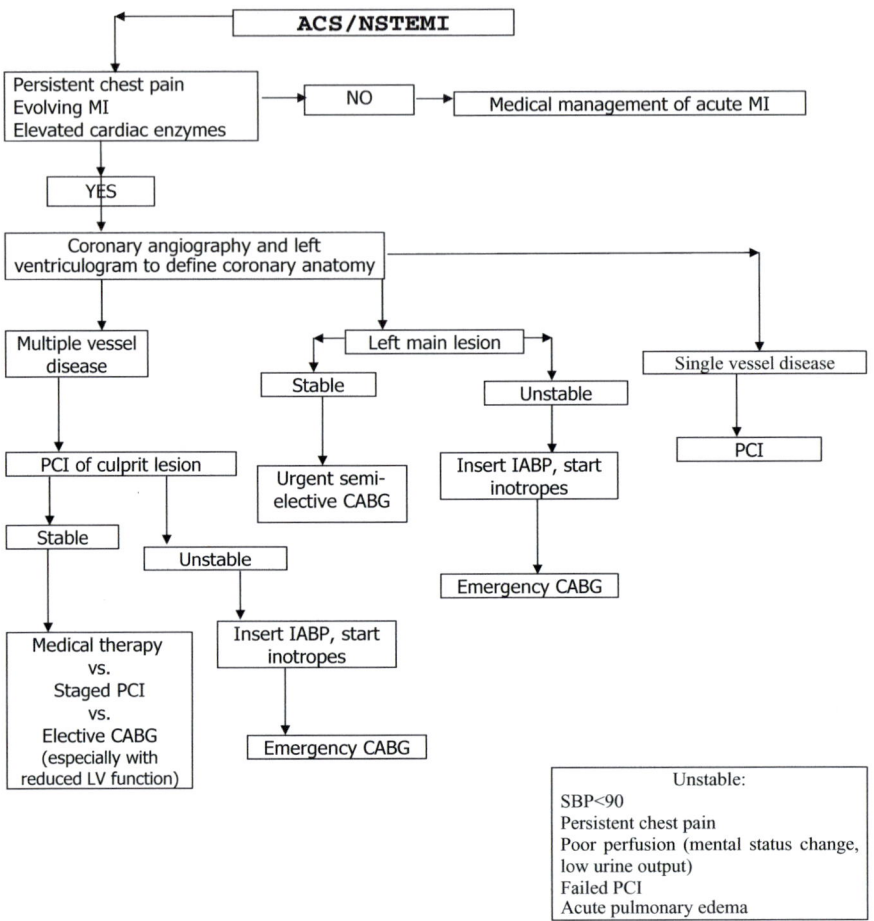

FIGURE 15.1. Algorithm 1: ACS-NSTEMI.

Timing is a critical and sometimes controversial aspect of surgical revascularization. On a cellular level, early reperfusion leads to less free-radical release and less interstitial edema, which may limit infarct size and prevent complications such as rupture or aneurysm formation. CABG provides complete revascularization in one setting. However, early surgical intervention also carries a risk of reperfusion injury, which may extend infarct size and increase scar development [7]. The main disadvantages of CABG include a high mortality with emergency surgery and a longer time to reperfusion when compared with PCI [8].

Data from the New York State Cardiac Surgery Registry show that after transmural AMI, patient mortality more than doubles from that of baseline when

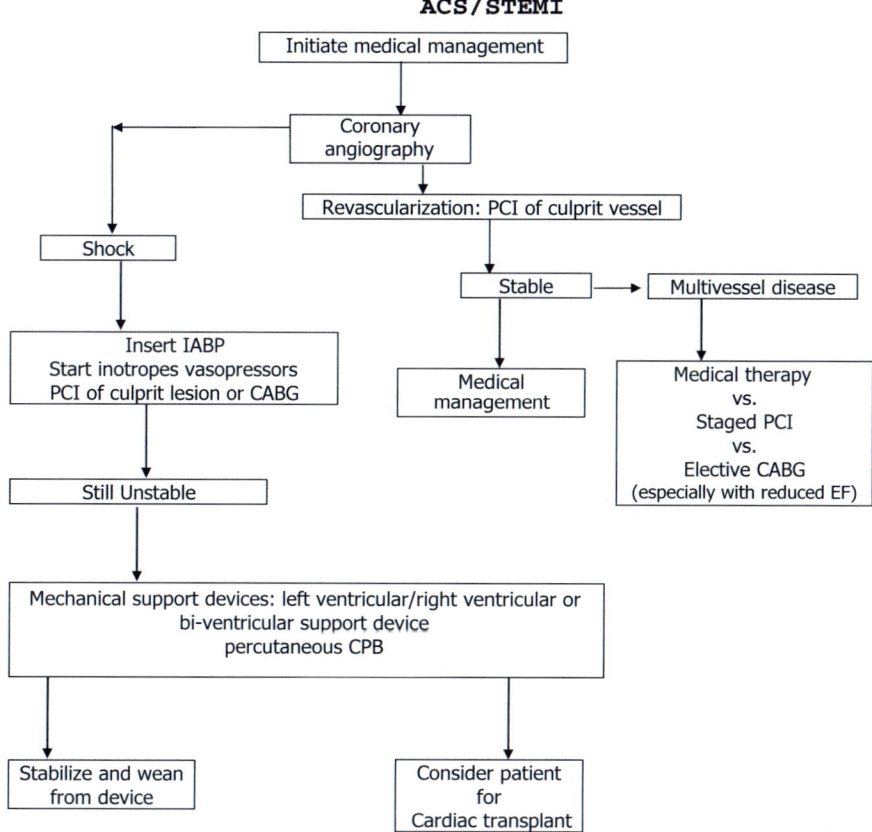

FIGURE **15.2.** Algorithm 2: ACS-STEMI.

surgery is performed within 3 days of the event [9]. Mortality for transmural AMI is 14% for those procedures performed within <24 hours and drops to 5% from 1 to 7 days and down to 3% in >7 days. Nontransmural AMI has a mortality of 13% when the timing of CABG was <6 hours, which dropped to 6% between 6 and 23 hours and 3% for those procedures performed after 7 days [9]. These data support stabilization of the patient if possible in the acute setting, with surgical intervention performed on a semiurgent or elective basis.

More recently, outcomes of patients with ACS were studied in-depth in a large European study. Evaluation of 10,484 patients who presented with ACS showed that 460 (4.5%) underwent CABG on initial hospitalization. Of these 460 patients, 15.2% had an associated PCI. Of the group with STEMI-ACS, surgical mortality was 3.4%. Those patients who underwent CABG who had NSTEMI-ACS had a mortality of 5.4%. The overall mortality was 3.7% among

TABLE 15.2. Indications for IABP.

1. Cardiogenic shock
2. Persistent ventricular arrhythmias
3. Refractory angina
4. Failed PCI
5. Bridge to assist device or transplant
6. Persistent angina after coronary intervention
7. Acute mitral regurgitation
8. Postoperative support
9. Acute ventricular septal defect
10. High-risk percutaneous intervention

those with CABG and 4.8% without surgical intervention [10]. At the present time, we can expect that hemodynamically stable patients that undergo surgical coronary revascularization for ACS will have acceptable immediate and long-term outcomes.

Cardiogenic Shock and Intraaortic Balloon Counterpulsation

The presence of cardiogenic shock significantly increases the morbidity and mortality of surgical intervention [11]. Adjunctive therapies used in the presence of shock include primary angioplasty, inotropes, vasopressors, glycoprotein IIb/IIIa inhibitors, and intraaortic balloon counterpulsation (IABP). The main goals for shock patients are to stabilize the patient using medical and percutaneous interventions, recover the immediately ischemic myocardium, and follow this with complete revascularization in the acute or subacute period [12].

The use of the IABP is critical for the patient with cardiogenic shock or persistent chest pain during coronary angiography. The placement of the balloon distal to the subclavian artery and its rapid collapse decreases impedance to aortic flow in the proximal aorta. The aortic valve opens to a 10% to 15% lower systolic pressure to decrease afterload, decrease myocardial work, and decrease oxygen consumption [13]. This decreases left ventricular end-diastolic pressure, increases cardiac output, decreases wall tension, and increases coronary blood flow. Table 15.2 outlines indications for placement of IABP.

Intraoperative Considerations

A number of techniques have evolved over the past 20 years that have improved outcomes for patients with ACS and both NSTEMI and STEMI. These include myocardial protection strategies, selection of conduits, the advent of off-pump surgery, and the use of ventricular assist devices.

Standard cardiac operations require a bloodless operative field and cardiac standstill. This is accomplished with a cross-clamp placed across the aorta to isolate the heart from the rest of the cardiopulmonary bypass circuit. The heart must be protected during this time from ischemic damage. The standard techniques of myocardial protection are hypothermia to decrease myocardial oxygen demand and myocardial preservation solution, called cardioplegia.

The basis of myocardial protection in CABG is to protect the ischemic myocardium during the time of cardiac arrest by decreasing myocardial consumption and providing oxygenated substrates to the tissue. The use of blood cardioplegia solutions is an important technical advance in limiting the amount of damage from decreased blood flow to the myocardium. After the myocardium shifts to anaerobic metabolism, reperfusion introduces oxygen free radicals, which can increase muscle damage and cellular edema. This is known as reperfusion injury. Blood cardioplegia provides oxygen recovery and helps replenish myocardial substrates. The advantages of blood cardioplegia lie in its ability to provide oxygenation during arrest, limit reperfusion injury, and provide endogenous factors such as oxygen radical scavengers and buffers to the ischemic myocardium [14].

Another important decision made by the surgeon is the choice of conduits for a particular patient. This decision is most often made with consideration of the patient's hemodynamic status. A hemodynamically unstable patient is less likely to tolerate the time required to dissect and prepare the left internal mammary artery for bypass. These patients often require immediate cardiopulmonary bypass for shock, and timing of revascularization in this setting is critical. However, in most clinical circumstances, the conduit choice is similar to that in a nonacute setting. Data show that the use of the internal mammary artery for hemodynamically stable patients does not increase morbidity even in emergency cases [15, 16]. Internal mammary arteries have been shown in multiple studies to improve long-term survival and have a decreased incidence of future intervention [17]. More recent articles suggest that bilateral internal mammary arteries can be used safely even in the acute setting [18].

Role of Off-Pump Surgery

An additional option to protect threatened myocardium is to avoid both cardiopulmonary bypass and ischemic cross-clamp time by performing off-pump surgery. This involves revascularization of the beating heart using special stabilization devices to allow for the construction of microanastomoses on the epicardial surface. An important technique used in off-pump surgery is to first

TABLE **15.3.** Selection criteria for insertion of circulatory support devices.

1. Reversibility of cardiac dysfunction
2. Etiology of cardiac dysfunction
3. Degrees of left and right cardiac dysfunction
4. Patient size
5. Degree of circulatory support required
6. Anticoagulation
7. Transplant candidate
8. Expected duration of support
9. Age and comorbid conditions

graft the vessel that supplies the myocardium at risk. A recent study of 638 patients with cardiogenic shock was performed: 124 patients underwent off-pump surgery and 116 underwent on-pump beating heart surgery. Those patients with left main lesions, circumflex lesions, or three-vessel disease were selected for standard ischemic arrest. Off-pump surgery demonstrated less time to culprit lesion revascularization, less incidence of stroke, less blood transfusion, less need for inotropes, and less renal failure [19]. IABP has also been used as a surgical adjunct to safely perform off-pump coronary surgery [20]. The complete role of off-pump surgery is not fully determined at present, but multiple studies suggest that it is a safe and effective option.

Use of Ventricular Assist Devices

Patients with persistent cardiogenic shock after AMI may be considered for a left ventricular assist device. These devices are available for either temporary use or as a long-term device prior to eventual transplant. Patients who are considered candidates for these devices have deteriorating hemodynamics. It is important that patients be considered for device implantation *before* they develop severe end-organ dysfunction. Intraoperatively, the decision to place an assist device comes with inability to wean from cardiopulmonary bypass despite the use of high-dose inotropes, cardiac index <2.0, and mixed venous saturation of less than 50%, despite the use of IABP therapy. The use of high-dose inotropes may prevent recovery of ischemic border zone myocardium after AMI. Table 15.3 includes selection criteria used for insertion of support devices [8].

References

1. Thornhill RE, Prato FS, Wisenberg G. The assessment of myocardial viability: a review of current diagnostic imaging approaches. J Cardiovasc Magn Reson 2002; 4:381–410.

2. Hannan EL, Wu C, Bennett EV, et al. Risk stratification of in-hospital mortality for coronary artery bypass graft surgery. J Am Coll Cardiol 2006;47:661–668.

3. Biancari F, Kangasniemi OP, Luukkonen J, et al. EuroSCORE predicts immediate and late outcome after coronary artery bypass surgery. Ann Thorac Surg 2006;82: 57–61.

4. DeRose JJ Jr, Toumpoulis IK, Balaram SK, et al. Preoperative prediction of long-term survival after coronary artery bypass grafting in patients with low left ventricular ejection fraction. J Thorac Cardiovasc Surg 2005;129:314–321.

5. Thielmann M, Massoudy P, Neuhauser M, et al. Prognostic value of preoperative cardiac troponin I in patients undergoing emergency coronary artery bypass surgery with non-ST-elevation or ST-elevation acute coronary syndromes. Circulation 2006; 114(1 Suppl):I448–453.

6. Eagle KA, Guyton RA, Davidoff R, et al. ACC/AHA guideline update for coronary artery bypass graft surgery: summary article. J Am Coll Cardiol 2004;44:1146–1154.

7. Roberts CS, Schoen FJ, Kloner RA. Effects of coronary reperfusion on myocardial hemorrhage and infarct healing. Am J Cardiol 1983;52:610.

8. Lee DC, Ting W, Oz MC. Myocardial revascularization after acute myocardial infarction. In: Cohn LH, Edmunds LH Jr, eds. Cardiac surgery in the adult. New York: McGraw-Hill; 2003:639–658.

9. Lee DC, Oz MC, Weinberg AD, et al. Optimal timing of revascularization: transmural versus nontransmural acute myocardial infarction. Ann Thorac Surg 2001;71: 1198–1204.

10. Solodky A, Behar S, Boyko V, et al. The outcome of coronary artery bypass grafting surgery among patients hospitalized with acute coronary syndrome: the Euro Heart Survey of acutecoronary syndrome experience. Cardiology 2005;103: 44–47.

11. Hochman JS, Sleeper LA, Webb JG, et al. Early revascularization in acute myocardial infarction complicated by cardiogenic shock. SHOCK Investigators. Should We Emergently Revascularize Occluded Coronaries for Cardiogenic Shock. N Engl J Med 1999;341:625–634.

12. Duvernoy CS, Bates ER. Management of cardiogenic shock attributable to acute myocardial infarction in the reperfusion era. J Intensive Care Med 2005;20(4): 188–198.

13. Ohman EM, George BS, White CJ, et al. Use of aortic counterpulsation to improve sustained coronary artery patency during acute myocardial infarction. Circulation 1994;90:792.

14. Baue AE, ed. Glenn's thoracic and cardiovascular surgery. 6th ed. Stamford, CT: Appleton and Lange.

15. Caes FL, Van Nooten GJ. Use of internal mammary artery for emergency grafting after failed coronary angioplasty. Ann Thorac Surg 1994;57:1295.

16. Zaplonski A, Rosenblum J, Myler RK, et al. Emergency coronary artery bypass surgery following failed balloon angioplasty: role of the internal mammary artery graft. J Cardiac Surg 1995;10:32.

17. Lytle BW, Loop FD. Superiority of bilateral internal thoracic artery grafting: it's been a long time comin. Circulation 2001;104:2152–2154.

18. Bonacchi M, Maiani M, Prifti E, et al. Urgent/emergent surgical revascularization in unstable angina: influence of different type of conduits. J Cardiovasc Surg 2006;47: 201–210.

19. Rastan AJ, Eckenstein JI, Hentschel B, et al. Emergency coronary artery bypass graft surgery for acute coronary syndrome:beating heart versus conventional cardioplegic cardiac arrest strategies. Circulation 2006;114(1 Suppl):I477–485.
20. Suzuki T, Okabe M, Handa M, et al. Usefulness of preoperative intraaortic balloon pump therapy during off-pump coronary artery bypass grafting in high-risk patients. Ann Thorac Surg 2004;77:2056–2059.

16
Arrhythmias Complicating Acute Myocardial Infarction–Bradyarrhythmias

Dan L. Musat, Delia Cotiga, Walter Pierce, and Aysha Arshad

In acute myocardial infarction (AMI) in addition to myocardium, the specialized conduction system can be affected directly by ischemia, necrosis, or autonomic imbalance [1]. Many serious arrhythmias develop within 1 hour of onset of symptoms, before presentation to the hospital and patient monitoring [2, 3]. It is important to recognize and treat them in this setting, as they may complicate the course and have prognostic significance [4–10].

Bradycardia is defined as a heart rate less than 60 beats per minute and is usually caused either by a failure of the sinus node (SN) impulse generation or failure of impulse propagation in distal conduction system [11]. The diagnosis of bradyarrhythmia starts with physical examination and is confirmed by electrocardiogram. The two most frequent bradycardic rhythms in the setting of AMI are sinus bradycardia, seen in 30% to 40 % of patients [12–14], and atrioventricular (AV) block, seen in 4% to 20% of patients with the following occurrence: 8% to 15 % first-degree, 5% to 12% second-degree, and 6% to 8% third-degree AV block [15–17]. Most of these arrhythmias are associated with inferior AMI [4–10, 16, 18]. The incidence of bradyarrhythmias has decreased in the era of thrombolysis and early invasive revascularization [4, 5, 8].

Anatomy of Conduction System

In order to better understand the pathophysiology of bradyarrhythmias in the setting of acute coronary syndrome (ACS), it is important to know the anatomy of the conduction system and its blood supply.

The conduction system has the following components [17, 19]:

- The sinoatrial (SA) node lies at the junction of the right atrium and superior vena cava and is richly innervated by both the sympathetic and parasympathetic nervous system.
- The AV node lies at the base of the interatrial septum just above the tricuspid annulus and anterior to the coronary sinus and is innervated by both divisions of the autonomic nervous system.

163

- The His bundle continues from the AV node, crosses the fibrous skeleton of the heart, and courses anteriorly across the membranous interventricular septum, adjacent to the noncoronary cusp of aortic valve.
- The right bundle branch (RBB) arises from the His bundle and continues its course subendocardial on the right ventricular part of the anterior interventricular septum toward the anterior papillary muscle of the right ventricle.
- The left bundle branch (LBB), following its origin from the His bundle, crosses the interventricular septum and splits into anterior and posterior fascicles:
  The anterior fascicle, the smaller one, passes along left ventricular outflow tract toward the anterior papillary muscle of the left ventricle.
  The posterior fascicle goes in a posteroinferior direction along the interventricular septum toward the posterior papillary muscle.
- The Purkinje fibers arise from arborization of both right and left bundle branches, are found deep in the myocardium, and extend throughout the endocardium of the right and left ventricles.

Physiologic Conduction

Under normal conditions, the dominant pacemaker is the SA node. After leaving the sinus node and perinodal tissue, the impulse traverses the atrium and reaches the AV node. Within the AV node there is a physiologic delay, and after propagation via the bundle of His, the impulse is conducted through the right and left bundle branches and reaches the myocardium via the Purkinje fibers [19].

Blood Supply of the Conduction System

The source of blood supply for each component plays an important role in ischemic hearts, and the type of bradycardia depends on which epicardial vessel is affected and the level of obstruction [1, 17, 19, 20].

1. The SA node is supplied by the sinus node artery, which arises from the proximal right coronary artery (RCA) in 50% to 60% of the cases and from the left circumflex coronary artery (LCX) in 35% to 45%, and a dual supply in up to 10%.
2. The AV node receives dual blood supply from the AV nodal artery, which originates from the distal RCA in about 90% of patients or from the distal LCX in the remainder, and a branch of the left anterior descending coronary artery (LAD), making it less vulnerable to ischemia.
3. The His bundle is supplied by the AV nodal branch with a minor contribution from the septal perforators of the LAD.

4. The LAD coronary artery provides most of the blood supply for the main or proximal left bundle branch, particularly for the initial portion. There may be some collateral flow from the RCA and LCX systems.

5. The left anterior and posterior fascicles are supplied by the AV nodal artery in the proximal part and by septal branches from the LAD and posterior septal perforating arteries in the distal portion.

6. The right bundle branch receives most of its blood supply from septal perforators from the LAD coronary artery, particularly in its initial course. It also receives some collateral supply from either the RCA or LCX coronary systems, depending upon the dominance of the coronary system.

Pathophysiology

Bradyarrhythmias arising in the setting of AMI occur in a significant number of patients. There are usually two main factors involved [3, 14, 16, 17]: (1) transient ischemia or irreversible necrosis of the dominant pacemaker or the specialized conduction system; (2) altered autonomic influence expressed by parasympathetic surge.

Other factors responsible for these bradyarrhythmias include [16, 17] systemic hypoxia, electrolyte disturbances (myocardial hyperkalemia), acid-based disorders (metabolic acidosis), local increases in adenosine, and complications of various medical therapies (beta and calcium channel blockers).

Bradyarrhythmias are frequently encountered with inferoposterior infarct due to occlusion of RCA or dominant LCX. This can be explained by a higher density of cardiac vagal afferent receptors in the inferoposterior portion of the left ventricle. Stimulation here results in increased vagal tone and cholinergic stimulation of the heart, with resultant bradycardia and possible hypotension [14, 16, 17]. Increased vagal tone can also be a result of pain in association with nausea and vomiting. The SA node, atrium, and AV node are significantly influenced by autonomic tone. Vagal influences depress the automaticity of the SA node, depress conduction, and prolong refractoriness in the tissue surrounding the SA node, slow atrial conduction, and prolong AV nodal conduction and refractoriness [19], whereas sympathetic influences exert the opposite effect. The typical underlying pathophysiology of bradyarrhythmias occurring early in the course of AMI (first 6 hours) is increased parasympathetic tone. The rhythm disturbance often develops abruptly, typically with slow ventricular escape rates and a good response to atropine or isoproterenol. Many such arrhythmias are of no prognostic significance [16, 17]. Also ischemia, as shown by Tjandrawijaja et al. [20], plays an important role as underlying mechanism in the context of early bradyarrhythmias due to AV block (up to 90 minutes post-fibrinolysis) when the AV nodal artery is compromised. When bradyarrhythmias develop after 6 hours of AMI, they tend to start gradually and ischemia is usually the underlying cause. The escape rhythm is frequently from the ventricle, with a relatively high rate and has a poor response to medical therapy. The return to normal sinus is slow as well.

One of the extreme autonomic reactions in this setting is Bezold-Jarisch cardioinhibitory reflex (BJR), arising from the ischemic left ventricle. It is mostly seen in the setting of reperfusion of an acutely occluded proximal RCA and may result in abrupt bradycardia and hypotension [21, 22]. Stimulation of vagal afferents in response to sympathetic overactivity may be the underlying pathogenic mechanism promoting a BJR response. The BJR in inferior AMI is considered by some authors to be a reliable prognosticator of timely reperfusion and sustained coronary patency [22, 23].

Types of Bradycardia in ACS and Their Management

Bradycardias encountered in AMI can be divided into two groups:

1. Pacemaker related (failure of impulse generation):
   (a) Sinus bradycardia
   (b) Junctional escape rhythm
   (c) Idioventricular rhythm.
2. Conduction related (delay or failure of impulse propagation):
   (a) First-degree AV block
   (b) High-degree AV block: second- or third-degree AV block
   (c) Intraventricular block.

Impulse Generation–Related Rhythm Disturbances

The SA node, in normal conditions, is the dominant pacemaker in the heart (normal rates 60 to 100 bpm). When the SA node fails to generate an impulse or the impulse cannot exit the SA node area due to a block, the AV node, which is a subsidiary pacemaker, generates a junctional (escape) rhythm (rates 40 to 60 bpm). If this site is also affected, then an impulse is generated in the ventricular tissue—idioventricular rhythm (rates 30 to 45 bpm).

Sinus Bradycardia

Sinus bradycardia is the most common bradyarrhythmia occurring in the early phases of acute myocardial infarction, seen in up to 40% of patients in the first 2 hours with decrease in incidence to about 20% after 4 hours [3, 16]:

• Is frequently associated with inferior and posterior wall infarct (due to involvement of the origin of SA node artery).
• Frequently resolves in 24 hours.
• Is generally caused by increased vagal tone, but ischemia of the SA node can also be a cause.
• It might represent a protective mechanism by decreasing the myocardial workload and oxygen demand [3].

- Can also be seen, in association with hypotension, after successful revascularization, and may be a useful noninvasive marker of successful reperfusion [23].

ECG findings:

- P wave with normal morphology.
- Normal, fixed-duration PR interval.
- Regular rhythm.
- Ventricular rate less than 60 bpm.
- Each P wave followed by a narrow QRS complex.

Management:

- When not accompanied by hypotension, sinus bradycardia does not require any specific treatment. Only close observation and avoidance of aggravating medication such as beta-blockers and nitroglycerin are sufficient.
- If severe bradycardia and hypotension occur, it usually responds to intravenous boluses of fluids, atropine 0.5 to 1 mg intravenously (maximum 2 mg) or isoproterenol.
- Persistent bradycardia with hemodynamic compromise despite medical therapy requires temporary cardiac pacing—transcutaneous or transvenous.

Junctional Bradycardia

Junctional bradycardia is an AV nodal area escape rhythm seen in up to 20% of the patients with AMI when the SA node fails to generate an impulse or there is a complete heart block and has a typical rate of 40 to 60 bpm [16]. It is commonly encountered with inferior AMI, especially in patients using digoxin or other AV nodal modifying drugs such as beta-blockers and calcium channel blockers. It is considered, as well, a protective rhythm in the setting of ACS [14]. It can also be seen in the context of a complete heart block.

ECG characteristics:

- No P waves are usually seen; if P waves are present, they may not have any relationship with QRS complexes. They may be retrograde, thus being negative in the inferior ECG leads (II, III, aVf). The atrial rate can be faster than junctional one.
- Regular rhythm.
- Narrow QRS complexes.

Management:

- In hemodynamically stable patients, close observation and avoidance of aggravating medication such as beta-blockers or calcium channel blockers are adequate.
- If severe bradycardia and hypotension occur, treatment with atropine (0.5 to 1 mg intravenously; maximum 2 mg), isoproterenol (2 to 10 µg/min), or glucagon (0.05 to 0.15 mg/kg) should be administered.
- Transvenous pacemaker is indicated if medical therapy is ineffective.

Idioventricular Rhythm

With failure of the dominant and subsidiary pacemaker, an escape rhythm at a rate of 30 to 45 bpm is seen in up to 15% of patients with AMI [16]. It is mostly seen as an escape rhythm in complete heart block. Most often an accelerated idioventricular rhythm with rates between 60 and 120 bpm is seen in the context of early reperfusion and is considered a marker of reperfusion [23].

ECG characteristics:

- Regular rhythm.
- Wide QRS complex.
- In the setting of complete heart block, the P waves are dissociated from the QRS impulses and the atrial rate is faster than the ventricular rate.

Management:

- Transvenous pacemaker is mainly indicated in conjunction with medical treatment.

Rhythm Disturbances Due to Impaired Impulse Propagation

AV conduction disturbances are characterized by a delay (as seen in first-degree AV block) or failure of the atrial impulse to be conducted through the AV conducting system (second- or third-degree AV block) [11]. Ischemia plays an important role, especially with compromise of the AV nodal artery [20] as well as the autonomic overstimulation. In the context of complete heart block, the escape rhythms generated in the distal part of the ventricular conduction system are usually unstable and the patient requires a pacemaker [11, 17]. Early AV conduction disturbances, appearing within 24 hours of AMI and usually associated with inferior ischemia, are easily reversible with revascularization and have a better prognosis than those occurring in the late phase of AMI, which are usually associated with anterior ischemia and most likely irreversible [7, 24].

First-Degree AV Block

First-degree AV block represents a delay in atrial conduction of the impulse and is defined as prolongation of PR interval duration more than 200 milliseconds. It can be seen in up to 15% of patients with AMI [16, 17] in the context of increased vagotonia or treatment with beta-blockers or non-dihydropyridine calcium channel blockers. It has no adverse prognosis; it is most commonly associated with AV node ischemia due to RCA involvement.

ECG characteristics:

- P wave and QRS complex have normal morphology with 1 : 1 relationship.
- Prolonged PR interval (>200 milliseconds) is constant.

Management [3]:

- No specific treatment is required if no hemodynamic compromise.
- The dose of beta-blockers or calcium channel blockers should be decreased if PR interval prolongs >240 milliseconds.
- These agents should be stopped if higher degree AV block or hemodynamic impairment occurs.
- When associated with sinus bradycardia and hypotension, administration of atropine may be helpful.
- Continued electrocardiographic monitoring is important in such patients in view of the possibility of progression to higher degrees of block.
- No need for temporary pacemaker.

Second-Degree Mobitz Type I AV Block (Wenckebach AV block)

Second-degree Mobitz type I AV block is characterized by an intermittent conduction failure of the atrial impulse to the ventricles following a progressive lengthening of the PR interval [14]. The site of block is usually at or above AV node as a result of ischemia at this level. It can be seen in 10% to 12 % of the AMI patients [16], frequently associated with inferior AMI [14] and has no prognostic implications.

ECG characteristics:

- Narrow QRS complex.
- Grouped beating.
- Progressive prolongation of PR interval, then a dropped beat/failed conduction.
- Progressive shortening of the R-R interval.
- The length of the R-R interval that includes the dropped beat is less than twice the shortest cycle.

Management:

- No specific therapy is required when the ventricular rate exceeds 50 beats/min and there are no premature ventricular contractions, heart failure, bundle branch block, or hemodynamic instability [3].
- Immediate treatment with atropine (0.5 to 1.0 mg intravenously) is indicated if the heart rate is <50 beats/min or the above coexisting conditions are present [14].
- Temporary pacing systems are almost never needed in the management of this arrhythmia [3, 14].

Second-Degree Mobitz Type II AV Block

Second-degree Mobitz type II AV block is defined as an intermittent failure of one or more atrial impulses to conduct to the ventricles, characterized by a fixed PR interval before the nonconducted atrial beat. The overall incidence is low (1%) and it represents 10% of the second-degree AV block seen in AMI. It usually originates from a lesion in the conduction system below the bundle of His reflecting impaired conduction distal to the bundle of His (trifascicular block) [3, 14] and is almost always associated with anterior infarction (LAD compromise). It is an unstable rhythm that often progresses suddenly to complete heart block and is associated with a poor prognosis.

ECG characteristics:

- In most instances, QRS complex is wide.
- PR interval is constant and can be normal or prolonged.
- R-R interval that contains the dropped beat is equal with two preceding R-R intervals.
- Magnitude of AV block is expressed as a ratio of P waves to QRS complexes (2:1, 3:2, etc.).
- Hard to differentiate from Wenckebach block when there is 2:1 conduction.

Management [3, 14]:

- Always needs to be treated
- Immediate treatment either with atropine (0.5 to 1.0 mg intravenously) or transcutaneous pacing is required
- Temporary transvenous pacemaker should be inserted, with the rate set at approximately 60 bpm.

Third-Degree AV Block (Complete Heart Block)

Third-degree AV block is characterized by a total failure of atrial impulses to penetrate the ventricles. The atria and ventricles are controlled by different pacemakers and are functioning independently. It can be seen in 5% to 15% [4, 6, 9, 14, 16, 20, 24, 25] and according to the escape site can be divided into:

1. Proximal escape at the level of AV node or upper His bundle:
   - Narrow QRS complex.
   - Stable rhythm, likely will not degenerate to asystole.
   - Higher heart rates 30 to 40 beats/min.
   - Responsive to atropine, isoproterenol, aminophylline, or glucagons.
   - Associated mostly with inferior MI due to AV node ischemia or vagotonic effect.
   - Appears early in the course of AMI and is usually reversible.
2. Distal escape below the His bundle or intraventricular:
   - Lower incidence.
   - Wide QRS complex with heart rates 20 to 30 beats/min.
   - Unstable rhythm; usually progress to asystole.
   - Not responsive to and usually worsened with atropine.
   - Develops later in the AMI course and most likely require permanent pacemaker placement.
   - Frequently associated with anterior MI.

Development of complete AV block usually implies that a bigger area of myocardium is jeopardized as shown by higher creatine phosphokinase (CPK) peaks and portends a poor prognosis [3, 4, 6, 9, 10, 26, 27]. Meine et al. identified inferior MI, older age, worse Killip class at presentation, female sex, current smoking, hypertension, and diabetes as independent predictors of AV block [9].

ECG features:

- Atrial rhythm can be sinus, ectopic, flutter, or fibrillation.
- Atrial rate is always greater than ventricular rate and usually is regular (if no fibrillation).
- No relationship between P waves and QRS complexes.
- Constant R-R intervals.
- QRS complexes could be narrow or wide depending on the level of pacemaker escape (proximal or distal).

Management:

- Immediate treatment with atropine, isoproterenol, aminophylline, glucagon (same doses as described above) if QRS complex is narrow.
- Immediate transcutaneous pacing.
- Transvenous pacemaker insertion.

Intraventricular Blocks

Bundle branch blocks (BBB) complicating the course of AMI represent a serious ischemia in their bed due to occlusion of bundle-related coronary artery [7]. Disturbances in one or more of the bundle branch fascicles can be encountered in 5% to 15% of the patients with AMI [3, 5, 16, 28]. BBB is frequently a marker of a multivessel disease as RBB and left posterior fascicular block have dual blood supply (from RCA and LAD); left anterior fascicular block is only supplied by LAD septal branches. A new BBB appearing in AMI, especially the RBB block, is considered a predictor for the development of a complete AV block [3, 7, 14].

1. Left anterior fascicular block (LAFB) occurs in 3% to 5% of the patients with AMI. It is unlikely to progress to complete AV block and does not need any specific treatment [14].

2. Left posterior fascicular block (LFPB) is encountered in 1% to 2% of the patients presenting with AMI. This bundle is larger than the anterior one and block at this level signifies a larger infarct, which heralds worse prognosis. It rarely progresses to complete AV block [3, 14].

3. Right bundle branch block (RBBB) is seen in approximately 2% of patients with AMI. It frequently progresses to complete heart block when it develops in this setting. It has been usually associated with large anteroseptal AMI and increased mortality due to higher frequency in cardiogenic shock [3, 14, 28, 29].

4. Bifascicular blocks are considered any combination of the above-mentioned blocks (RBBB + LAFB, RBBB + LPFB, LAFB + LPFB = LBBB). The risk of developing complete AV block is quite high, as is the mortality, due to occurrence of severe pump failure, secondary to the extensive myocardial necrosis, and arrhythmias [3, 14].

Conclusion

Bradyarrhythmias occur frequently in patients in the context of AMI. Symptoms and hemodynamic sequelae are important determinants of the management strategy in these patients. Asymptomatic arrhythmias do not need treatment; however, close observation is warranted. Temporary pacing is indicated prophylactically in patients at risk of developing higher degree AV block, severe sinus node dysfunction, or asystole in acute myocardial infarction.

References

1. Zimetbaum PJ, Arnsdorg MF, Josephson ME. Conduction abnormalities after myocardial infarction. In: Rose DB, ed. Up to date. 14.2 ed. 2006.
2. O'Doherty M, Tayler DI, Quinn E, et al. Five hundred patients with myocardial infarction monitored within one hour of symptoms. Br Med J 1983;286:1405–1408.
3. Antman EM. ST-elevation myocardial infarction: pathology, pathophysiology, and clinical features; arrhythmias. In: Braunwald E, Zipes DP, eds. Zipes: Braunwald's heart disease: a textbook of cardiovascular medicine. 7th ed. Philadelphia: WB Saunders; 2005:1207–1218.
4. Melgarejo MA, Galcera TJ, Garcia AA, et al. The prognostic significance of complete atrioventricular block in patients with acute inferior myocardial infarct. A study in the era thrombolytics. Rev Esp Cardiol 1997;50:397–405.
5. Archbold RA, Sayer JW, Ray S, et al. Frequency and prognostic implications of conduction defects in acute myocardial infarction since the introduction of thrombolytic therapy. Eur Heart J 1998;19:893–898.
6. Ben AY, Mghaieth F, Ouchallal K, et al. Prognostic significance of second and third degree atrioventricular block in acute inferior wall myocardial infarction. Ann Cardiol Angeiol (Paris) 2003;52:30–33.
7. Jurkovicova O, Cagan S. Supraventricular arrhythmias and disorders of atrioventricular and intraventricular conduction in patients with acute myocardial infarct. Bratisl Lek Listy 1998;99:172–180.
8. Petrina M, Goodman SG, Eagle KA. The 12-lead electrocardiogram as a predictive tool of mortality after acute myocardial infarction: current status in an era of revascularization and reperfusion. Am Heart J 2006;152:11–18.
9. Meine TJ, Al-Khatib SM, Alexander JH, et al. Incidence, predictors, and outcomes of high-degree atrioventricular block complicating acute myocardial infarction treated with thrombolytic therapy. Am Heart J 2005;149:670–674.
10. Melgarejo MA, Galcera TJ, Garcia AA, et al. Prognostic significance of advanced atrioventricular block in patients with acute myocardial infarction. Med Clin (Barc) 2000;114:321–325.

11. Durham D, Worthley LI. Cardiac arrhythmias: diagnosis and management. The bradycardias. Crit Care Resusc 2002;4:54–60.
12. Rotman M, Wagner GS, Wallace AG. Bradyarrhythmias in acute myocardial infarction. Circulation 1972;45:703–722.
13. Adgey AA, Geddes JS, Mulholland HC, et al. Incidence, significance, and management of early bradyarrhythmia complicating acute myocardial infarction. Lancet 1968;2:1097–1101.
14. Aufderheide TP. Arrhythmias associated with acute myocardial infarction and thrombolysis. Emerg Med Clin North Am 1998;16:583–600, viii.
15. Arnsdorf MF. Etiology of atrioventricular block. In: DB R, ed. Up to date. 14.2 ed. 2006.
16. Brady WJ Jr, Harrigan RA. Diagnosis and management of bradycardia and atrioventricular block associated with acute coronary ischemia. Emerg Med Clin North Am 2001;19:371–84, xi–xii.
17. Brady WJ Jr, Harrigan RA. Evaluation and management of bradyarrhythmias in the emergency department. Emerg Med Clin North Am 1998;16:361–388.
18. George M, Greenwood TW. Relationship between bradycardia and the site of myocardial infarction. Lancet 1967;1:739.
19. Josephson ME, Zimetbaum P. The bradyarrhythmias: disorders of sinus node function and av conduction disturbances. In: Kasper DLB, Braunwald E, Fauci AS, Hauser SL, et al., eds. Harrison's principles of internal medicine. 16th ed. New York: McGraw-Hill; 2006:1333–1341.
20. Tjandrawidjaja MC, Fu Y, Kim DH, et al. Compromised atrial coronary anatomy is associated with atrial arrhythmias and atrioventricular block complicating acute myocardial infarction. J Electrocardiol 2005;38:271–278.
21. Goldstein JA, Lee DT, Pica MC, et al. Patterns of coronary compromise leading to bradyarrhythmias and hypotension in inferior myocardial infarction. Coron Artery Dis 2005;16:265–274.
22. Chiladakis JA, Patsouras N, Manolis AS. The Bezold-Jarisch reflex in acute inferior myocardial infarction: clinical and sympathovagal spectral correlates. Clin Cardiol 2003;26:323–328.
23. Goldberg S, Greenspon AJ, Urban PL, et al. Reperfusion arrhythmia: a marker of restoration of antegrade flow during intracoronary thrombolysis for acute myocardial infarction. Am Heart J 1983;105:26–32.
24. Garcia GC, Curos AA, Serra FJ, et al. Duration of complete atrioventricular block complicating inferior wall infarction treated with fibrinolysis. Rev Esp Cardiol 2005;58:20–26.
25. Nguyen N, Reddy PC. Management of cardiac arrhythmias in acute coronary syndromes. J La State Med Soc 2001;153:300–305.
26. Harpaz D, Behar S, Gottlieb S, et al. Complete atrioventricular block complicating acute myocardial infarction in the thrombolytic era. SPRINT Study Group and the Israeli Thrombolytic Survey Group. Secondary Prevention Reinfarction Israeli Nifedipine Trial. J Am Coll Cardiol 1999;34:1721–1728.
27. Ruiz-Bailen M, de Hoyos EA, Issa-Khozouz Z, et al. Clinical implications of acute myocardial infarction complicated by high grade atrioventricular block. Med Sci Monit 2002;8:CR138–147.
28. Melgarejo MA, Galcera TJ, Garcia AA. Prognostic significance of bundle-branch block in acute myocardial infarction: the importance of location and time of appearance. Clin Cardiol 2001;24:371–376.

29. Abidov A, Kaluski E, Hod H, et al. Influence of conduction disturbances on clinical outcome in patients with acute myocardial infarction receiving thrombolysis (results from the ARGAMI-2 study). Am J Cardiol 2004;93:76–80.

17
Arrhythmias Complicating Acute Myocardial Infarction: Atrial Tachyarrhythmias Including Atrial Fibrillation and Atrial Flutter

Dan L. Musat, Jonathan S. Steinberg, Delia Cotiga, and Eyal Herzog

In patients presenting with acute coronary syndrome (ACS), supraventricular tachyarrhythmias (SVTs) are relatively common in the peri-infarction period. Their occurrence often heralds significant myocardial ischemia with ventricular dysfunction or cardiogenic shock and may, in themselves, cause congestive heart failure and exacerbate ongoing myocardial ischemia. They also are a predictor of short- and long-term complications and prognosis [1–4].

Atrial tachyarrhythmias or narrow QRS complex tachycardias are defined as tachyarrhythmias with a rate faster than 100 beats per minute (bpm) and a QRS duration of less than 120 milliseconds (0.12 second), as demonstrated on the electrocardiogram (ECG) or cardiac monitor [5]. SVT is considered any tachyarrhythmia that requires atrial or atrioventricular junctional tissue for its initiation and maintenance [6].

The most frequent SVT is sinus tachycardia occurring in approximately 30% to 40% of acute myocardial infarctions (AMIs) [2, 7]. The incidence of atrial tachyarrhythmias, excluding sinus tachycardia, in the peri-infarct period ranges from 6% to 20% [1, 8–12], with the highest incidence of these being atrial fibrillation and flutter, 7% to 12% in various series [1, 10–16].

Mechanisms of Supraventricular Tachyarrhythmias

All cardiac tachyarrhythmias are produced by one or more mechanisms, including disorders of impulse initiation (*automatic*), abnormalities of impulse conduction (*reentrant*), or disturbances of recovery or repolarization (*triggered*) [17, 18].

The apparent increase in prevalence of SVT during AMI has been ascribed to one or more of the following factors [7]:

- Atrial dysfunction (due to atrial ischemia or atrial stretching from heart failure).
- Congestive heart failure with increased pressure in all cardiac chambers.

- Increased sympathetic nervous system activity (due to persistent pain, anxiety, hypoxemia, anemia, or pericarditis) with increased concentrations of circulating catecholamines and local release of catecholamines from nerve endings within the heart [19, 20].
- Iatrogenic factors (atropine, inotropes, and vasopressors for cardiogenic shock treatment).

In the setting of AMI, the underlying cause for cellular electrophysiologic inhomogeneity resulting in early-onset SVT is ischemia of the atria [10, 21, 22], while the substrate for late-onset (i.e., days) atrial tachyarrhythmias is related to ventricular dysfunction [10, 13, 23, 24]. Most of the patients with early-onset SVT are found to have an inferior AMI [10, 21, 22, 25], whereas the patients with late-onset SVT and sinus tachycardia have had predominantly anterior AMI [3, 25]. Heart rhythm disorders related to AMI are also accompanied with a profound increase in plasma free fatty acids, sympatho-adrenal and kallikrein-kinin activity, and carboxycathepsin as shown by Latoguz et al. in 49 patients with AMI. These metabolic and neurohumoral changes were eventually reversed and tended to normalize as soon as sinus rhythm resumed [26].

Angiographic Anatomy of Atrial Blood Supply

Anatomical compromise of the principal atrial branches can precipitate various degrees of atrial ischemia according to the location of the culprit lesion relative to the origins of these branches. The following principal atrial coronary branches have been characterized [10, 27–29] (Fig. 17.1):

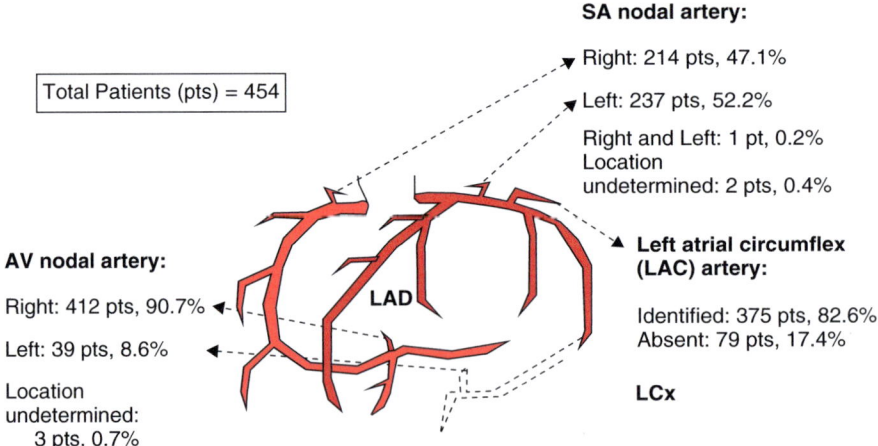

FIGURE 17.1. Anatomical distribution of the SA nodal, LAC, and AV nodal arteries relative to the major epicardial coronary arteries among the 454 patients with AMI studied. (Reproduced from Tjandrawidjaja MC, Fu Y, Kim DH, et al. Compromised atrial coronary anatomy is associated with atrial arrhythmias and atrioventricular block complicating acute myocardial infarction. J Electrocardiol 2005;38:271–278.)

1. *Sinus nodal (SA nodal) artery*: Arises from the proximal right coronary artery (RCA) in 50% to 60% of persons and from the proximal left circumflex artery (LCX) in the remainder; it supplies most of the right atrium and part of the left atrium. Rarely, the SA nodal artery arises from the left main (LM) coronary artery.

2. *Left atrial circumflex (LAC) artery*: Originates from the proximal LCX and supplies most of the left atrium. Rarely, the LAC artery arises from either LM or proximal left anterior descending (LAD) artery.

3. *Atrioventricular nodal (AV) artery*: Originates from distal RCA in about 90% of persons and from distal LCX in the remainder and supplies the AV nodal region predominantly and part of the left atrium directly and/or indirectly by anastomoses with other left atrial branches.

In 454 patients who presented with AMI, Tjandrawidjaja et al. observed anatomical compromise of at least 1 principal atrial branch in 49% of the patients, the majority of the cases being AV nodal artery. In 96% of these patients, ECG showed evidence of an inferior myocardial infarction (MI) with RCA angiographically involved in 89% of cases. Overall, 57 (13%) patients had an atrial arrhythmia evident on at least one ECG from baseline to discharge. Compromise of either the SA nodal or LAC artery, which together supply the majority of the atrial myocardium, was associated with the development of early atrial arrhythmias (evident only up to the 90-minute ECG). This abnormality accounted for approximately two thirds of all patients with atrial arrhythmias. Compared with their counterparts without compromise, patients with compromised anatomy of at least one principal atrial branch sustained a higher incidence of early atrial arrhythmias (12.6% vs. 4.3%). Similar findings were not observed for the occurrence of either late or intermediate atrial arrhythmias. In contrast, compromise of the AV nodal artery, which supplies the AV nodal region predominantly, was associated with the development of early AV block and, to a lesser extent, early atrial arrhythmias [10]. These findings provide support for the pathophysiologic role of atrial ischemia in the development of atrial arrhythmias and AV block complicating AMI as shown by other series as well [10, 21].

ECG Criteria for Atrial Infarction

Major and minor criteria for atrial infarction were defined by Nielsen et al. using PR displacements on hospital presentation ECG obtained from 277 patients with AMI [30].

1. Major criteria suggested for atrial infarction are
   (a) PR segment elevation greater than 0.5 mm in leads V_5 and V_6 with reciprocal PR segment depression in leads V_1 and V_2.
   (b) PR segment elevation greater than 0.5 mm in lead I with reciprocal PR segment depression in leads II and III.
   (c) PR segment depression greater than 1.5 mm in precordial leads and greater than 1.2 mm in leads I, II, and III.
2. Abnormal P waves are classified as minor criteria.

The occurrence of PR segment displacements on the admission ECG was shown by the author to predict the risk of developing supraventricular arrhythmias during hospitalization for myocardial infarction [30].

Types of Atrial Tachyarrhythmias in ACS and Their ECG Definitions

The most frequent atrial tachyarrhythmias in the setting of ACS are

1. *Sinus tachycardia* in an adult is defined as a sinus node rate faster than 100 bpm and usually less than 180 bpm (may be higher with extreme exertion). Features include:
   - Gradual onset and termination.
   - P-P interval can vary slightly from cycle to cycle.
   - P waves appear before each QRS complex with a stable PR interval unless concomitant atrioventricular (AV) block ensues [31].
   - Typically associated with augmented sympathetic activity.
   - May be associated with transient hypertension or hypotension.
   In the setting of ACS, common causes are anxiety, persistent pain, left ventricular failure, pericarditis, hypovolemia, and the administration of cardioaccelerator drugs such as atropine, epinephrine, or dopamine; rarely, it occurs in patients with atrial infarction. Sinus tachycardia is particularly common in patients with anterior infarction, especially if there is significant accompanying left ventricular dysfunction [20].
2. *Premature atrial complexes* is indicated on the ECG by a premature P wave with a PR interval exceeding 120 milliseconds:
   - Premature P wave generally differs in morphology from a normal sinus P wave.
   - Conduction may not be completely normal when beat occurs early in diastole: blocked/nonconducted when AV junction is still refractory from preceding beat, prolonged PR interval if conduction is slowed [31].
   - Often can herald the development of paroxysmal supraventricular tachycardia, atrial flutter, or atrial fibrillation [19].
3. *Unifocal atrial tachycardia* is a supraventricular tachycardia arising from atrial muscle that does not include the sinus node with an atrial rate of generally 150 to 200 bpm (usually less than 250 bpm) (Fig. 17.2):
   - Single P-wave morphologic pattern: configuration depends entirely on the atrial site from which the tachycardia originates and the spread of activation [6, 31].
   - Rate "warming up" at the onset: slight increase in heart rate over the initial several complexes.
   - Occur in short, recurrent bursts with spontaneous termination.
   - Isoelectric intervals between P waves (in contrast with atrial flutter) are usually present in all leads, although at rapid atrial rates, the distinction between atrial tachycardia with block and atrial flutter can be difficult.
   - Each P wave can conduct to the ventricles if the atrial rate is not excessive and AV conduction is intact.

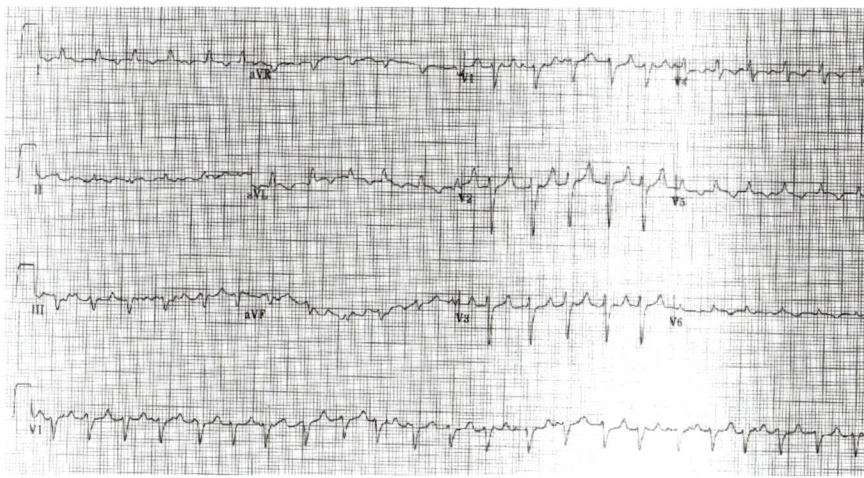

FIGURE 17.2. Focal atrial tachycardia with 2:1 AV block.

- *Atrial tachycardia with block* emerges if the atrial rate increases and AV conduction becomes impaired (Wenckebach/Mobitz type 1 second-degree AV block can ensue).

4. *Multifocal atrial tachycardia* is an enhanced automaticity or triggered activity atrial tachycardia, in which there are three or more different morphologic patterns of P waves on ECG and an irregular atrial rate averaging 100 bpm or more:
   - PR intervals are variable.
   - Atrioventricular block of variable degree is common.
   - Isoelectric periods between adjacent P waves help distinguish this arrhythmia from atrial fibrillation.
   - 60% of patients have also associated pulmonary disease [6].

5. *Atrial fibrillation* is an arrhythmia characterized by disorganized atrial depolarizations of variable amplitude and morphology (called f *waves* on ECG) (Fig. 17.3) at a rate of 350 to 600 bpm, without effective atrial contraction through the atria [31]:
   - "Irregularly irregular" ventricular response due to concealed AV node conduction of the wavefronts.
   - Ventricular rates usually between 100 and 160 bpm in an untreated patient with normal AV conduction, depending on refractory period and conductivity of the AV node.
   - Supraventricular complexes at an irregular rhythm with no obvious P waves on ECG.

6. *Atrial flutter* is a macro-reentrant atrial arrhythmia, the most frequent (*type I*) being found in the right atrium, constrained anteriorly by the tricuspid annulus and posteriorly by the crista terminalis and eustachian ridge:

- Typical flutter circulates in a counterclockwise direction around the tricuspid annulus in the frontal plane and atypical in a clockwise direction.
- Atrial rate during typical atrial flutter is usually 250 to 350 bpm (slower around 200 bpm, when treated with antiarrhythmic drugs).
- Ordinarily, atrial rate is about 300 bpm, and usually ventricular rate is half the atrial rate, 150 bpm: slower ventricular rate (in the absence of drugs) suggests abnormal AV conduction or drug effect.
- ECG diagnosis:
  Identically recurring regular sawtooth flutter waves (Fig. 17.4).
  Lack of an isoelectric interval between flutter waves.
  Flutter waves are best visualized in leads II, III, aVF, or V_1.
  In typical atrial flutter, the flutter waves are inverted (negative) in leads II, III, aVF with positive waves in V_1.
  In atypical atrial flutter, the waves are positive and often notched in leads II, III, aVF, and negative in V_1.
  The ratio of flutter waves to conducted ventricular complexes is most often an even number (e.g., 2:1, 4:1, and so on) [31].

  Atrial flutter and atrial fibrillation are the most common supraventricular arrhythmias early in the setting of AMI and are thought to be due to atrial ischemia [10].

7. *Nonparoxysmal AV junctional tachycardia* is an *accelerated automatic discharge* in or near the His bundle at a fairly regular rate of 70 to 130 bpm or faster:

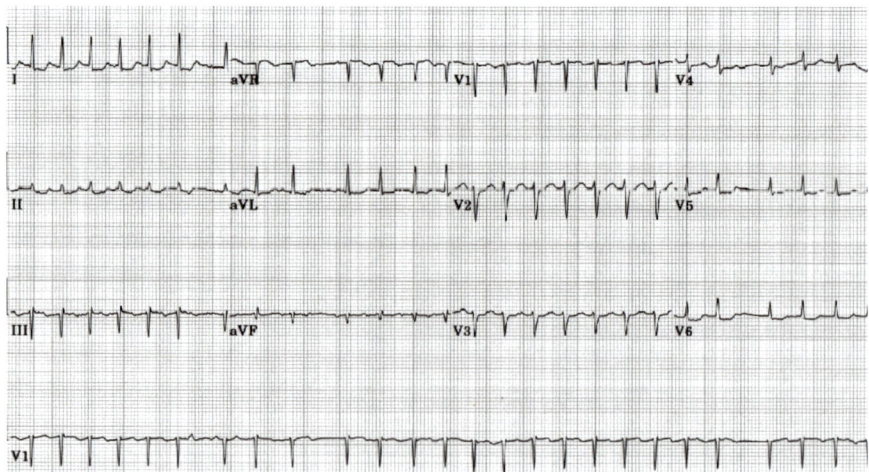

FIGURE 17.3. Atrial fibrillation with no organized atrial activity and irregular R-R intervals.

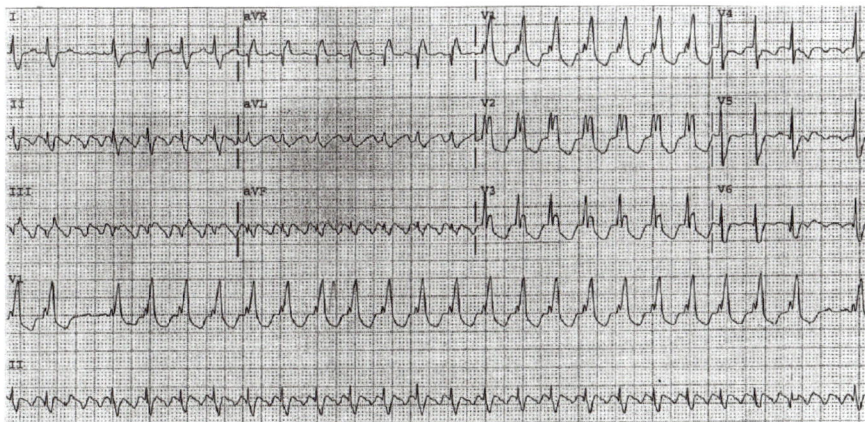

FIGURE 17.4. Twelve-lead ECG from a patient with counterclockwise flutter with negative flutter waves in inferior leads and positive in V_1.

- QRS of supraventricular configuration.
- Usually no P waves are seen; when retrograde activation of the atria occur, P wave can precede or follow the QRS; occasionally an independent sinus or atrial focus discharge results in AV dissociation.
- Enhanced vagal tone can slow while vagolytic agents can speed up the discharge rate [31].

Hemodynamic Consequences of Supraventricular Tachyarrhythmias

Patients presenting with ACS have at least two reasons for low cardiac output [20], with up to 20% of the patients with early SVT developing hemodynamic compromise in a series of 208 patients reported by Berisso [32]:

1. Left ventricular dysfunction (systolic and diastolic) due to ischemic myocardium, which will give a relatively low, fixed stroke volume.
2. Loss of the atrial contribution to ventricular preload in particular arrhythmias. In patients with ST-segment elevation MI (STEMI), atrial systole can boost end-diastolic volume by 15%, end-diastolic pressure by 29%, and stroke volume by 35% [20].

There is a narrow range of heart rate over which the cardiac output is maximal, with significant reductions occurring at both faster and slower rates. Thus, all forms of bradycardia and tachycardia can depress the cardiac output in patients with STEMI. In patients with ACS, the optimal heart rate is usually in the 60 bpm range, leading to decreased myocardial oxygen consumption and myocardial energy needs, even though this can affect the cardiac output [20].

Symptoms and Physical Examination Findings

SVT in a patient with ACS can start before arrival to the hospital or during hospitalization, after reperfusion. Symptoms due to tachycardia usually are confounding with the ones induced by myocardial infarction and can range from asymptomatic or mildly symptomatic to moderate or severe:

- Palpitations felt as a rapid heart rate, skipped beats, or pounding in the neck
- Persistent chest pain/pressure
- Shortness of breath
- Nausea
- Symptoms of shock: altered mental status, agitation, sluggishness

Physical examination findings could include:

- Mild to moderate distress due to pain or shortness of breath
- Jugular venous distension
- Neck arterial pounding
- Auscultation:
   Heart: tachycardia: regular or irregular, S3, S4, systolic ejection murmur of mitral regurgitation
   Lungs: crackles
- Diaphoresis
- Signs of cardiogenic shock: cold extremities, lung crackles

Initial Evaluation and Treatment

Every patient who presents with signs and symptoms of AMI should be evaluated as soon as possible and have an ECG within the first 10 minutes of arrival [33]. When there is ECG evidence of AMI, the treatment should start immediately.

   If the tachycardia is noticed, this should be addressed as well. There are few basic treatment goals.

- Optimize oxygenation of the blood by oxygen supplementation.
- Optimize the cardiac output and myocardial oxygen consumption by heart rate control (optimal around 60 bpm) and blood pressure control (SBP less than 130 mm Hg) using beta-blockers, if no contraindication.
- Antiplatelet and antithrombotic therapy.
- Decrease sympathetic surge with analgesics for pain and anxiolytics.
- Close electrolyte monitoring with prompt replenishment when K^+ < 4.0 mmol/L.

   Atrial tachyarrhythmias including sinus tachycardia are undesirable rhythms in patients with STEMI, because they can result in an augmentation of myocardial oxygen consumption as well as a reduction in the time available for coronary perfusion, thereby intensifying myocardial ischemia and/or myocardial necrosis [7, 20]. Also SVT, either early or late onset, is associated with increased risk of complications, such as pulmonary edema, cardiogenic shock, and ventricular tachyarrhythmias with higher short- and long-term mortalities. In some studies, however, SVT had no independent prognostic significance [1, 2, 8, 12, 25].

Persistent sinus tachycardia can signify persistent heart failure and under these circumstances is a poor prognostic sign associated with an excess mortality [3]. An underlying cause should be sought and appropriate treatment instituted, such as analgesics for pain; diuretics for heart failure; oxygen, beta-blockers, and nitroglycerin for ischemia; and aspirin for fever or pericarditis [19, 20].

Premature atrial complexes generally do not require therapy but should be monitored as they are a sign of irritable atrial tissue that can precipitate atrial tachyarrhythmias [19].

Other paroxysmal supraventricular tachycardia (PSVT) occurs in less than 10% of patients after an AMI but may require aggressive management due to a rapid ventricular rate [6, 7]. The 2004 American College of Cardiology/American Heart Association (ACC/AHA) guidelines recommended the following sequence of therapeutic measures for PSVT in this setting [7, 34]:

- Carotid sinus massage (if no carotid bruit heard).
- Intravenous adenosine (6 mg over 1 to 2 seconds; if no response, 12 mg 1 to 2 minutes later; may repeat 12 mg dose if needed) (Fig. 17.5)
- Intravenous beta blockade with metoprolol (2.5 to 5.0 mg every 2 to 5 minutes to a total of 15 mg over 10 to 15 minutes), or atenolol (2.5 to 5.0 mg over 2 minutes to a total of 10 mg in 10 to 15 minutes).
- Intravenous diltiazem (20 mg [or 0.25 mg/kg] over 2 minutes followed by an infusion of 10 mg/hour).
- Intravenous digoxin (8 to 15 μg/kg, or 0.6 to 1.0 mg in a patient weighing 70 kg). A delay of at least one hour may occur before the onset of pharmacological effects with digoxin.

Nonparoxysmal junctional tachycardia is an uncommon arrhythmia associated with AMI. It is typically transient, occurring within the first 48 hours of infarction and terminating gradually. No specific antiarrhythmic therapy is indicated [34].

Atrial Fibrillation/Flutter

Special attention should be given to atrial fibrillation and atrial flutter, as they are the most common early and late tachyarrhythmias and portend, as an independent factor, an increased risk for complications, stroke, and overall worse prognosis [1, 2, 8, 12, 35]. Aggressive treatment should be instituted for rate control, and electrical cardioversion should be considered if no spontaneous cardioversion to sinus rhythm occurs within the first 48 hours of onset, or if rapid heart rates with unstable hemodynamics are noted.

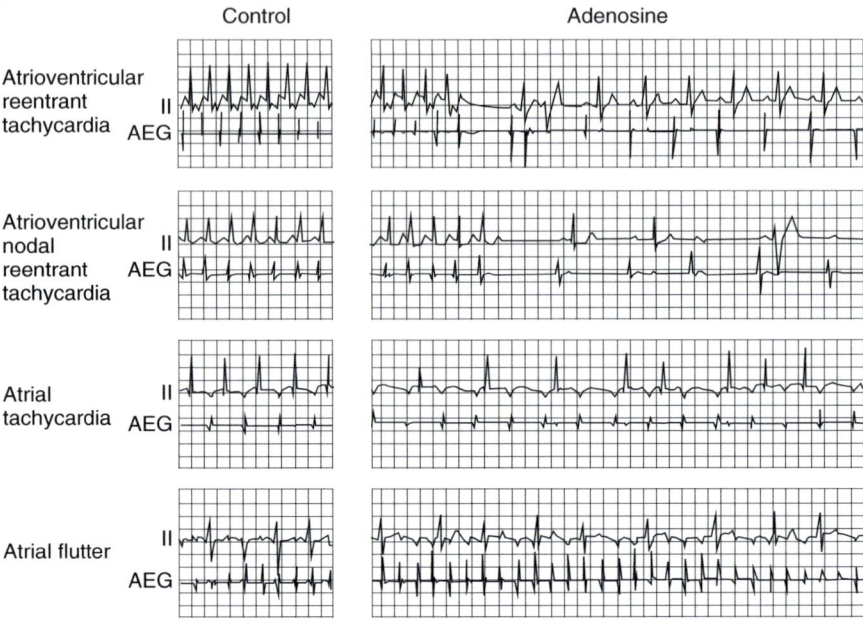

FIGURE 17.5. Effect of adenosine on atrioventricular reentrant tachycardia, atrioventricular nodal reentrant tachycardia, atrial tachycardia, and atrial flutter. Each panel shows the tracings for surface electrocardiographic lead II and an intracardiac bipolar high right atrial electrogram (AEG) that shows the position of the P waves. Retrograde P waves and QRS complexes are registered simultaneously during atrioventricular nodal reentrant tachycardia, whereas retrograde P waves are registered shortly after each QRS during atrioventricular reentrant tachycardia but with RP < PR. In both atrioventricular reentrant tachycardia and atrioventricular nodal reentrant tachycardia, adenosine blocks anterograde conduction in the atrioventricular node, causing termination of the tachycardia after a retrograde P wave. During atrial tachycardia, the RP interval is greater than the PR interval. Adenosine causes transient 2 : 1 atrioventricular conduction without affecting the atrial rate or interrupting the tachycardia, thus ruling out an accessory pathway as part of the mechanism of the tachycardia. During atrial flutter, there is 2 : 1 atrioventricular conduction, but only alternate P waves are visible on the surface electrocardiogram, with the RP interval apparently greater than the PR interval. Adenosine causes transient atrioventricular block, revealing typical flutter waves. (Reproduced from Ganz LI, Friedman PL. Supraventricular tachycardia. N Engl J Med 1995;332:162–173.)

Direct Current Cardioversion

Transthoracic electrical cardioversion is preferred in the setting of AMI over pharmacological cardioversion, with overall success rate of 75% to 93% (inversely related to the duration of atrial fibrillation, chest wall impedance, and left atrial size) [35–37] and lower risk of proarrhythmia [38]. The antero-posterior position is recommended as several studies have shown that less energy is required and higher success rate is achieved [35, 39, 40]. The energy required for cardioversion of atrial fibrillation is often ≥200 joules and 50 joules for atrial flutter, and biphasic devices have been shown to be more effective and require less energy than monophasic devices [35, 41, 42].

Rate Control with Medication

Usually in patients with AMI and atrial fibrillation, a fast ventricular rate is observed and symptoms are usually present depending upon the rapidity of the ventricular response [35]. Acute ventricular rate control is the primary goal initially, because patient's symptoms and degree of ischemia are chiefly governed by the rapid ventricular rate. Correction of ischemia, adrenergic surge, and pain often helps in controlling ventricular rates in addition to enhancing the chances for conversion to sinus rhythm. Rate control in ACS patients should ideally be a resting ventricular rate around 60 to 65 bpm. Atrioventricular node blocking agents including beta-adrenergic blockers, non–dihydropyridine calcium channel blockers, and digoxin are usually effective in controlling ventricular rate [35, 43]. The agent of first choice is usually individualized depending upon the clinical situation. Intravenous beta-blocker and non–dihydropyridine calcium channel blockers are equally effective in rapidly controlling the ventricular rate:

- Options include *metoprolol* (2.5 to 5.0 mg every 2 to 5 minutes to a total of 15 mg over 10 to 15 minutes), or *atenolol* (2.5 to 5.0 mg over 2 minutes to a total of 10 mg in 10 to 15 minutes), or *esmolol* in relative beta-blocker contraindication situations, starting with a bolus of up to 500 μg/kg, followed by continuous infusion of 50 to 200 μg kg^{-1} min^{-1}, to be titrated to a desirable heart rate [44].
- When beta-blockers are contraindicated (Table 17.1), intravenous *diltiazem* (20 mg [or 0.25 mg/kg] over 2 minutes followed by an infusion of 10 mg/hour), or intravenous *verapamil* (2.5 to 10 mg over 2 minutes; may repeat a 5 to 10 mg dose after 15 to 30 minutes) can be used.

TABLE **17.1.** Contraindications to beta-blocker therapy in STEMI.

Relative contraindications to beta-blocker therapy in patients with AMI	
1. Bradycardia	Heart rate less than 60 bpm
2. Hypotension	Blood pressure less than 100 mm Hg
3. Heart failure	Moderate or severe left ventricular failure
	Signs of peripheral hypoperfusion
	Shock
4. AV blocks	First-degree AV block with PR >240 milliseconds
	Second- or third-degree AV block
5. Reactive airway disease	Active asthma
	Severe chronic obstructive pulmonary disease
6. Myocardial infarction precipitated by cocaine use	

Source: Adapted from Antman EM, Anbe DT, Armstrong PW, et al. ACC/AHA guidelines for the management of patients with ST-elevation myocardial infarction—executive summary: a report of the American College of Cardiology/American Heart Association Task Force on Practice Guidelines (Writing Committee to Revise the 1999 Guidelines for the Management of Patients With Acute Myocardial Infarction). Circulation 2004;110:588–636.

The addition of *digoxin* to the regimen is helpful but digoxin as a single agent is generally less effective. Magnesium and amiodarone have also been used for acute ventricular rate control in atrial fibrillation [43, 45].

Anticoagulation

Continuation of the anticoagulation, which is initially started as part of the treatment for AMI, is a controversial issue. There are opinions that long-term therapy is generally not necessary if atrial fibrillation has been precipitated by a myocardial infarction, as this arrhythmia occurs in less than 1% of patients with chronic coronary disease [7, 16, 46, 47]. Other studies showed high recurrence of atrial tachyarrhythmias up to 30% in the first 30 days after myocardial infarction [48], and long-term oral anticoagulation for atrial fibrillation showed a 29% relative and 7% absolute reduction in 1-year mortality as reported by Stenestrand et al. [49] compared with antiplatelet therapy alone. Our recommendation would be to continue long-term oral anticoagulation with follow-up noninvasive monitoring and, if no recurrences, to stop after approximately 3 months.

Conclusion

Supraventricular tachyarrhythmias, in the setting of acute myocardial infarction, are relatively common and are associated with increased complication rates and higher short- and long-term mortality. This category of patients warrants more aggressive monitoring and management for rate control and anticoagulation therapy when indicated, which can lead to an improved outcome.

References

1. Bandiera A, Rosanio S, Tocchi M, et al. Supraventricular hyperkinetic arrhythmias in acute myocardial infarct: their prognostic assessment and correlation with the echocardiographic evolution. Cardiologia 1994;39:633–639.
2. Brazdzionyte J, Baksyte G. Risk assessment in acute myocardial infarction. Medicina (Kaunas) 2004;40:121–126.
3. Crimm A, Severance HW, Coffey K, et al. Prognostic significance of isolated sinus tachycardia during first three days of acute myocardial infarction. Am J Med 1984; 76:983–988.
4. Becker RC, Burns M, Gore JM, et al. Early assessment and in-hospital management of patients with acute myocardial infarction at increased risk for adverse outcomes: a nationwide perspective of current clinical practice. The National Registry of Myocardial Infarction (NRMI-2). Am Heart J 1998;135:786–796.
5. Arnsdorf MF, Ganz LI. Approach to narrow QRS complex tachycardias. Up to date. 14.2 ed. 2006.
6. Olgin JE, Zipes DP. Specific arrhythmias: diagnosis and treatment. In: Braunwald E, Zipes DP, eds. Zipes: Braunwald's heart disease: a textbook of cardiovascular medicine, 7th ed. Philadelphia: WB Saunders; 2005:803–836.

7. Podrid PJ. Supraventricular arrhythmias after myocardial infarction. Up to date. 14.2 ed. 2006.
8. Madias JE, Patel DC, Singh D. Atrial fibrillation in acute myocardial infarction: a prospective study based on data from a consecutive series of patients admitted to the coronary care unit. Clin Cardiol 1996;19:180–186.
9. Blumlein SL, Armstrong R, Haywood LJ. Atrial flutter associated with acute myocardial infarction. West J Med 1981;135:97–103.
10. Tjandrawidjaja MC, Fu Y, Kim DH, et al. Compromised atrial coronary anatomy is associated with atrial arrhythmias and atrioventricular block complicating acute myocardial infarction. J Electrocardiol 2005;38:271–278.
11. Goldberg RJ, Seeley D, Becker RC, et al. Impact of atrial fibrillation on the in-hospital and long-term survival of patients with acute myocardial infarction: a community-wide perspective. Am Heart J 1990;119:996–1001.
12. Galcera TJ, Melgarejo MA, Garcia AA, et al. Incidence, clinical characteristics and prognostic significance of supraventricular tachyarrhythmias in acute myocardial infarction. Rev Esp Cardiol 1999;52:647–655.
13. Crenshaw BS, Ward SR, Granger CB, et al. Atrial fibrillation in the setting of acute myocardial infarction: the GUSTO-I experience. J Am Coll Cardiol 1997;30:406–413.
14. Wong CK, White HD, Wilcox RG, et al. New atrial fibrillation after acute myocardial infarction independently predicts death: the GUSTO-III experience. Am Heart J 2000;140:878–885.
15. Pizzetti F, Turazza FM, Franzosi MG, et al. Incidence and prognostic significance of atrial fibrillation in acute myocardial infarction: the GISSI-3 data. Heart 2001;86:527–532.
16. Eldar M, Canetti M, Rotstein Z, et al. Significance of paroxysmal atrial fibrillation complicating acute myocardial infarction in the thrombolytic era. SPRINT and Thrombolytic Survey Groups. Circulation 1998;97:965–970.
17. Blomström-Lundqvist, Scheinman MM, Aliot EM. ACC/AHA/ESC guidelines for the management of patients with supraventricular arrhythmias. J Am Coll Cardiol 2003;42:1493–1531.
18. Fogoros R. Abnormal heart rhythms. In: Forgoros R, ed. Electrophysiologic testing. Massachusetts: Blackwell; 2006:12–21.
19. Aufderheide TP. Arrhythmias associated with acute myocardial infarction and thrombolysis. Emerg Med Clin North Am 1998;16:583–600.
20. Antman EM, Braunwald E. ST-elevation myocardial infarction: pathology, pathophysiology, and clinical features; arrhythmias. In: Braunwald E, Zipes DP, eds. Zipes: Braunwald's heart disease: a textbook of cardiovascular medicine. 7th ed. Philadelphia: WB Saunders; 2005:1207–1218.
21. Kyriakidis M, Barbetseas J, Antonopoulos A, et al. Early atrial arrhythmias in acute myocardial infarction. Role of the sinus node artery. Chest 1992;101:944–947.
22. Hod J, Lew AS, Keltai M. Early atrial fibrillation during evolving myocardial infarction: a consequence of impaired left atrial perfusion. Circulation 1987;75:146–150.
23. Lokshyn S, Mewis C, Kuhlkamp V. Atrial fibrillation in coronary artery disease. Int J Cardiol 2000;72:133–136.
24. Celik S, Erdol C, Baykan M, et al. Relation between paroxysmal atrial fibrillation and left ventricular diastolic function in patients with acute myocardial infarction. Am J Cardiol 2001;88:160–162.

25. Serrano CV Jr, Ramires JA, Mansur AP, et al. Importance of the time of onset of supraventricular tachyarrhythmias on prognosis of patients with acute myocardial infarction. Clin Cardiol 1995;18:84–90.

26. Latoguz IK, Ovcharenko LI, Shapkin EI, et al. Pathogenetic mechanisms of the development of cardiac rhythm disorders in the acute period of myocardial infarction. Kardiologiia 1988;28:38–41.

27. Kyriakidis M, Vyssoulis G, Barbetseas J, et al. A clinical angiographic study of the arterial blood supply to the sinus node. Chest 1988;94:1054–1057.

28. James TN, Burch GE. The atrial coronary arteries in man. Circulation 1958;17:90–98.

29. Gensini GG, Buonanno C, Palacio A. Anatomy of the coronary circulation in living man. Dis Chest 1967;52:125.

30. Nielsen FE, Andersen HH, Gram-Hansen P, et al. The relationship between ECG signs of atrial infarction and the development of supraventricular arrhy-thmias in patients with acute myocardial infarction. Am Heart J 1992;123:69–72.

31. Olgin JE, Zipes DP. Specific arrhythmias: diagnosis and treatment. In: Braunwald DPZE, ed. Zipes: Braunwald's heart disease: a textbook of cardiovascular medicine. 7th ed. Philadelphia: WB Saunders; 2005:803–863.

32. Berisso MZ, Ferroni A, Molini D, et al. Supraventricular tachyarrhythmias during acute myocardial infarction: short- and mid-term clinical significance, therapy and prevention of relapse. G Ital Cardiol 1991;21:49–58.

33. Herzog E, Saint-Jacques H, Rozanski A. The PAIN pathway as a tool to bridge the gap between evidence and management of acute coronary syndrome. Crit Pathways Cardiol 2004;3:20–24.

34. Antman EM, Anbe DT, Armstrong PW, et al. ACC/AHA guidelines for the management of patients with ST-elevation myocardial infarction—executive summary: a report of the American College of Cardiology/American Heart Association Task Force on Practice Guidelines (Writing Committee to Revise the 1999 Guidelines for the Management of Patients With Acute Myocardial Infarction). Circulation 2004; 110:588–636.

35. Herzog E, Steinberg JS. Management of atrial fibrillation and atrial flutter. In: Cannon CPOGP, ed. Critical pathways in cardiovascular medicine. 2nd ed: Philadelphia: Lippincott Williams & Wilkins; 2006:181–189.

36. Dalzell GW, Anderson J, Adgey AA. Factors determining success and energy requirement for cardioversion of atrial fibrillation. Q J Med 1990;76:903–913.

37. Gallagher MM, Guo XH, Poloniecki JD, et al. Initial energy sitting, outcome and efficiency in direct current cardioversion of atrial fibrillation. J Am Coll Cardiol 2001;38:1498–1504.

38. Boriani G, Diemberger I, Biffi M, et al. Pharmacological cardioversion of atrial fibrillation: current management and treatment options. Drugs 2004;64:2741–2762.

39. Kirchhof O, Eckardt L, Loh P, et al. Anterior-posterior versus anterior-lateral electrode positions for external cardioversion of atrial fibrillation. Lancet 2002;360:1275–1279.

40. Myerburg RJ, Castellanos A. Electrode positioning for cardioversion of atrial fibrillation. Lancet 2002;360:1263–1264.

41. Page RL, Kerber RE, Russell JK, et al. Biphasic versus monophasic shock waveform for conversion of atrial fibrillation. The result of an international randomized, double-blind multicenter trial. J Am Coll Cardial 2002;39:1956–1963.

42. Ricard P, Levy S, Trigamo J, et al. Prospective assessment of the minimum energy needed for external cardioversion of atrial fibrillation. Am J Cardiol 1997;79:815–816.
43. Herzog E, Fischer A, Steinberg JS. The rate control, anticoagulation therapy, and electrophysiology/antiarrhythmic medication pathway for the management of atrial fibrillation and atrial flutter. Crit Pathways Cardiol 2005:121–126.
44. Barbier GH, Shettigar UR, Appunn DO. Clinical rationale for the use of an ultra-short acting beta-blocker: esmolol. Int J Clin Pharmacol Ther 1995;33:212–218.
45. Cybulski J, Kulakowski P, Makowska E, et al. Intravenous amiodarone is safe and seems to be effective in termination of paroxysmal supraventricular tachyarrhythmias. Clin Cardiol 1996;19:563–566.
46. Cameron A, Schwartz MJ, Kronmal RA, et al. Prevalence and significance of atrial fibrillation in coronary artery disease (CASS Registry). Am J Cardiol 1988;61:714–717.
47. Sakata K, Kurihara H, Iwamori K, et al. Clinical and prognostic significance of atrial fibrillation in acute myocardial infarction. Am J Cardiol 1997;80:1522–1527.
48. Huikuri HV, Mahaux V, Bloch-Thomsen PE. Cardiac arrhythmias and risk stratification after myocardial infarction: results of the CARISMA pilot study. Pacing Clin Electrophysiol 2003;26:416–419.
49. Stenestrand U, Lindback J, Wallentin L. Anticoagulation therapy in atrial fibrillation in combination with acute myocardial infarction influences long-term outcome: a prospective cohort study from the Register of Information and Knowledge About Swedish Heart Intensive Care Admissions (RIKS-HIA). Circulation 2005;112:3225–3231.

18
Ventricular Arrhythmias in Patients After Myocardial Infarction

Delia Cotiga, Tina Sichrovsky, Kataneh Maleki, and Suneet Mittal

Ventricular arrhythmias, ranging from premature ventricular contractions (PVCs) to ventricular fibrillation (VF), occur frequently in patients after acute myocardial infarction (AMI) [1]. The prognostic significance of these arrhythmias as well as their optimal management is largely dependent on several factors (Table 18.1): time from AMI, type of ventricular arrhythmia, and extent of myocardial dysfunction. In this chapter, we discuss specific ventricular arrhythmias observed in patients after MI and their significance, the impact of current medical therapy on the incidence of sudden cardiac death, and the role of antiarrhythmic drugs and implantable cardioverter-defibrillators in the management of post-MI patients.

Specific Arrhythmias

Premature Ventricular Contractions

Premature ventricular contractions are seen in most patients after AMI. In the thrombolytic era, predischarge 24-hour ambulatory electrocardiographic recordings demonstrate some degree of ventricular ectopy in up to 64% of patients [1]. When observed >48 hours after an AMI, frequent PVCs (>10/h) appear to be associated with adverse prognosis [1, 2]. In the GISSI-2 trial, PVCs were an independent predictor of overall and sudden mortality within the first 6 months after AMI, with a relative risk (RR) of 1.62 and 2.24, respectively [1].

Accelerated Idioventricular Rhythm

Accelerated idioventricular rhythm (AIVR) is characterized by a wide QRS complex, with a regular rate higher than the atrial rate and lower than 100 beats per minute (bpm) [3]; this can represent an escape rhythm or an accelerated ectopic focus from the ventricle. Although AIVR is frequently found in the first 12 hours of AMI, it does not appear to be a risk factor for the development of VF [4]. In patients who receive thrombolytics, AIVR has been shown to be a

TABLE **18.1.** Ventricular arrhythmias in AMI.

	Time			
	AMI 24 hrs	48 hrs		40 days
	●————————————|—|————————————➤		
Pathophysiology	↓ATP, local electrolyte imbalance→ ↑automaticity, ↑triggered activity (transient)	Abnormal gap junctions in border zone of healing infarct and viable myocardium→ slow, inhomogeneous conduction→ reentry (substrate starts to form within 2 weeks after MI and remains indefinitely)		
Dominant ventricular arrhythmia	PVCs, AIVR, VF	PVCs, NSVT, monomorphic VT		Monomorphic VT
Therapy	Revascularization, beta-blockers, ACE-inhibitors, statins	Rule out/ treat ischemia Beta-blockers, ACE inhibitors, statins, ICDs (if sustained arrhythmia)		ICD

AMI, acute myocardial infarction; ATP, adenosinetriphosphate; PVC, premature ventricular contraction; AIVR, accelerated idioventricular rhythm; VF, ventricular fibrillation; NSVT, non-sustained ventricular tachycardia; VT, ventricular tachycardia; ICD, implantable cardiac defibrillator.

marker for both myocardial necrosis and reperfusion of the infarct vessel. In fact, the QRS morphology of the AIVR may be useful for the noninvasive identification of the infarct vessel [5].

Nonsustained Ventricular Tachycardia

Nonsustained ventricular tachycardia (NSVT) is defined as ≥3 consecutive ventricular ectopic beats at a rate of >100 bpm lasting <30 seconds and not accompanied by hemodynamic collapse [6]. Its incidence after AMI ranges from 1% to 7% [7, 8]. In the early postinfarct period, electrical instability caused by abnormal automaticity within surviving Purkinje fibers, triggered activity arising from Purkinje fibers, or reentry involving either the Purkinje fibers or within the ischemic myocardium is the likely mechanism [9]; NSVT that occurs later is likely due to reentry involving a fixed substrate [6]. The prognostic significance of NSVT depends on its time of occurrence with respect to the AMI. Likely benign in the early peri-infarct period, its association with early mortality increases as time progresses, becoming significant at 13 hours after infarction and plateauing at approximately 24 hours (relative risk 7.5) [9].

Sustained Ventricular Tachycardia

Sustained ventricular tachycardia (VT) is defined as a regular, wide-complex tachycardia of ventricular origin lasting ≥30 seconds or accompanied by hemodynamic instability requiring cardioversion or defibrillation. Sustained monomorphic VT can occur in nearly 2% of patients within 48 hours of AMI [10]. Its occurrence during the first 48 hours of myocardial infarction (MI) is often a sign of extensive myocardial damage and is an independent predictor of in-hospital mortality [10]. Beyond 48 hours of MI, sustained VT is considered a marker of a fixed arrhythmic substrate and a marker of long-term risk of recurrence of ventricular tachyarrhythmia and sudden cardiac death.

Ventricular Fibrillation

Ventricular fibrillation is a rapid, disorganized rhythm originating in the ventricles, which is not accompanied by organized ventricular contraction and results in hemodynamic collapse. It is the most frequent cause of sudden cardiac death. It can occur de novo; more commonly, it degenerates from preceding monomorphic VT. Primary VF occurs in ~4% to 6% of patients with AMI with a peak incidence in the first 4 hours after AMI [11–13]. As such, it is a frequent cause of out-of-hospital cardiac arrest in the early postinfarct period. The risk of primary VF is influenced by the cumulative ST-segment deviation during AMI and family history of sudden death [14]. Once VF occurs, rapid restoration of the normal rhythm via unsynchronized electrical shock (defibrillation) with at least 200 to 360 joules monophasic or 120 to 200 joules biphasic shock is necessary. When VF persists, administration of epinephrine intravenously (1 mg) may facilitate subsequent defibrillation attempts. Shock-refractory VF may be treated with amiodarone bolus (300 mg or 5 mg/kg) followed by repeat defibrillation [4]. The arrhythmia may indicate ongoing myocardial ischemia and often requires effective anti-ischemic interventions, including revascularization.

Therapeutic Approach

Ventricular arrhythmias occur during the acute (within 48 hours), late (days to weeks), and chronic (months to years) phases of MI. In the early days of modern coronary care units, lidocaine was used widely in an attempt to prevent VF during the acute phase of MI. However, analysis of available pooled data suggests that although prophylactic administration of lidocaine does reduce the incidence of VT and VF, its use is associated with excess mortality [15]. The latter may in part be due to a higher likelihood of developing asystole and atrioventricular block in patients treated with lidocaine. As a result, the prophylactic use of lidocaine in AMI is no longer recommended. Today, interventions are mainly targeted at reducing the incidence of ventricular arrhythmias occurring during the late and chronic phases of MI.

Medical Therapy

Beta-Blockers

The first class of drugs shown to reduce the incidence of sudden death after AMI were beta-blockers, which have become an essential component in the treatment of acute coronary syndromes. Beta-blockers effectively suppress a wide spectrum of ventricular arrhythmias, ranging from isolated PVCs to VF [16–18] and reduce mortality due to sudden death by 32% to 50% and overall mortality by 25% to 40% [19–22]. An overview including more than 26,000 patients demonstrated that beta-blockers given early intravenously in AMI conclusively reduced mortality [23], at least to some extent by preventing VF [24]. More recently, two studies have evaluated the effect of beta-blockers on sudden death reduction in a post-MI population in the angiotensin-converting enzyme (ACE) inhibitor era. The carvedilol postinfarct survival control in LV dysfunction (CAPRICORN) study randomized 1,959 postinfarct patients (3 to 21 days after MI) with left ventricular dysfunction (ejection fraction ≤40%) to receive either carvedilol or placebo. All patients were already receiving an ACE inhibitor. Treatment with carvedilol was associated with a non-significant 26% reduction in incidence of sudden death [25]. Of note, therapy with carvedilol reduced the incidence of VT/VF from 3.9% to 0.9% during the follow-up period [26]. The metoprolol CR/XL randomized intervention trial in congestive heart failure (MERIT-HF) found that addition of long-acting metoprolol in patients with left ventricular dysfunction (ejection fraction ≤40%) and overt congestive heart failure (New York Heart Association [NYHA] class II to IV) to a medical regiment that already included an ACE inhibitor and a diuretic reduced the primary end point of total mortality or all-cause hospitalization by 19% [27]. The study included a prespecified substudy of 1,926 patients with history of hospitalization for AMI. In most patients, the MI had occurred more than 1 year prior to enrollment into the study. Active treatment was shown to reduce sudden death by 50% [28]. In sum, these data demonstrate the profound impact of beta-blockers in the prevention of sudden death, especially in patients with concomitant congestive heart failure.

ACE Inhibitors

Although a cornerstone in the therapy in patients with heart failure and left ventricular dysfunction, the efficacy of ACE inhibitors in reducing the incidence of sudden death in these patients has been difficult to demonstrate. In fact, in a heart failure population, the major benefit of ACE inhibitors appears to be to slow progression of heart failure [29]. A number of studies have evaluated the role of ACE inhibitors specifically in the post-MI setting. The survival and ventricular enlargement (SAVE) trial randomized 2,231 post-MI patients (3 to 16 days after infarction) with left ventricular ejection fraction

≤40% without overt heart failure or myocardial ischemia to receive either captopril or placebo. Although captopril reduced all-cause mortality by 19%, no significant reduction in incidence of sudden death could be demonstrated [30]. The survival of myocardial infarction long-term evaluation (SMILE) study randomized 1,556 patients to receive either zofenopril or placebo within 24 hours of AMI. Patients were treated for only 6 weeks. Again, zofenopril reduced major cardiovascular events (death or severe congestive heart failure) by 34% but did not lead to a significant reduction in likelihood of sudden death [31]. The trandolapril cardiac evaluation (TRACE) study randomized 1,749 postinfarct patients (3 to 7 days after MI) with left ventricular dysfunction (ejection fraction ≤35%) to receive either trandolapril or placebo. In contrast with the prior studies, in addition to a 22% reduction in overall mortality, treatment with trandolapril was associated with a 24% reduction in sudden death [32]. Of note, survival curves for freedom from sudden death began to diverge within the first few weeks of active treatment. Finally, the acute infarction ramipril efficacy (AIRE) study evaluated 2,006 postinfarct patients (3 to 10 days after MI) who developed transient or persistent evidence of congestive heart failure. Patients were randomized to receive either ramipril or placebo. Sudden death accounted for 54% of all deaths and 93% of out-of-hospital deaths. Treatment with ramipril reduced the risk of sudden death by 30% [33]. In sum, these data support the routine use of ACE inhibitors after MI. In this patient population, reductions in total mortality can be accounted for by reduction in sudden death, as well as reduction in death due to pump failure.

3-Hydroxy-3-Methyglutaryl Coenzyme A Reductase Inhibitors (Statins)

Statins and other lipid-lowering drugs have impressive beneficial effects on cardiovascular and all-cause mortality [34–37]. In addition, it has been suggested that these drugs have antiarrhythmic properties [34, 36]. Although a number of putative mechanisms have been proposed, no one mechanism has been identified to explain the observed antiarrhythmic effect of these medications. A post hoc analysis of the antiarrhythmics versus implantable defibrillator (AVID) trial found that statin therapy was associated with a 40% reduction in the incidence of VT/VF in the patients randomized to receive an implantable cardioverter-defibrillator (ICD) [38]. Similar findings were reported from a primary prevention ICD trial. Specifically, in the multicenter automatic defibrillator implantation trial (MADIT)-II study, statin use was associated with a 28% reduction in risk for first episode of VT/VF [39]. Given the demonstrated efficacy of statins in a post-MI population, it is unlikely that a randomized, placebo-controlled trial will ever be performed to specifically address the issue of antiarrhythmic effects of statin therapy.

Aldosterone Antagonists

Aldosterone blockade with spironolactone has been shown to reduce the burden of ventricular ectopy as assessed by 24-hour ambulatory ECG recordings and improve heart rate variability [29]. The eplerenone post–acute myocardial infarction heart failure efficacy and survival (EPHESUS) study randomized 6,632 postinfarct patients (3 to 14 days after MI) with left ventricular systolic dysfunction (ejection fraction ≤40%) and heart failure (or diabetes mellitus) to receive either eplerenone, a selective aldosterone receptor antagonist, or placebo. Eplerenone, added to optimal medical therapy (which included beta-blockers in 75% of patients), reduced overall mortality by 15% and sudden cardiac death (SCD) by 21% [40]. The reduction in sudden death was even greater (33%) in patients with an ejection fraction ≤30% [41].

Antiarrhythmic Drug Therapy

A number of observational studies have shown an association between ventricular ectopy and excess mortality in a post-MI population. Because antiarrhythmic drugs effectively suppress ventricular ectopy, it was natural to assume that these agents would be highly efficacious in a post-MI population with underlying ventricular ectopy. A number of trials have evaluated the utility of various antiarrhythmic drugs for the prophylaxis against sudden cardiac death in a post-MI patient population. However, none of these antiarrhythmic drugs has been shown to favorably impact on the reduction of sudden cardiac death.

Type I Antiarrhythmic Drugs

The cardiac arrhythmia suppression trial (CAST) enrolled patients with prior MI (between 6 days and 2 years prior to enrollment), ≥6 PVCs/h, and reduced left ventricular ejection fraction (≤40%; ≤55% if the MI occurred within 3 months of enrollment). Patients underwent open titration with a type I antiarrhythmic drug (encainide, flecainide, or moricizine); patients who tolerated the medication and in whom the ventricular ectopy was suppressed were then randomized to one of these medications or placebo. Active therapy was associated with *excess* mortality, including an excess of arrhythmic deaths [42]. This trial effectively ended the use of these medications in patients with ischemic heart disease.

Sotalol

Sotalol is a racemic mixture of the *d-* (pure type III antiarrhythmic drug) and *l-* (beta-blocker) stereoisomers. The survival with oral *d*-sotalol (SWORD) trial evaluated 3,121 postinfarct patients (6 to 42 days after MI or >42 days after MI if heart failure was present) with left ventricular dysfunction (ejection fraction ≤40%). At the time the trial was designed, it was believed that patients with depressed ventricular function and symptomatic heart failure would not be able to tolerate beta blockade; hence, the *d*-isomer of sotalol was chosen for the study. The trial was terminated prematurely because of a 65% increase in risk of death in patients randomized to active treatment [43]. One trial evaluated sotalol at a dose of 320 mg once daily versus placebo in 1,456 postinfarct patients (5 to 14 days after MI). All patients were followed for a year. No difference in overall mortality was observed between the two groups [44].

Dofetilide

The Danish investigators of arrhythmia and mortality on dofetilide (DIAMOND)-MI study was designed to evaluate the efficacy of dofetilide (another type III antiarrhythmic drug) in post-MI patients with left ventricular dysfunction. The study enrolled 1,510 patients with left ventricular dysfunction (ejection fraction ≤35%). Dofetilide effectively suppressed atrial arrhythmias in these patients; however, no effect on arrhythmic or all-cause mortality was observed [45].

Azimilide

Azimilide in a unique antiarrhythmic drug that blocks both the slow and rapid components of the delayed rectifier potassium current. The azimilide postinfarct survival evaluation (ALIVE) investigators enrolled 3,717 postinfarct patients (5 to 21 days after MI) with an ejection fraction between 15% and 35% and randomized them to receive either azimilide 100 mg or placebo. No difference in overall mortality was observed in the two groups [46]. Azimilide reduced the incidence of atrial arrhythmias; however, active therapy was associated with increased risk of torsades de pointes and neutropenia.

Amiodarone

Initial observational studies suggested that amiodarone may have a favorable effect on total mortality in patients at high risk for sudden death. Two trials, the European myocardial infarction amiodarone trial (EMIAT) and the Canadian amiodarone myocardial infarction arrhythmia trial (CAMIAT), have specifically evaluated the utility of amiodarone in post-MI patients [47, 48]. CAMIAT enrolled 1,202 postinfarct patients (6 to 45 days after MI) with ≥10 PVCs/h; EMIAT enrolled 1,486 postinfarct patients (5 to 21 days after MI) and left ventricular ejection fraction ≤40%. Neither study showed a favorable impact on total mortality with amiodarone; importantly, however, amiodarone was not associated with excess mortality. More recently, the sudden cardiac death in heart failure trial (SCD-HeFT) evaluated the role of amiodarone (in comparison with an ICD and placebo) in patients with a cardiomyopathy (ejection fraction ≤35%) and NYHA class II or III congestive heart failure [49]. No benefit was observed with amiodarone as compared with placebo.

Implantable Cardioverter-Defibrillator

Secondary Prevention

In postinfarct patients, an ICD should be considered in all patients with a sustained ventricular arrhythmia, especially when the event is not related to acute ischemia and occurs in the setting of left ventricular dysfunction. The AVID trial randomized 1,016 patients who were resuscitated from hemodynamically significant VT or VF to either an ICD or an antiarrhythmic drug, which was almost always amiodarone [50]. ICD implantation was associated with a significant increase in survival. These findings were corroborated by the cardiac arrest study Hamburg (CASH) and the Canadian implantable defibrillator study (CIDS) [51, 52].

Primary Prevention

Given the association of sudden cardiac death with underlying structural heart disease, most commonly coronary artery disease, it is not surprising that a great deal of effort has been spent in trying to identify appropriate candidates for ICD implantation to *prevent* sudden death (Table 18.2). Toward this end, a number of trials have recently been completed.

The multicenter automatic defibrillator implantation trial (MADIT) enrolled patients with history of MI (≥3 weeks before entry), documented nonsustained VT (asymptomatic) and left ventricular dysfunction (ejection fraction ≤35%). All patients underwent electrophysiologic testing. Patients in whom a sustained ventricular arrhythmia was inducible and not suppressible acutely with intravenous procainamide were randomized to receive either an ICD or continued conventional medical therapy [53]. In this study, ICD implantation was associated with a 54% reduction in mortality. Of note, in three-fourths of the patients, the most recent MI had occurred more than 6 months prior to enrollment in the study.

The multicenter unsustained tachycardia trial (MUSTT) enrolled patients with prior MI and a left ventricular ejection fraction ≤40%. All patients needed to demonstrate at least one episode of nonsustained VT, ≥96 hours after MI or revascularization. Of note, in ≥80% of patients, the qualifying MI had occurred

TABLE 18.2. ICD trials for primary prevention in post-MI patients.

Study	n	Days after MI	Qualifying arrhythmia	EF (%)	EPS	Hazard ratio (range)
MADIT [53]	196	>21	Yes (NSVT)	≤35	Yes	0.46 (0.26–0.82)
MUSTT [54]	704	>4	Yes (NSVT)	≤40	Yes	0.42 (0.28–0.62)
MADIT-II [55]	1,232	>28	Not required	≤30	No	0.69 (0.51–0.93)
DINAMIT [57]	674	6–40	Not required*	≤35	No	No benefit

ICD, implantable cardioverter-defibrillator; MI, myocardial infarction; EF, ejection fraction; EPS, electrophysiologic study; NSVT, nonsustained ventricular tachycardia.
*Depressed heart rate variability was required.

≥1 month prior to enrollment, and in ~60% of patients, the qualifying MI had occurred ≥1 year prior to enrollment. The primary objective of the this trial was to evaluate the efficacy of antiarrhythmic therapy guided by electrophysiologic testing in reducing the risk of sudden death and cardiac arrest in this patient population. A secondary goal was to evaluate the usefulness of electrophysiologic testing for risk stratification [54]. All patients underwent electrophysiologic testing. Patients in whom a sustained ventricular arrhythmia was not inducible were followed in a registry. Inducible patients were randomized to no therapy or to electrophysiology-guided therapy, which included ICD implantation in patients in whom ventricular tachycardia could not be suppressed with antiarrhythmic medications. In essence, patients implanted with an ICD derived maximal benefit. Importantly, noninducible patients still had a 12% risk of cardiac arrest/arrhythmic death during 2 years of follow-up [54].

The relatively high event rate in noninducible patients raised the issue of whether electrophysiologic testing was an appropriate method to risk-stratify postinfarct patients. Toward this end, the multicenter automatic defibrillator implantation trial (MADIT)-II enrolled patients with prior MI (≥4 weeks before entry) and left ventricular ejection fraction ≤30%. Of note, in this trial, 88% of patients had suffered their MI more than 6 months prior to enrollment. Patient having undergone percutaneous coronary revascularization or coronary artery bypass grafting surgery within 3 months were specifically excluded. Once again, ICD implantation was associated with improved overall survival [55].

Although MADIT, MUSTT, and MADIT-II clearly demonstrated the utility of prophylactic ICD implantation in patients with an ischemic cardiomyopathy, these studies either excluded patients early post-MI or did not actually enroll patients who had recently suffered a MI. This is of importance because sudden death frequently occurs in the early post-MI period. The valsartan in acute myocardial infarction trial (VALIANT) enrolled 14,703 patients with a MI complicated by heart failure, left ventricular dysfunction (ejection fraction ≤40%), or both. Patients were randomized to receive captopril, valsartan, or both. The highest risk of sudden death (1.4% per month) was observed in the first 30 days of MI; patients with severe left ventricular dysfunction (ejection fraction ≤30%) were at highest risk (2.3% per month event rate) [56].

Although these data suggest that there may be an opportunity to intervene with ICDs early after MI, the available data do not support their efficacy in this patient population. The defibrillators in acute myocardial infarction trial (DINAMIT) randomized 674 postinfarct patients (6 to 40 days after MI) with left ventricular dysfunction (ejection fraction ≤35%) and depressed heart rate variability to receive either an ICD or continued medical therapy. No difference in overall mortality was observed in the two groups [57]. Although ICDs were associated with a reduction in the rate of arrhythmic death, this was offset by an increase in the rate of death from nonarrhythmic causes [57].

Finally, it has been asked whether electrophysiologic testing in the early post-MI setting can identify patients most likely to benefit from ICD implantation. The beta-blocker strategy plus ICD (BEST-ICD) trial evaluated 1,060 postinfarct patients (5 to 30 days after MI) with left ventricular dysfunction (ejection fraction $\leq$35%) and one other high-risk marker of sudden death. The latter included $\geq$10 PVCs/h, depressed heart rate variability or an abnormal signal-averaged electrocardiogram. Patients were randomized in a 2:3 manner to either conventional management or an electrophysiology study–guided approach, in which patients with inducible VT/VF underwent ICD implantation. Ultimately, only 138 patients were randomized, and no difference in outcome was observed between the two strategies [58].

Conclusion

Ventricular arrhythmias remain an important concern after AMI. Appropriate revascularization followed by evidence-based medical therapies, including beta-blockers, ACE inhibitors, statins, and (when appropriate) aldosterone antagonists, remain a cornerstone of therapy. However, some patients remain at risk for sudden death, most commonly due to a sustained ventricular arrhythmia.

The ICD has been demonstrated to be the most effective intervention against sudden death. However, ICDs do not appear to be of benefit within the first 40 days of MI (and are generally excluded within 3 months of revascularization). Currently available data show that patients in whom ventricular function remains depressed (ejection fraction $\leq$35%) 3 months after MI and revascularization benefit from ICD implantation. Whether an electrophysiologic testing–guided approach is warranted in certain high-risk patients during this "waiting period" remains to be determined. In the future, additional tools for risk stratification will be necessary and welcomed.

References

1. Maggioni AP, Zuanetti G, Franzosi MG, et al. Prevalence and prognostic significance of ventricular arrhythmias after acute myocardial infarction in the fibrinolytic era. GISSI-2 results. Circulation 1993;87:312–322.
2. Andresen D, Bethge KP, Boissel JP, et al. Importance of quantitative analysis of ventricular arrhythmias for predicting the prognosis in low-risk postmyocardial infarction patients. European Infarction Study Group. Eur Heart J 1990;11:529–536.
3. Antman EM, Anbe DT, Armstrong PW, et al. ACC/AHA guidelines for the management of patients with ST-elevation myocardial infarction—executive summary. A report of the American College of Cardiology/American Heart Association Task Force on Practice Guidelines (Writing Committee to revise the 1999 guidelines for the management of patients with acute myocardial infarction). J Am Coll Cardiol 2004;44:671–719.
4. Dhurandhar RW, MacMillan RL, Brown KW. Primary ventricular fibrillation complicating acute myocardial infarction. Am J Cardiol 1971;27:347–351.
5. Gorgels AP, Vos MA, Letsch IS, et al. Usefulness of the accelerated idioventricular rhythm as a marker for myocardial necrosis and reperfusion during thrombolytic therapy in acute myocardial infarction. Am J Cardiol 1988;61:231–235.

6. Zipes DP, Camm AJ, Borggrefe M, et al. ACC/AHA/ESC 2006 guidelines for management of patients with ventricular arrhythmias and the prevention of sudden cardiac death: a report of the American College of Cardiology/American Heart Association Task Force and the European Society of Cardiology Committee for Practice Guidelines (Writing Committee to Develop Guidelines for Management of Patients With Ventricular Arrhythmias and the Prevention of Sudden Cardiac Death). J Am Coll Cardiol 2006;48:e247–346.
7. Eldar M, Sievner Z, Goldbourt U, et al. Primary ventricular tachycardia in acute myocardial infarction: clinical characteristics and mortality. The SPRINT Study Group. Ann Intern Med 1992;117:31–36.
8. Heidbuchel H, Tack J, Vanneste L, et al. Significance of arrhythmias during the first 24 hours of acute myocardial infarction treated with alteplase and effect of early administration of a beta-blocker or a bradycardiac agent on their incidence. Circulation 1994;89:1051–1059.
9. Cheema AN, Sheu K, Parker M, et al. Nonsustained ventricular tachycardia in the setting of acute myocardial infarction: tachycardia characteristics and their prognostic implications. Circulation 1998;98:2030–2036.
10. Mont L, Cinca J, Blanch P, et al. Predisposing factors and prognostic value of sustained monomorphic ventricular tachycardia in the early phase of acute myocardial infarction. J Am Coll Cardiol 1996;28:1670–1676.
11. Volpi A, Cavalli A, Santoro L, et al. Incidence and prognosis of early primary ventricular fibrillation in acute myocardial infarction—results of the Gruppo Italiano per lo Studio della Sopravvivenza nell'Infarto Miocardico (GISSI-2) database. Am J Cardiol 1998;82:265–271.
12. Henkel DM, Witt BJ, Gersh BJ, et al. Ventricular arrhythmias after acute myocardial infarction: a 20-year community study. Am Heart J 2006;151:806–812.
13. Campbell RW, Murray A, Julian DG. Ventricular arrhythmias in first 12 hours of acute myocardial infarction. Natural history study. Br Heart J 1981;46:351–357.
14. Dekker LR, Bezzina CR, Henriques JP, et al. Familial sudden death is an important risk factor for primary ventricular fibrillation: a case-control study in acute myocardial infarction patients. Circulation 2006;114:1140–1145.
15. Sadowski ZP, Alexander JH, Skrabucha B, et al. Multicenter randomized trial and a systematic overview of lidocaine in acute myocardial infarction. Am Heart J 1999; 137:792–798.
16. Norris RM, Barnaby PF, Brown MA, et al. Prevention of ventricular fibrillation during acute myocardial infarction by intravenous propranolol. Lancet 1984;2: 883–886.
17. Reiter MJ, Reiffel JA. Importance of beta blockade in the therapy of serious ventricular arrhythmias. Am J Cardiol 1998;82:9I–19I.
18. Ellison KE, Hafley GE, Hickey K, et al. Effect of beta-blocking therapy on outcome in the Multicenter UnSustained Tachycardia Trial (MUSTT). Circulation 2002;106: 2694–2699.
19. A randomized trial of propranolol in patients with acute myocardial infarction. I. Mortality results. JAMA 1982;247:1707–1714.
20. Hjalmarson A. Effects of beta blockade on sudden cardiac death during acute myocardial infarction and the postinfarction period. Am J Cardiol 1997;80:35J–39J.
21. Yusuf S, Wittes J, Friedman L. Overview of results of randomized clinical trials in heart disease. I. Treatments following myocardial infarction. JAMA 1988;260: 2088–2093.

22. Janosi A, Ghali JK, Herlitz J, et al. Metoprolol CR/XL in postmyocardial infarction patients with chronic heart failure:experiences from MERIT-HF. Am Heart J 2003;146:721–728.
23. Teo KK, Yusuf S, Furberg CD. Effects of prophylactic antiarrhythmic drug therapy in acute myocardial infarction. An overview of results from randomized controlled trials. JAMA 1993;270:1589–1595.
24. Ryden L, Ariniego R, Arnman K, et al. A double-blind trial of metoprolol in acute myocardial infarction. N Engl J Med 1983;308:614–618.
25. The CAPRICORN investigators. Effect of carvedilol on outcome after myocardial infarction in patients with left ventricular dysfunction: the CAPRICORN randomised trial. Lancet 2001;357:1385–1390.
26. McMurray J, Kober L, Robertson M, et al. Antiarrhythmic effect of carvedilol after acute myocardial infarction:results of the Carvedilol Post-Infarct Survival Control in Left Ventricular Dysfunction (CAPRICORN) trial. J Am Coll Cardiol 2005;45: 525–530.
27. Hjalmarson A, Goldstein S, Fagerberg B, et al., for the MERIT-HF study group. Effects of controlled-release metoprolol on total rortality, hospitalizations, and well-being in patients with heart failure: the metoprolol CR/XL randomized intervention trial in congestive heart failure (MERIT-HF) JAMA 2000;283:1295–1302.
28. Janosi A, Ghali JK, Herlitz J, et al., on behalf of the MERIT-HF study group. Metoprolol XL/CR in post-myocardial infarction patients with chronic heart failure: Experiences from MERIT-HF. Am Heart J 2003;146:721–728.
29. Squire I. Neurohormonal intervention to reduce sudden cardiac death in heart failure: what is the optimal pharmacologic strategy? Heart Fail Rev 2004;9: 337–345.
30. Pfeffer MA, Braunwald E, Moye LA, et al. Effect of captopril on mortality and morbidity in patients with left ventricular dysfunction after myocardial infarction. Results of the survival and ventricular enlargement trial. The SAVE investigators. N Engl J Med 1992;327:669–677.
31. Ambrosioni E, Borghi C, Magnani B, for the survival of myocardial infarction long-term evaluation (SMILE) investigators. The effect of the angiotensin-converting-enzyme inhibitor zofenopril on mortality and morbidity after anterior myocardial infarction. N Engl J Med 1995;332:80–85.
32. Kober L, Torp-Pedersen C, Carlsen JE, et al., for the trandolapril cardiac evaluation (TRACE) study group. A clinical trial of the angiotensin-converting-enzyme inhibitor trandolapril in patients with left ventricular dysfunction after myocardial infarction. N Engl J Med 1995;333:1670–1676.
33. Cleland JG, Erhardt L, Murray G, et al., on behalf of the AIRE study investigators. Effect of ramipril on morbidity and mode of death among survivors of acute myocardial infarction with clinical evidence of heart failure. Eur Heart J 1997;18: 41–51.
34. Randomised trial of cholesterol lowering in 4444 patients with coronary heart disease: the Scandinavian Simvastatin Survival Study (4S). Lancet 1994;344:1383–1389.
35. Sacks FM, Pfeffer MA, Moye LA, et al. The effect of pravastatin on coronary events after myocardial infarction in patients with average cholesterol levels. Cholesterol and recurrent events trial investigators. N Engl J Med 1996;335:1001–1009.
36. The Long-term Intervention with Pravastatin in Ischaemic Disease (LIPID) study group. Prevention of cardiovascular events and death with pravastatin in patients

with coronary heart disease and a broad range of initial cholesterol levels. N Engl J Med 1998;339:1349–1357.

37. Downs JR, Clearfield M, Weis S, et al. Primary prevention of acute coronary events with lovastatin in men and women with average cholesterol levels: results of AFCAPS/TexCAPS. Air Force/Texas coronary atherosclerosis prevention study. JAMA 1998;279:1615–1622.

38. Mitchell LB, Powell JL, Gillis AM, et al. Are lipid-lowering drugs also antiarrhythmic drugs? An analysis of the antiarrhythmics versus implantable defibrillators (AVID) trial. J Am Coll Cardiol 2003;42:81–87.

39. Vyas AK, Guo H, Moss AJ, et al., for the MADIT-II research group. Reduction in ventricular tachyarrhythmias with statins in the multicenter automatic defibrillator implantation trial (MADIT)–II. J Am Coll Cardiol 2006;47:769–773.

40. Pitt B, Remme W, Zannad F, et al. Eplerenone, a selective aldosterone blocker, in patients with left ventricular dysfunction after myocardial infarction. N Engl J Med 2003;348:1309–1321.

41. Pitt B, Zannad F, Bittman R, et al. The EPHESUS Trial: evaluation of eplerenone in the subgroup of patients with baseline left ventricular ejection fraction ≤30%. J Cardiac Fail 2003;9(Suppl 1):S57.

42. Echt DS, Liebson PR, Mitchell LB, et al. Mortality and morbidity in patients receiving encainide, flecainide, or placebo. The Cardiac Arrhythmia Suppression Trial. N Engl J Med 1991;324:781–788.

43. Waldo AL, Camm AJ, de Ruyter H, et al., for the SWORD investigators. Effect of d-sotalol on mortality in patients with left ventricular dysfunction after recent and remote myocardial infarction. Lancet 1996;348:7–12.

44. Julian DG, Prescott RJ, Jackson FS, et al. Controlled trial of sotalol for one year after myocardial infarction. Lancet 1982;1(8282):1142–1147.

45. Kober L, Thomsen PEB, Moller M, et al., on behalf of the Danish investigators of arrhythmia and mortality on dofetilide (DIAMOND) study group. Effect of dofetilide in patients with recent myocardial infarction and left-ventricular dysfunction: a randomized trial. Lancet 2000;356:2052–2058.

46. Camm AJ, Pratt CM, Schwartz PJ, et al., on behalf of the azimilide post infarct survival evaluation (ALIVE) investigators. Mortality in patients after a recent myocardial infarction. A randomized, placebo-controlled trial of azimilide using heart rate variability for risk stratification. Circulation 2004;109: 990–996.

47. Julian DG, Camm AJ, Frangin G, et al., for the European myocardial infarct amiodarone trial investigators. Randomised trial of effect of amiodarone on mortality in patients with left-ventricular dysfunction after recent myocardial infarction. Lancet 1997;349:667–674.

48. Cairns JA, Connolly SJ, Roberts R, et al., for the Canadian amiodarone myocardial infarction arrhythmia trial investigators. Randomised trial of outcome after myocardial infarction in patients with frequent or repetitive ventricular premature depolarisations: CAMIAT. Lancet 1997;349:675–682.

49. Bardy GH, Lee KL, Mark DB, et al. Amiodarone or an implantable cardioverter-defibrillator for congestive heart failure. N Engl J Med 2005;352:225–237.

50. The Antiarrhythmics versus Implantable Defibrillators (AVID) Investigators. A comparison of antiarrhythmic-drug therapy with implantable defibrillators in patients resuscitated from near-fatal ventricular arrhythmias. N Engl J Med 1997; 337:1576–1583.

51. Kuck KH, Cappato R, Siebels J, et al. Randomized comparison of antiarrhythmic drug therapy with implantable defibrillators in patients resuscitated from cardiac arrest: the Cardiac Arrest Study Hamburg (CASH). Circulation 2000;102:748–754.
52. Connolly SJ, Gent M, Roberts RS, et al. Canadian implantable defibrillator study (CIDS): a randomized trial of the implantable cardioverter defibrillator against amiodarone. Circulation 2000;101:1297–1302.
53. Moss AJ, Hall WJ, Cannom DS, et al. Improved survival with an implanted defibrillator in patients with coronary disease at high risk for ventricular arrhythmia. Multicenter Automatic Defibrillator Implantation Trial Investigators. N Engl J Med 1996;335:1933–1940.
54. Buxton AE, Lee KL, Fisher JD, et al. A randomized study of the prevention of sudden death in patients with coronary artery disease. Multicenter Unsustained Tachycardia Trial Investigators. N Engl J Med 1999;341:1882–1890.
55. Moss AJ, Zareba W, Hall WJ, et al. Prophylactic implantation of a defibrillator in patients with myocardial infarction and reduced ejection fraction. N Engl J Med 2002;346:877–883.
56. Solomon SD, Zelenkofske S, McMurray JJ, et al. Sudden death in patients with myocardial infarction and left ventricular dysfunction, heart failure, or both. N Engl J Med 2005;352:2581–2588.
57. Hohnloser SH, Kuck KH, Dorian P, et al. Prophylactic use of an implantable cardioverter-defibrillator after acute myocardial infarction. N Engl J Med 2004;351:2481–2488.
58. Raviele A, Bongiorni MG, Brignole M, et al. Early EPS/ICD strategy in survivors of acute myocardial infarction with severe left ventricular dysfunction on optimal beta-blocker treatment. The BEta-blocker STrategy plus ICD trial. Europace 2005;7:327–337.

19
Management of Cocaine-Induced Chest Pain

Olivier Frankenberger, Tseday Sirak, Sripal Bangalore,
and Henry H. Greenberg

Cocaine is the most commonly used illicit drug among individuals seeking care in hospital emergency departments or drug treatment centers. More than 30% of men and 20% of women between the ages of 26 and 34 years, representing an estimated 25 million Americans, report that they have used cocaine at least once [1–3]. Of those, 3.7 million had used it within the previous year, and 1.5 million were current users [1–3]. As cocaine use reaches epidemic proportions, the number of cocaine-related cardiovascular events, including angina pectoris, myocardial infarction (MI), cardiomyopathy, and sudden death from cardiac causes, has increased multifold. It has become the most frequent cause of drug-related deaths reported by medical examiners [1–3].

Pharmacology and Mechanism of Action

Cocaine (benzoylmethylecgonine; $C_{17}H_{21}NO_4$) is an alkaloid extract from the leaf of the *Erythroxylum coca* plant, which mainly grows in South America [4]. It is available in two forms: the free base and the hydrochloride salt. The free base is the heat-stable form that melts with heating, allowing it to be smoked as "crack" and is considered the most addictive form. The hydrochloride salt is water soluble and decomposes when heated. This form can be taken orally, intranasally, or intravenously. Depending on the route of administration, peak effects are reached within 1 to 90 minutes [5, 6]. The serum half-life of cocaine ranges from 45 to 90 minutes and the duration of action ranges from 15 minutes to 3 hours [5, 6].

Cocaine is metabolized to its inactive water-soluble form (benzoylecgonine and ecgonine methyl ester) by liver and plasma cholinesterase as well as by nonenzymatic hydrolysis and eliminated via the urinary system [7]. Metabolites of cocaine are detectible in urine or blood for up to 24 to 72 hours after ingestion, providing clues to recent use of cocaine.

Cocaine acts as a local anesthetic by inhibiting membrane permeability to sodium during depolarization and thus blocking the initiation and transmission of electrical signals. Cocaine also blocks the presynaptic reuptake of norepinephrine and dopamine, producing an excess of these neurotransmitters at the site of the postsynaptic receptor. Cocaine is a potent sympathomimetic agent, and its actions at the cellular level are mediated by stimulation of both the alpha and beta adrenergic receptors [8].

Pathophysiology of Cocaine on the Cardiovascular System

Vagotonic response or bradycardia predominates with initial use of cocaine [9]. However, this episode is rapidly followed by an increase in sympathetic stimulation producing tachycardia and hypertension [9]. By the same token, the initial effect of cocaine on the coronary arteries is vasodilation, which decreases coronary perfusion pressure by 13% to 68% [10]. This vasodilatory effect is rapidly replaced by sustained vasoconstriction, which is associated with a 5% to 20% reduction in epicardial coronary artery diameter [10]. In addition, cocaine indirectly causes vasoconstriction by inhibiting the production of nitric oxide, a potent vasodilator [11]. There is also evidence that cocaine increases blood viscosity by increasing red blood cells (RBCs) by 4% to 6% and increases platelet aggregation and in situ thrombus formation [12, 13]. It also results in a 40% increase in von Willebrand factor and increased plasminogen activator inhibitor levels facilitating further thrombus formation [12, 13].

Cardiovascular Effects of Cocaine

Chest pain, cardiac ischemia, and acute coronary syndrome (ACS) are the most common findings in patients with recent use of cocaine, independent of the route of intake of cocaine [14, 15]. Other common cardiac problems include arrhythmias, cardiomyopathy, and myocarditis.

Cocaine-Related Chest Pain and Myocardial Infarction

Complications from cocaine abuse involve nearly all organ systems, and thus, when a patient presents with symptoms of chest pain, or dyspnea, anxiety, palpitations, dizziness and/or nausea, the initial evaluation should be directed toward ruling out MI [5, 16]. ACS and MI can occur minutes to a few days after cocaine use [17]. However, the risk of MI is increased up to 24 times over the baseline in the first hour after cocaine administration irrespective of the route of use [14, 18]. In one study, 1% of the patients who had an acute MI had used cocaine within the previous year and 25% of these had used cocaine 60 minutes before the infarct [18, 19]. Two prospective studies report that only 6% of cocaine-induced chest pains are attributable to MI [20, 21], with 77% of cocaine-induced MI involving the anterior wall [21, 22].

The typical patient with cocaine-associated MI is a young, tobacco-smoking male with a history of repetitive cocaine use but few other cardiac risk factors

[23, 24]. In these young patients, ECGs in the setting of cocaine-induced MI are difficult to interpret, because they have a higher incidence of early repolarization and left ventricular hypertrophy with associated repolarization changes. The reported ECG sensitivity for detecting an MI is only 36% with a specificity of 90% [14, 25]. In addition, increased concentration of creatine kinase (CK) and CK-MB occurs in 50% of patients after cocaine use, even in the absence of MI, primarily due to increased motor activity, hyperthermia, and rhabdomyolysis [26, 27]. Thus, serum CK is not a reliable indicator of myocardial injury. In contrast, the immunoassay for cardiac troponin I has no detectible cross-reactivity with human skeletal muscle troponin I, making it more a specific and sensitive test for assessing myocardial injury even when coexistent skeletal muscle injury exists [26].

Cardiac Arrhythmias

Although the exact arrhythmogenic potential of cocaine is poorly defined, several benign and malignant arrhythmias have been reported with cocaine use, including sinus tachycardia and bradycardia, supraventricular arrhythmias, bundle branch block, ventricular fibrillation or asystole, ventricular tachycardia, and torsade de pointes [14, 27–29]. Cocaine is known to reduce vagal activity, which may potentiate cocaine's sympathomimetic effects, thereby increasing ventricular irritability and lowering the threshold for fibrillation [30]. Its sodium channel blocking properties inhibit the generation and conduction of the action potentials, which prolong the duration of the QRS and QTc, much like class I agents [31, 32]. Therefore, concomitant use of class I antiarrhythmic drugs, such as quinidine, procainamide, and disopyramide, should be avoided and could increase the risk in cocaine users, because they exacerbate the prolongation of the QRS and QT intervals and slow the metabolism of cocaine and its metabolites [33].

Aortic Dissection

Acute aortic dissection or rupture, albeit an uncommon cause of chest pain, is commonly associated with antecedent cocaine use in most inner-city hospitals as reviewed by Hsue et al. [34]. Cocaine, especially crack cocaine, seems to initiate dissection very infrequently, but when it does, it occurs in the descending aorta and afflicts predominately young, black and Hispanic, hypertensive individuals [34]. The profound sympathetic stimulation related to cocaine use is presumed to cause sheer stress on the aorta's intimal surface, causing a "nick" or a tear [35]. Such tears are said to occur in the region of the ligamentum arteriosum, where the aorta is fixed anatomically and hence less able to withstand the accelerating aortic pressure wave generated after contraction of the left ventricle [36]. It is also believed that chronic use makes the endothelium more permeable to atherogenic low-density lipoprotein and facilitates the migration of leukocytes into the aortic wall, leading to premature and accelerated atherosclerosis [37].

Cardiomyopathy, Myocarditis, and Endocarditis

Long-term cocaine abuse has been reported to cause dilated cardiomyopathy, left ventricular hypertrophy, systolic dysfunction, as well as profound myocardial depression after binge cocaine use [38–40]. The direct toxic effect of cocaine on the heart induces the transcription of genes responsible for changes in the composition of myocardial collagen and myosin, induces myocyte apoptosis leading to myofibril destruction, interstitial fibrosis, and myocardial dilation and systolic dysfunction [41]. Repetitive sympathetic stimulation, similar to that seen in pheochromocytoma, is associated with cardiomyopathy and characteristic subendocardial contraction band necrosis [42].

Myocarditis was reported in 20% to 30% of patients dying from cocaine abuse as well as in active users after myocardial biopsies. The mechanism for the myocarditis is believed to be due in part from concomitant administration of adulterants or infectious agents, especially in intravenous cocaine users and in part from hypersensitivity reactions leading to vasculitis in cocaine abusers [19, 43].

Cocaine-related endocarditis, unlike the endocarditis associated with other intravenous drug use, often involves the left-sided cardiac valves [44]. Cocaine use seems to be a greater independent risk factor for developing endocarditis than the use of other illicit drugs [44]. Although the reason for this is unknown, it is presumed that the increase in interventricular, and arterial pressure related to cocaine use may lead to valvular and vascular injury that predisposes users to bacterial invasion of the left-sided heart valves [45].

Takotsubo Cardiomyopathy

Takotsubo in Japanese means "an octopus fishing pot with a round bottom and a narrow neck." This reversible left ventricular cardiomyopathy exhibits both apical akinesis and basal hyperkinesis in the left ventriculography in the acute phase and normalizes within hours to a few weeks [46]. Although the exact mechanism of this dysfunction has not been clarified, several case studies have elucidated that coronary spasms or catecholamine cardiotoxicity, especially cocaine use, are suspected as possible causes of this disease [46]. This cardiomyopathy has a clinical course associated with an acute MI-like ST-segment change, usually acute heart failure, but mostly good prognosis with no sequelae and is not associated with atherosclerotic coronary arterial disorder [46].

Treatment of Cocaine-Related Chest Pain

There are no well-designed, randomized, prospective clinical trials to compare treatment algorithms for cocaine-associated ischemia. However, there is a general agreement that treatment of cocaine-induced myocardial ischemia differs in several ways from that of acute MI due to other causes. According to the American College of Cardiology/American Heart Association (ACC/AHA) guidelines, the first-line treatment in patients with cocaine-related chest pain and ECG changes is focused on benzodiazepines, aspirin, and nitrates [9, 47]. The benefit of benzodiazepines results from a reduction in blood pressure, tachycardia, or anxiety, and thus a reduction in myocardial oxygen demand [48]. Aspirin prevents thrombus formation, and nitrates reverse cocaine-induced vasoconstriction [49].

Second-line treatments include calcium channel blockers and alpha-blockers [50–52]. Calcium channel blockers such as diltiazem, nifedipine, and verapamil have beneficial effects on cocaine-induced ischemia, but all three have been associated with an increased risk of seizures in animal models [53]. Hence, these second-line treatments must be administered after benzodiazepines have been given. Beta-blockers have commonly been avoided in the acute stage of cocaine use, because they may worsen vasospasm by permitting unopposed stimulation of alpha receptors [54]. The use of combination alpha/beta blockers such as labetalol was shown to reduce the cocaine-induced rise in mean arterial pressure with no effect on coronary vasoconstriction [55].

Thrombolytic therapy in patients with cocaine-induced MI remains controversial. Factors that mitigate the use of thrombolytics in the management of cocaine-induced MI include the overall difficulty in making a reliable diagnosis, the low mortality of patients with cocaine-induced infarction, and higher risk of treatment complications in this population, especially the risk of intracranial hemorrhage and the fact that a large proportion of patients is markedly hypertensive at the time of presentation [56, 57]. Therefore, thrombolytic therapy should only be considered when immediate coronary angiography and angioplasty are not available [56, 57].

Cocaine-induced ventricular arrhythmias shortly after ingestion of the drug may safely be treated with sodium bicarbonate, because it reverses cocaine-induced QRS prolongation [58]. Although limited data in humans suggest that lidocaine is safe to use several hours after cocaine use, some concern exists about its use, because both cocaine and lidocaine have proarrhythmic and proconvulsant effects mediated through sodium-channel blockade [59]. Hence, cautious use of lidocaine several hours after cocaine use may be reasonable.

Conclusion

Early recognition and understanding of cocaine-related cardiovascular complications are crucial for their optimal management. Cocaine use should always be considered in a young patient with myocardial ischemia or infarction, arrhythmias, myocarditis, or dilated cardiomyopathy. Primary prevention such as educating the public about the considerable risks of cocaine use and encouraging the young to refrain from cocaine use are paramount, as cocaine-related visits to the emergency departments continue to rise dramatically.

References

1. Lange RA, Hillis LD. Cardiovascular complications of cocaine use. N Engl J Med 2001;345:351–358.
2. Office of Applied Studies. Year-end 1999 emergency department data from the Drug. Abuse Warning Network. DHHS Publication No.(SMA) 00-3462. Rockville, MD: Substance Abuse and Mental Health Services Administration; 2000.
3. Leikin JB, Morris RW, Warren M, et al. Trends in a decade of drug abuse presentations to an inner city ED. Am J Emerg Med 2001;19:37–39.
4. Kosten TR, Hollister LE. Drugs of abuse. In: Katzung BG, ed. Basic and clinical pharmacology. New York: Lange MedicalBooks/McGraw-Hill; 2001:532–547.
5. Goldfrank LR, Hoffman RS. The cardiovascular effects of cocaine. Ann Emerg Med 1991;20:165–175.
6. Pitts WR, Lange RA, Cigarroa JE, et al. Cocaine-Induced myocardial ischemia and infarction: pathophysiology, recognition, and management. Prog Cardiovasc Dis 1997;40:65–76.
7. Jeffcoat AR, Perez-Reyes M, Hill JM, et al. Cocaine disposition in humans after intravenous injection, nasal insufflation (snorting), or smoking. Drug Metab Dispos 1989;17:153–159.
8. Lange RA, Flores ED, Cigarroa RG, et al.Cocaine-induced myocardial ischemia and infarction. Cardiology 1990;7:74–81.
9. Hollander J. The management of cocaine associated myocardial ischemia. N Engl J Med 1995;333:1267–1272.
10. Benzaquen BS, Cohen V, Eisenberg MJ. Effects of cocaine on coronary arteries. Am Heart J 2001;142:402–410.
11. Mo W, Singh AK, Arruda JA, et al. Role of nitric oxide in cocaine-induced acute hypertension. Am J Hypertens 1998;11:708–714.
12. Siegel AJ, Sholar MB, Mendelson JH, et al. Cocaine-induced erythrocytosis and increase in von Willebrand factor: evidence for drug-related blood doping and prothrombotic effects. Arch Intern Med 1999;159:1925–1929.
13. Moliterno DJ, Lange RA, Gerard RD, et al. Influence of intranasal cocaine on plasma constituents associated with endogenous thrombosis and thrombolysis. Am J Med 1994;96:492–496.
14. Isner JM, Estes NA, Thompson PD, et al. Acute cardiac events temporally related to cocaine abuse. N Engl J Med 1986;315:1438–1443.
15. Hollander JE, Hoffman RS. Cocaine-induced myocardial infarction: an analysis and review of the literature. J Emerg Med 1992;10:169–177.
16. Brody SL, Slovis CM, Wrenn KD. Cocaine-related medical problems: consecutive series of 233 patients. Am J Med 1990;88:325–331.
17. Fendrich M, Johnson TP, Sudman S, et al. Validity of drug use reporting in a high-risk community sample: a comparison of cocaine and heroin survey reports with hair tests. Am J Epidemiol 1999;149:955–962.
18. Isner JM, Estes NA, Thompson PD, et al. Acute cardiac events temporally related to cocaine abuse. N Engl J Med 1986;315:1438–1443.

19. Minor RL Jr, Scott BD, Brown DD, et al. Cocaine-induced myocardial infarction in patients with normal coronary arteries. Ann Intern Med 1992;115:797–806.
20. Hollander JE, Hoffman RS, Gennis P, et al. Prospective multicenter evaluation of cocaine associated chest pain. Acad Emerg Med 1994;1:330–339.
21. Tokarski GF, Paganussi P, Urbanski R, et al. An evaluation of cocaine-induced chest pain. Ann Emerg Med 1990;19:1088–1092.
22. Lange RA, Willard JE. The cardiovascular effects of cocaine. Heart Dis Stroke 1993; 2:136–141.
23. Moliterno DJ, Willard JE, Lange RA, et al. Coronary-artery vasoconstriction induced by cocaine, cigarette smoking, or both. N Engl J Med 1994;330:454–459.
24. Inaba T, Stewart DJ, Kalow W. Metabolism of cocaine in man. Clin Pharmacol Ther 1978;23:547–552.
25. Hollander JE, Lozano M, Fairweather P, et al. "Abnormal" electrocardiograms in patients with cocaine associated chest pain are due to "normal" variants. J Emerg Med 1994;12:199–120.
26. Adams JE III, Bodor GS, Davila-Roman VG, et al. Cardiac troponin I: a marker with high specificity for cardiac injury. Circulation 1993;88:101–106.
27. Bauman JL, Grawe JJ, Winecoff AP, et al. Cocaine-related sudden cardiac death: a hypothesis correlating basic science and clinical observations. J Clin Pharmacol 1994;34:902–911.
28. Om A, Ellenbogen KA, Vetrovec GW. Cocaine-induced bradyarrhythmias. Am Heart J 1992;124:232–234.
29. Nanji AA, Filipenko JD. Asystole and ventricular fibrillation associated with cocaine intoxication. Chest 1984;85:132–133.
30. Kanani PM, Guse PA, Smith WM, et al. Acute deleterious effects of cocaine on cardiac conduction, hemodynamics, and ventricular fibrillation threshold: effects of interaction with a selective dopamine D1 antagonist SCH 39166. J Cardiovasc Pharmacol 1998;32:42–48.
31. Perera R, Kraebber A, Schwartz MJ. Prolonged QT interval and cocaine use. J Electrocardiol 1997;30:337–339.
32. Kerns W II, Garvey L, Owens J. Cocaine-induced wide complex dysrhythmia. J Emerg Med 1997;15:321–329.
33. Bailey DN. Amitriptyline and procainamide inhibition of cocaine and cocaethylene degradation in human serum in vitro. J Anal Toxicol 1999;23:99–102.
34. Hsue PY, Salinas CL, Bolger AF, et al. Acute aortic dissection related to crack cocaine. Circulation 2002;105:1592–1595.
35. Nallamothu BK, Saint S, Kolias TJ, et al. Of nicks and time. N Engl J Med 2001;345: 359–363.
36. Eagle KA, Isselbacher EM, DeSanctis RW. Cocaine-related aortic dissection in perspective. Circulation 2002;105:1529–1530.
37. Kolodgie FD, Virmani R, Cornhill JF, et al. Increase in atherosclerosis and adventitial mast cells in cocaine abusers: an alternative mechanism of cocaine-associated coronary vasospasm and thrombosis. J Am Coll Cardiol 1991;17:1553–1560.
38. Wiener RS, Lockhart JT, Schwartz RG. Dilated cardiomyopathy and cocaine abuse: report of two cases. Am J Med 1986;81:699–701.
39. Bertolet BD, Freund G, Martin CA, et al. Unrecognized left ventricular dysfunction in an apparently healthy cocaine abuse population. Clin Cardiol 1990;13:323–328.
40. Chokshi SK, Moore R, Pandian NG, et al. Reversible cardiomyopathy associated with cocaine intoxication. Ann Intern Med 1989;111:1039–1040.

41. Xiao Y, He J, Gilbert RD, et al. Cocaine induces apoptosis in fetal myocardial cells through a mitochondria-dependent pathway. J Pharmacol Exp Ther 2000;292: 8–14.
42. Tazelaar HD, Karch SB, Stephens BG, et al. Cocaine and the heart. Hum Pathol 1987; 18:195–199.
43. Virmani R, Robinowitz M, Smialek JE, et al. Cardiovascular effects of cocaine: an autopsy study of 40 patients. Am Heart J 1988;115:1068–1076.
44. Chambers HF, Morris DL, Tauber MG, et al. Cocaine use and the risk for endocarditis in intravenous drug users. Ann Intern Med 1987;106:833–836.
45. Mao JT, Zhu LX, Sharma S, et al. Cocaine inhibits human endothelial cell IL-8 production: the role of transforming growth factor-beta. Cell Immunol 1997;181: 38–43.
46. Akashi YJ, Nakazawa K, Sakakibara M, et al. Reversible left ventricular dysfunction "Takotsubo" cardiomyopathy related to catecholamine cardiotoxicity. J Electrocardiol 2002;35:351–356.
47. Braunwald E, Antman E, Beasley J, et al. ACC/AHA 2002 guideline update for the management of patients with unstable angina and non-ST-segment elevation infatcrion-summary article. A report of the American College of Cardiology/American Heart Association task force on practice guidelines (Committee on the Management of Patients With Unstable Angina). J Am Coll Cardiol 2002;40:1366–1374.
48. Guinn MM, Bedford JA, Wilson MC. Antagonism of intravenous cocaine lethality in nonhuman primates. Clin Toxicol 1980;16:499–508.
49. Brogan WC III, Lange RA, Kim AS, et al. Alleviation of cocaine induced coronary vasoconstriction by nitroglycerin. J Am Coll Cardiol 1991;18:581–586.
50. Lange RA, Cigarroa RG, Flores ED, et al. Cocaine-induced coronary artery vasoconstriction. N Engl J Med 1989;321:1557–1562.
51. Hollander JE, Carter WA, Hoffman RS. Use of phentolamine for cocaine induced myocardial ischemia. N Engl J Med 1992;327:361.
52. Negus BH, Willard JE, Hillis LD, et al. Alleviation of cocaine-induced coronary vasoconstriction with intravenous verapamil. Am J Cardiol 1994;73:510–513.
53. Derlet RW, Albertson TE. Potentiation of cocaine toxicity with calcium channel blockers. Am J Emerg Med 1989;7:464–468.
54. Lange RA, Cigarroa RG, Flores ED, et al. Potentiation of cocaine-induced coronary vasoconstriction by beta-blockade. Ann Intern Med 1990;112:897–903.
55. Boehrer JD, Moliterno DJ, Willard JE, et al. Influence of labetalol on cocaine induced coronary vasoconstriction in humans. Am J Med 1993;94:608–610.
56. Hoffman RS, Hollander JE. Thrombolytic therapy and cocaine-induced myocardial infarction. Am J Emerg Med 1996;14:693–695.
57. Hollander JE, Burstein JL, Hoffman RS, et al. Cocaine-associated myocardial infarction: clinical safety of thrombolytic therapy. Chest 1995;107:1237–1241.
58. Beckman KJ, Parker RB, Hariman RJ, et al. Hemodynamic and electrophysiological actions of cocaine: effects of sodium bicarbonate as an antidote in dogs. Circulation 1991;83:1799–1807.
59. Heit J, Hoffman RS, Goldfrank LR. Lidocaine is protective against lethalityin mice. Acad Emerg Med 1994;1:438–442.

20
Acute Coronary Syndrome in Women and the Elderly

Jacqueline E. Tamis-Holland, Catherine R. Weinberg, Simbo Chiadika, and Bette Kim

Cardiovascular disease (CVD), specifically coronary heart disease (CHD), is the leading cause of death in women and men. Approximately 6 million females in the United States have CHD, and more than 250,000 women die each year from CHD [1]. Over a lifetime, 1 in 2.6 women will die of CVD, and 1 in 30 women will die of breast cancer [1].

In women, there is a 10-year delay in the incidence of obstructive coronary artery disease (CAD) compared with aged-matched males and a 20-year delay in the incidence of major CHD events such as myocardial infarction (MI) and death [1]. The prevalence of CAD is low in women before menopause, but it begins to equal the prevalence in men at about the seventh decade of life [1]. Over the years, overall deaths from CVD have progressively declined [2]. In men, the decline in CVD deaths has been steady; however, in women, death rates from CVD actually increased over time until the year 2000, after which they began to decline [1].

Overall, CHD incidence and mortality increase with increasing age. In the 2006 Heart and Stroke Statistics, the annual incidence of a first myocardial infarction steadily increased with increasing age [1]. Approximately 83% of deaths from CHD occur in patients over age 65 years [1].

Risk Factors

Traditional Risk Factors

The presence of traditional CVD risk factors will confer an increased risk for developing CHD in both women and men. However, there are sex and age differences in the prevalence and significance of these risk factors. For example, among patients presenting to the hospital with acute coronary syndromes (ACS), women are older and more likely to have a history of hypertension, diabetes, and high cholesterol but are less likely to have a history of cigarette smoking [3–7]. Hypertension appears more prevalent in older patients with ACS, but smoking history is less often noted in older patients [8, 9].

In addition, the presence of CVD risk factors may confer a different degree of risk in women and men. Women with diabetes are at a higher risk for CHD compared with age-matched diabetic men [10]. The relative risk for developing nonfatal cardiovascular events in young women smokers is higher than that for young male smokers [11]. High-density lipoprotein (HDL) cholesterol, an important CVD risk predictor, is considered low in women if levels are less than 50 mg/dL, whereas in men levels less than 40 mg/dL are abnormal. A low HDL cholesterol has been shown to predict fatal CHD events in women and young men, but it has not been shown to affect fatal CHD outcomes in older men [12]. Elevated triglycerides appear to be an independent risk factor for CHD events in women, but not in men [13].

Risk Assessment Tools and Unique Risk Factors

The Framingham risk score, a useful tool for assessing long-term CVD risk, largely underestimates risk in young females and has been shown to be a poor predictor of cardiovascular risk in many female subsets. Several recent studies have demonstrated that approximately 30% to 50% of "low risk women" as measured by the Framingham risk score actually had evidence of CHD as demonstrated by elevated coronary calcium scores on electron-beam computed tomography (CT) [14, 15]. In young women with multiple risk factors, an alternative approach to risk assessment needs to be considered. On the other hand, older patients are often placed in a high-risk category for CVD events when assessed using the Framingham risk score, just by virtue of the large number of "points" allotted for advanced age.

The metabolic syndrome is a constellation of findings that has been shown to contribute to increased CVD risk. The NCEP III defines the metabolic syndrome as three of the following risk factors [16]: central obesity, hypertension, insulin resistance, hypertriglyceridemia, low HDL, or small low-density lipoprotein (LDL) particles. The metabolic syndrome is the most common risk factor for women with premature CHD and is more common among women with documented premature CHD than among men with premature CHD [17]. The WISE study demonstrated that among women with angiographically significant CHD, the presence of the metabolic syndrome increased the risk for CVD events by nearly fivefold when compared with women with a normal metabolic status [18].

In the WISE study, endogenous estrogen deficiency as is seen in hypoestrogenemia of hypothalamic origin was associated with a 7.4-fold higher incidence of CHD in premenopausal women with suspected ischemia [19] while prior oral contraceptive use conveys a protective effect on postmenopausal atherosclerosis [20]. In another study examining women with CAD, polycystic ovaries were associated with more severe and extensive disease on cardiac catheterization [21].

Presentation

Presenting Signs and Symptoms

Although chest pain is the most common presenting symptom for women and men with ACS [22–24], some studies [6, 22, 24], but not all [25, 26] have shown that women are less likely than men to present with this symptom. Overall, more women than men have atypical symptoms [24, 27]. This is particularly apparent in younger women, who tend to have dyspnea more often than younger men [6, 22]. Among patients with atypical symptoms, women are more likely than men to present with dyspnea or congestive heart failure, back pain, nausea and/or vomiting, and indigestive symptoms [23, 25]. After adjustment for other potentially confounding variables, dyspnea does not appear to be significantly more notable in women than men [22, 23]. Older patients are more likely to have no chest pain or atypical symptoms when compared with younger patients [28].

Some studies of women with ACS have demonstrated that women tend to present to the hospital after a longer delay than men [6, 7, 24, 25, 27, 29–35], whereas others have not demonstrated longer delay times in women [3, 26, 36]. The longer delay times, when present, may reflect a misperception by women that their symptoms are not a result of a serious cardiac disorder, because of either the atypical nature of symptoms in some women or the lack of CVD awareness [37]. The latter has resulted in the development of large nationwide campaigns created by the National Heart, Lung, and Blood Institute (NHLBI) and American Heart Association (AHA) focused on improving heart disease awareness in women. Alternatively, some studies demonstrated that women were more likely to consult their physician by phone to discuss symptoms, whereas men were more likely to go directly to the emergency room (ER) [27, 32]. In one study, consultation with a physician by phone prior to an ER visit seemed to be responsible for the delay in presentation to the ER [27].

Women with ACS are older than men and significantly more likely to have a history of hypertension, diabetes, and prior congestive heart failure [4–7, 31, 38, 39]. They are less likely than men to have ever smoked, or have a history of prior MI, prior angioplasty (PCI), or coronary artery bypass surgery (CABG) [3–6, 31]. On presentation to the ER, women with ACS are sicker than men. They have faster heart rates [4, 6, 40], higher blood pressure [4, 29, 40], and are more likely to be in congestive heart failure [4–6, 31, 33] or shock [25, 27, 30, 36] than their male counterparts. This is particularly notable among younger women when compared with younger men [6].

Elderly patients with ACS also tend to have a greater burden of comorbid conditions, including hypertension, diabetes mellitus, congestive heart failure, and prior cardiac disease compared with younger patients [9, 41, 42]. The incidence of cardiac hypertrophy and ventricular dysfunction, particularly diastolic dysfunction, is higher in the elderly in part due to decreased beta-sympathetic response, arterial compliance, and arterial hypertension [43]; hence, the elderly are more likely to have congestive heart failure on presentation to the hospital [42].

Electrocardiogram and Cardiac Biomarkers

Women presenting to the hospital with ACS tend to present with less severe syndrome. When examining patients with all forms of ACS, women are less likely than men to have ST elevation on 12-lead ECG [4, 6, 31]. This is particularly more notable in younger women compared with younger men [6]. When ST elevation is present, the magnitude of ST changes is less pronounced than that seen in men [44]. Among patients with no ST-segment elevation on ECG, women have more T-wave inversions [40, 45, 46] and are less likely to have cardiac enzyme elevations [4, 5, 40, 45–47]. Older patients (>65 years) are also less likely to have ST elevations when compared with younger patients [9, 42], but they are more likely to have positive cardiac markers [42].

Hospital Management and Treatment

Sex and Age Differences in Management of ACS

Women and men are not created equal, and therefore response to treatment administered may differ. The reasons for such differences are not entirely understood but may relate to sex differences in thrombotic and fibrinolytic activity, enzymatic activities, glomerular filtration, levels of endogenous hormones, body surface area, and proportion of body fat. As a result, women may have an increased risk for untoward events from certain therapies used in treating ACS. However, most studies have demonstrated a favorable treatment response in women, justifying the use of such therapies. Therefore, the overall management of women with ACS should parallel that given to men with focus on instances where differences may play a role in increasing risk related to therapy and modifying therapy when indicated to attenuate this risk.

Drug responses in the elderly are influenced by decreased cardiac output, plasma volume, and perfusion and function of the kidneys and liver, as well as lower vasomotor tone, baroreceptor and beta-adrenergic responses [43]. Because the elderly are more prone to hypotension and medication toxicity, medications used for the treatment of ACS should be initiated at lower doses and patients should be observed for toxicity [5, 43]. Despite the potential for increased side effects from certain therapies, older patients have a higher risk for events after ACS, and hence, they actually derive a larger absolute benefit from such therapies.

Unfortunately, despite the favorable risk/benefit ratio of most therapies, women and the elderly are generally less aggressively treated with American College of Cardiology/American Heart Association (ACC/AHA) guideline recommended therapy for ACS [5–7, 27, 31, 33, 42, 48–50]. This may in part be related to the presence of other comorbidities, including advanced age, and the higher incidence of hypertension and congestive heart failure, which might raise a concern by physicians regarding the increased risk related to certain therapies. In addition, the less specific symptoms seen in women and older patients, and the less pronounced ST changes on ECG can often lead to a misdiagnosis on initial presentation. Another reason for gender and age disparities is that women and the elderly are less likely to be treated by a cardiologist during hospitalization [5, 24, 51]. Cardiologists use a higher proportion of procedures and medications associated with improved survival, and treatment by a cardiologist is associated with a better outcome [51].

Antithrombotic Therapy

Unfractionated heparin (UFH) is commonly used in the treatment of ACS. Bleeding is a recognized complication from UFH and appears to be related to activated partial thromboplastin time (aPTT) levels [52]. Studies have demonstrated that female sex and age are independent predictors of a high aPTT level and bleeding complications after use with UFH [52, 53]. Bleeding complications in patients with ACS may be related to excess dosing of antiplatelet and anticoagulant therapies. In the CRUSADE registry, excess dosing of UFH, low-molecular-weight heparin, and glycoprotein (GP) IIb/IIIa agents occurred in 42% of patients and was associated with higher rates of bleeding. Women and older patients were more likely to get excess dosing of these therapies [42]. In an attempt to minimize the bleeding risk from UFH, the ACC/AHA guidelines recommend that UFH be administered as a weight-based drip [54]. Although there are no specific guidelines on dosing in women and older patients, some authors have suggested even lower dosing of UFH in these subsets of patients, especially when GP IIb/IIIa agents are anticipated during PCI [55].

Glycoprotein IIb/IIIa Agents

Glycoprotein IIb/IIIa agents have been shown to decrease the likelihood for adverse outcomes among high-risk patients with unstable angina (UA)/non–ST-elevation myocardial infarction (NSTEMI) [56–58]. The benefit of these agents is particularly notable for patients with elevated troponin levels, high TIMI risk scores, or for those patients with a planned early invasive strategy. Tirofiban has been shown to be equally efficacious in women and men, and older and younger patients in the early days after UA/NSTEMI [56, 57]. However, the benefit of eptifibatide in women and older patients with UA/NSTEMI is less apparent [58]. Both of these agents when used for extended periods of time result in an increased risk of bleeding complications [56, 57, 59]. Bleeding complications are higher in women and older patients and are independent of baseline variables [59, 60]. In view of the increased risk of bleeding in women and older patients associated with upstream use, these agents should be reserved for high-risk patients, who will derive the most benefit [56–58].

Acute Reperfusion Therapy

Thrombolytic Therapy

Thrombolytic therapy is a commonly used method for acute reperfusion in the treatment of ST-elevation myocardial infarction (STEMI). The introduction of thrombolytic therapy has resulted in a 25% to 35% reduction in all-cause mortality associated with acute myocardial infarction (AMI). The benefits of thrombolytic therapy in terms of myocardial salvage, infarct-related artery patency, and improvement in left ventricular function have been shown to be similar in women and men [61, 62].

The elderly also benefit from the use of thrombolytic therapy. For every 1,000 patients treated, 34 lives are saved in patients older than 75 years versus only 28 lives in younger patients; however, the relative benefit of this therapy is equal or lower in the older population [54]. Compared with younger patients, the elderly patients are less likely to achieve normal flow after fibrinolytic therapy and have a higher mortality whether they receive therapy or not [54].

Bleeding complications after thrombolytic therapy, including intracerebral hemorrhage (ICH), are more prevalent in women and older patients [29, 39, 61–66]. Much of this sex/age difference in bleeding risk is attenuated by adjustment for baseline variables, including age, history of hypertension, and (in some studies) body weight [29, 61]. Despite adjustment, some studies still demonstrate that female gender is an independent predictor of ICH [63] and bleeding [29, 52, 63, 67]. Older age has also been shown to be an independent predictor of bleeding after fibrinolytic therapy [63, 67]. Bleeding may be attenuated by altering the dosing of adjunctive anticoagulation or choosing a different fibrinolytic agent [29, 52, 53].

Primary Angioplasty

Primary angioplasty (primary PCI) is the preferred approach of reperfusion therapy for the treatment of AMI in most hospitals with cardiac catheterization laboratories and PCI facilities [54]. It has been shown to be superior to thrombolytic therapy in many large-scale studies. Potential benefits include a lower early mortality, less nonfatal disabling stroke, lower rates of re-myocardial infarction (MI), and shorter hospital stays [68–70]. Several studies have demonstrated that women may derive a larger absolute benefit from treatment with primary PCI [39, 64]. Treatment with primary PCI instead of fibrolytic therapy prevents an estimated 56 events for every 1,000 women treated compared with 42 events for every 1,000 men treated [39]. Therefore, in women, primary PCI is the recommend treatment for STEMI if available [55].

The benefits of primary PCI in older patients are not as well understood. Subgroup analysis of the randomized trials of primary PCI to fibrinolytic therapy has suggested improved outcomes with primary PCI for older patients

[69] although these data are limited by the small number of elderly patients enrolled in these studies. In a recent randomized clinical trial of primary PCI and fibrinolytic therapy for older patients with STEMI (Grines, 2005; unpublished data), primary PCI was not found to be superior in decreasing the primary end point of death, or nonfatal stroke, although the composite of death, nonfatal disabling stroke, and re-MI was reduced with primary PCI.

Women and men seem to be referred for primary PCI at equal rates [62, 71], and most studies report that the time to reperfusion therapy with primary PCI is similar in women and men [35, 62, 71]. Angiographic and procedural variables including initial and final TIMI flow, extent of coronary artery disease, left ventricular ejection fraction on left ventricle (LV) angiogram, and success of PCI are not significantly different in women and men undergoing primary PCI [30, 35, 36, 39, 62, 64, 72].

Time to reperfusion therapy with primary PCI also appears similar in older and younger patients [73]. The elderly have smaller reference vessel diameters during primary PCI, but they have similar success rates as younger patients, with no significant differences by age in final TIMI flow or percent diameter stenosis [73, 74].

Subsequent Diagnostic Studies and Revascularization

Cardiac Catheterization and Percutaneous Coronary Intervention

Cardiac catheterization is an important tool to assess coronary anatomy and help to determine subsequent management options. Women with ACS are more likely than men to have normal coronary arteries or insignificant disease at cardiac catherization [4, 40, 47, 75]. This is noted among patients with STEMI, NSTEMI, and UA [4]. Women also tend to have less extensive disease than men [40, 45–47, 75].

Women have significantly more major bleeding after PCI than men [30, 36, 38, 47, 76–78]. This is noted even after adjustment for baseline characteristics and mean activated clotting time [38, 47]. Women are also more likely to have other vascular access–related complications [36, 79–81]. Major bleeding rates with PCI are reduced in women with the use of bivalirudin instead of the combination of GP IIb/IIIa inhibitors and UFH [82]. In the REPLACE 2 study, the higher bleeding risk associated with PCI in women was no longer apparent when bivalirudin was used [82].

In older patients, coronary disease at cardiac cath is more extensive [73] and reference vessel diameters are smaller [73, 74]. Older patients undergoing PCI with balloon angioplasty have more adverse events and less successful revascularization compared with younger patients [83]. Access for PCI is more difficult in the elderly with peripheral vascular disease and with tortuous aorto-iliac or subclavian vessels [83]. Bleeding [8, 83, 84], vascular complications [79, 80], and renal failure [83] after PCI are also more common in older patients.

Coronary Artery Bypass Grafting Surgery

Coronary artery bypass grafting (CABG) surgery is recommended when feasible for patients with ACS, who have left main disease, triple-vessel disease, or complex single- or double-vessel disease [85]. CABG improves long-term survival in moderate- to high-risk patients with a risk reduction of approximately 40% compared with medical therapy alone [85]. On average, women who undergo CABG tend to be older, have smaller body surface area, more unstable angina, congestive heart failure, and other comorbid conditions, as well as worse LV function, smaller vessels, and less multivessel disease than their male counterparts [85–87]. Elderly patients have a higher rate of urgent revascularization and more severe disease than younger patients [88].

Complications after CABG including neurologic events [89, 90] and bleeding [91] are higher in women than in men. Surgical mortality has also been shown to be higher in women [89, 80, 92, 93]. After adjustment for other confounding variables and body surface area, mortality is equal in women and men [92–94]. Perioperative morbidity and morality rates are also higher in the elderly [88].

The Role of Early Invasive Strategy Versus Early Conservative Strategies

An early invasive strategy with catheterization within 48 hours and appropriate revascularization are preferable in patients with UA/NSTEMI who are at high risk for death and MI [43]. Multiple studies have demonstrated benefits for men; however, controversy arises with early invasive versus early conservative strategies in women [40, 45, 47]. In TACTICS-TIMI 18 [47], women and men had a similar reduction in risk of death, re-MI, or rehospitalization from an early invasive strategy. This benefit was further enhanced in women after adjusting for baseline variables and was particularly marked in those women with an elevated baseline troponin T. Treatment of women in the early invasive arm resulted in similar outcome compared with men, including death and MI after PCI or CABG, although rates of major bleeding were independently associated with female gender. In this study, women at lower risk and those with negative troponins had more events in the invasive strategy than in the conservative strategy. On the other hand, in the RITA-3 and FRISC II studies, an early invasive strategy did not appear to offer any significant improvement in outcome for women [40, 45], although outcome was better for men treated with this approach.

The CRUSADE registry allows us to explore outcomes from each approach in a large, nonrandomized population of patients during a more contemporary era of revascularization. In this registry of patients with UA/NSTEMI, an early invasive strategy (catheterization within 48 hours) was associated with a lower in-hospital mortality than a strategy of deferred catheterization and revascularization. These findings were similarly evident in women and men [95].

So, what is the most appropriate management strategy for women with UA/STEMI? Certain conclusions can be drawn from looking at these studies as a whole. It seems that women in the RITA-3 and FRISC II studies were at lower risk than those enrolled in TACTICS-TIMI 18 or the CRUSADE registry [96]. Women who are at lower risk for MI and death are exposed to an early upfront risk, with little to gain from an invasive procedure, therefore allowing the procedural risk to influence the ultimate outcome. On the other hand, high-risk women with UA/NSTEMI should be referred for early catheterization and revascularization when appropriate, whereas women with low-risk features will likely benefit from a conservative strategy.

Death or nonfatal MI rates are lower in elderly patients who receive early invasive versus early conservative therapy [8]. Although outcome is worse in older patients compared with younger patients, early invasive therapy with percutaneous or surgical revascularization is still beneficial in elderly patients with ACS. Despite these findings, older patients are less often treated with this aggressive therapy [95].

Outcome

Nearly all studies examining women and men with ACS have demonstrated that women have higher unadjusted early mortality compared with men [5, 6, 97–100] and higher long-term mortality rates [101, 102]. The increase in mortality in women is largely related to the higher incidence of other comorbidities, such as older age, higher prevalence of congestive heart failure on presentation, systemic hypertension, and diabetes mellitus. After adjustment for age and these other comorbidities, there is a diminution in risk in women so that short-term mortality rates [5, 7, 103] and long-term mortality rates [25, 36, 38, 63] appear similar in women and men. However, some studies still show a higher mortality in women that is independent of baseline variables [24, 29, 32, 34, 104].

Why is there such a discrepancy in the literature regarding outcomes in women? Most of the variability in results relates to differences in study design and the populations that are examined in the various reports. Sex difference in outcomes among different studies may vary with age, type of ACS, and era in which the study was conducted.

Younger women as a subset appear to be at higher risk of increased mortality [6, 98]. Analysis of the National Registry of Myocardial Infarction (NRMI-2) showed a higher mortality in women compared with men for patients less than 75 years of age. There was an 11% greater risk of death in women than men for every 5-year decrease in age. After adjusting, younger women were more than 2 times more likely to die in the hospital after MI compared with younger men, whereas older women and men had similar outcomes. Similarly, in another paper of hospitalized patients with an acute MI [98], adjusted in-hospital and long-term mortality was significantly higher among younger women compared with younger men, but older women actually had a lower adjusted mortality when compared with older men.

It has been hypothesized that young women may have more aggressive CHD or other "unknown" risk factors that override the protective effects of estrogen. Psychosocial variables including depression, poorer access to health care resources, and lifestyle variables that might limit women's ability to comply with standard post-MI care may also contribute to differences in outcome in younger women and men. It has been reported that younger women have a lower rate of use of established treatments for myocardial infarction such as aspirin, beta-blockers, and thrombolytic therapy [6]. Alternative mechanism for the increased risk in younger women may relate to sex differences in the pathophysiology of disease, which may interfere with standard therapies provided for patients with ACS including antiplatelet agents and anticoagulants (see Chapter 5).

The outcome by gender for patients with ACS may also depend on the type of presenting syndrome. In the GUSTO II-B study [4], overall event-free survival at 30 days was worse in women than in men. However, when stratified by the type of presenting ACS and adjusted for differences in comorbidities, women with unstable angina actually had a better outcome than men with unstable angina, women and men with NSTEMI had similar outcome, and women with STEMI tended to have a worse outcome than men with STEMI. Similarly, in another study examining outcomes by type of acute coronary syndrome [33], the investigators found that adjusted short-term outcomes were higher among women than men with a first Q-wave infarction, but similar for women and men with a non–Q-wave MI or unstable angina. Other studies examining only patients with unstable angina have demonstrated better outcome in women when compared with men [48].

Finally, differences in outcome for women and men in various studies may reflect difference in management. In this era of aggressive medical therapy, overall outcomes have improved for women and men, and this improvement parallels the changes in practice patterns resulting from evidence-based guidelines. When examining contemporary studies of patients aggressively treated with ACC/AHA guideline therapies, there are no reported differences in mortality in women and men [5, 30, 38].

Advanced age has always been a predictor of poor outcome [9, 24, 74, 105]. The elderly have a higher overall rate of mortality from ACS compared with younger patients despite successful intervention [46, 54]. The risk increases with increasing age [9]. Although some of this increased risk may be related to differences in baseline variables, advanced age has been shown to be an independent predictor of mortality with ACS [9].

In summary, women and older patients with ACS should receive an individualized approach to management, with early recognition of disease potential and aggressive administration of guideline-recommended therapies. Modification of such therapies should be instituted when indicated to avoid the potential for increased risk. It is essential that these subgroups of patients are given appropriate treatment to ensure optimal outcomes.

References

1. Thom T et al. Heart disease and stroke statistics—2006 update: a report from the American Heart Association Statistics Committee and Stroke Statistics Subcommittee. Circulation 2006;113(6):e85–151.
2. Gerber Y et al. Secular trends in deaths from cardiovascular diseases: a 25-year community study. Circulation 2006;113(19):2285–2292.
3. Anand SS et al. Differences in the management and prognosis of women and men who suffer from acute coronary syndromes. J Am Coll Cardiol 2005;46(10): 1845–1851.
4. Hochman JS et al. Sex, clinical presentation and outcome in patients with acute coronary syndromes. Global Use of Strategies to Open Occluded Coronary Arteries in Acute Coronary Syndromes IIb Investigators. N Engl J Med 1999;341(4): 226–232.
5. Blomkalns AL et al. Gender disparities in the diagnosis and treatment of non-ST-segment elevation acute coronary syndromes: large-scale observations from the CRUSADE (Can Rapid Risk Stratification of Unstable Angina Patients Suppress Adverse Outcomes With Early Implementation of the American College of Cardiology/American Heart Association Guidelines) National Quality Improvement Initiative. J Am Coll Cardiol 2005;45(6):832–837.
6. Vaccarino V et al. Sex-based differences in early mortality after myocardial infarction. National Registry of Myocardial Infarction 2 Participants. N Engl J Med 1999;341(4):217–225.
7. Gan SC et al. Treatment of acute myocardial infarction and 30-day mortality among women and men. N Engl J Med 2000;343(1):8–15.
8. Bach RG et al. The effect of routine early invasive management on outcome for elderly patients with non-ST-segment elevation acute coronary syndromes. Ann Intern Med 2004;141(3):186–195.
9. Avezum A et al. Impact of age on management and outcome of acute coronary syndrome: observations from the Global Registry of Acute Coronary Events (GRACE). Am Heart J 2005;149(1):67–73.
10. Zandbergen AA et al. Normotensive women with type 2 diabetes and microalbuminuria are at high risk for macrovascular disease. Diabetes Care 2006;29(8): 1851–1855.
11. Mahonen MS et al. Current smoking and the risk of non-fatal myocardial infarction in the WHO MONICA Project populations. Tob Control 2004;13(3):244–250.
12. Manolio TA et al. Cholesterol and heart disease in older persons and women. Review of an NHLBI workshop. Ann Epidemiol 1992 2(1-2):161–176.
13. Sharrett AR et al. Coronary heart disease prediction from lipoprotein cholesterol levels triglycerides lipoprotein(a) apolipoproteins A-I and B and HDL density subfractions: The Atherosclerosis Risk in Communities (ARIC) Study. Circulation 2001;104(10):1108–1113.
14. Michos ED et al. Framingham risk equation underestimates subclinical atherosclerosis risk in asymptomatic women. Atherosclerosis 2006;184(1):201–206.
15. Michos ED et al. Women with a low Framingham risk score and a family history of premature coronary heart disease have a high prevalence of subclinical coronary atherosclerosis. Am Heart J 2005;150(6):1276–1281.
16. Executive Summary of The Third Report of The National Cholesterol Education Program (NCEP) Expert Panel on Detection Evaluation And Treatment of High

Blood Cholesterol In Adults (Adult Treatment Panel III). JAMA 2001;285(19): 2486–2497.

17. Turhan H et al. High prevalence of metabolic syndrome among young women with premature coronary artery disease. Coron Artery Dis 2005;16(1):37–40.

18. Marroquin OC et al. Metabolic syndrome modifies the cardiovascular risk associated with angiographic coronary artery disease in women: a report from the Women's Ischemia Syndrome Evaluation. Circulation 2004;109(6):714–721.

19. Bairey Merz CN et al. Hypoestrogenemia of hypothalamic origin and coronary artery disease in premenopausal women: a report from the NHLBI-sponsored WISE study. J Am Coll Cardiol 2003;41(3):413–419.

20. Merz CN et al. Past oral contraceptive use and angiographic coronary artery disease in postmenopausal women: data from the National Heart Lung and Blood Institute-sponsored Women's Ischemia Syndrome Evaluation. Fertil Steril 2006; 85(5):1425–1431.

21. Birdsall MA, Farquhar CM, White HD. Association between polycystic ovaries and extent of coronary artery disease in women having cardiac catheterization. Ann Intern Med 1997;126(1):32–35.

22. Milner KA et al. Gender and age differences in chief complaints of acute myocardial infarction (Worcester Heart Attack Study). Am J Cardiol 2004;93(5):606–608.

23. Goldberg RJ et al. Sex differences in symptom presentation associated with acute myocardial infarction: a population-based perspective. Am Heart J 1998;136(2): 189–195.

24. Kober L et al. Influence of gender on short- and long-term mortality after acute myocardial infarction. TRACE study group. Am J Cardiol 1996;77(12):1052–1056.

25. Karlson BW, Herlitz J, Hartford M. Prognosis in myocardial infarction in relation to gender. Am Heart J 1994;128(3):477–483.

26. Kudenchuk PJ et al. Comparison of presentation treatment and outcome of acute myocardial infarction in men versus women (the Myocardial Infarction Triage and Intervention Registry). Am J Cardiol 1996;78(1):9–14.

27. Tunstall-Pedoe H et al. Sex differences in myocardial infarction and coronary deaths in the Scottish MONICA population of Glasgow 1985 to 1991. Presentation, diagnosis, treatment, and 28-day case fatality of 3991 events in men and 1551 events in women. Circulation 1996;93(11):1981–1992.

28. Stern S et al. Presenting symptoms admission electrocardiogram management and prognosis in acute coronary syndromes: differences by age. Am J Geriatr Cardiol 2004;13(4):188–196.

29. Weaver WD et al. Comparisons of characteristics and outcomes among women and men with acute myocardial infarction treated with thrombolytic therapy. GUSTO-I investigators. JAMA 1996;275(10):777–782.

30. Cheng CI et al. Comparison of baseline characteristics clinical features angiographic results and early outcomes in men vs women with acute myocardial infarction undergoing primary coronary intervention. Chest 2004;126(1):47–53.

31. Vaccarino V et al. Sex and racial differences in the management of acute myocardial infarction, 1994 through 2002. N Engl J Med 2005;353(7):671–682.

32. Clarke KW et al. Do women with acute myocardial infarction receive the same treatment as men? BMJ 1994;309(6954):563–566.

33. Marrugat J et al. Short-term (28 days) prognosis between genders according to the type of coronary event (Q-wave versus non-Q-wave acute myocardial infarction versus unstable angina pectoris). Am J Cardiol 2004;94(9):1161–1165.

34. Jenkins JS et al. Causes of higher in-hospital mortality in women than in men after acute myocardial infarction. Am J Cardiol 1994;73(5):319–322.
35. Mehilli J et al. Gender and myocardial salvage after reperfusion treatment in acute myocardial infarction. J Am Coll Cardiol 2005;45(6):828–831.
36. Antoniucci D et al. Sex-based differences in clinical and angiographic outcomes after primary angioplasty or stenting for acute myocardial infarction. Am J Cardiol 2001;87(3):289–293.
37. Lefler LL, Bondy KN. Women's delay in seeking treatment with myocardial infarction: a meta-synthesis. J Cardiovasc Nurs 2004;19(4):251–268.
38. Lansky AJ et al. Gender differences in outcomes after primary angioplasty versus primary stenting with and without abciximab for acute myocardial infarction: results of the Controlled Abciximab and Device Investigation to Lower Late Angioplasty Complications (CADILLAC) trial. Circulation 2005;111(13):1611–1618.
39. Tamis-Holland JE et al. Benefits of direct angioplasty for women and men with acute myocardial infarction: results of the Global Use of Strategies to Open Occluded Arteries in Acute Coronary Syndromes Angioplasty (GUSTO II-B) Angioplasty Substudy. Am Heart J 2004;147(1):133–139.
40. Clayton TC et al. Do men benefit more than women from an interventional strategy in patients with unstable angina or non-ST-elevation myocardial infarction? The impact of gender in the RITA 3 trial. Eur Heart J 2004;25(18):1641–1650.
41. Liistro F et al. Early invasive strategy in elderly patients with non-ST elevation acute coronary syndrome: comparison with younger patients regarding 30 day and long term outcome. Heart 2005;91(10):1284–1288.
42. Alexander KP et al. Evolution in cardiovascular care for elderly patients with non-ST-segment elevation acute coronary syndromes: results from the CRUSADE National Quality Improvement Initiative. J Am Coll Cardiol 2005;46(8):1479–1487.
43. Braunwald E et al. ACC/AHA 2002; guideline update for the management of patients with unstable angina and non-ST-segment elevation myocardial infarction—summary article: a report of the American College of Cardiology/American Heart Association task force on practice guidelines (Committee on the Management of Patients With Unstable Angina). J Am Coll Cardiol 2002;40(7):1366–1374.
44. Dellborg M et al. ECG changes during myocardial ischemia. Differences between men and women. J Electrocardiol 1994;27(Suppl):42–45.
45. Lagerqvist B et al. Is early invasive treatment of unstable coronary artery disease equally effective for both women and men? FRISC II Study Group Investigators. J Am Coll Cardiol 2001;38(1):41–48.
46. Mueller C et al. Women do have an improved long-term outcome after non-ST-elevation acute coronary syndromes treated very early and predominantly with percutaneous coronary intervention: a prospective study in 1,450 consecutive patients. J Am Coll Cardiol 2002;40(2):245–250.
47. Glaser R et al. Benefit of an early invasive management strategy in women with acute coronary syndromes. JAMA 2002;288(24):3124–3129.
48. Roger VL et al. Sex differences in evaluation and outcome of unstable angina. JAMA 2000;283(5):646–652.
49. Gottlieb S et al. Sex differences in management and outcome after acute myocardial infarction in the 1990s: a prospective observational community-based study. Israeli Thrombolytic Survey Group. Circulation 2000;102(20):2484–24890.

50. Rosengren A et al. Age clinical presentation and outcome of acute coronary syndromes in the Euroheart acute coronary syndrome survey. Eur Heart J 2006; 27(7):789–795.
51. Jollis JG et al. OutcHome of acute myocardial infarction according to the specialty of the admitting physician. N Engl J Med 1996;335(25):1880–1887.
52. Granger CB et al. Activated partial thromboplastin time and outcome after thrombolytic therapy for acute myocardial infarction: results from the GUSTO-I trial. Circulation 1996;93(5):870–878.
53. Lee MS et al. The determinants of activated partial thromboplastin time relation of activated partial thromboplastin time to clinical outcomes and optimal dosing regimens for heparin treated patients with acute coronary syndromes: a review of GUSTO-IIb. J Thromb Thrombolysis 2002;14(2):91–101.
54. Antman EM et al. ACC/AHA guidelines for the management of patients with ST-elevation myocardial infarction—executive summary. A report of the American College of Cardiology/American Heart Association Task Force on Practice Guidelines (Writing Committee to revise the 1999 guidelines for the management of patients with acute myocardial infarction). J Am Coll Cardiol 2004;44(3):671–719.
55. Lansky AJ et al. Percutaneous coronary intervention and adjunctive pharmacotherapy in women: a statement for healthcare professionals from the American Heart Association. Circulation 2005;111(7):940–953.
56. A comparison of aspirin plus tirofiban with aspirin plus heparin for unstable angina. Platelet Receptor Inhibition in Ischemic Syndrome Management (PRISM) Study Investigators. N Engl J Med 1998;338(21):1498–1505.
57. Platelet Receptor Inhibition in Ischemic Syndrome Management in Patients Limited by Unstable Signs and Symptoms (PRISM-PLUS) Study Investigators. Inhibition of the platelet glycoprotein IIb/IIIa receptor with tirofiban in unstable angina and non-Q-wave myocardial infarction. N Engl J Med 1998;338(21):1488–1497.
58. The PURSUIT Trial Investigators. Platelet glycoprotein IIb/IIIa in unstable angina: receptor suppression using integrilin therapy. Inhibition of platelet glycoprotein IIb/IIIa with eptifibatide in patients with acute coronary syndromes. N Engl J Med 1998;339(7):436–443.
59. Alexander KP et al. Sex differences in major bleeding with glycoprotein IIb/IIIa inhibitors: results from the CRUSADE (Can Rapid risk stratification of Unstable angina patients Suppress ADverse outcomes with Early implementation of the ACC/AHA guidelines) initiative. Circulation 2006;114(13):1380–1387.
60. Huynh T et al. Analysis of bleeding complications associated with glycoprotein IIb/IIIa receptors blockade in patients with high-risk acute coronary syndromes: insights from the PRISM-PLUS study. Int J Cardiol 2005;100(1):73–78.
61. Lincoff AM et al. Thrombolytic therapy for women with myocardial infarction: is there a gender gap? Thrombolysis and Angioplasty in Myocardial Infarction Study Group. J Am Coll Cardiol 1993;22(7):1780–1787.
62. Cariou A et al. Sex-related differences in eligibility for reperfusion therapy and in-hospital outcome after acute myocardial infarction. Eur Heart J 1997;18(10): 1583–1589.
63. White HD et al. After correcting for worse baseline characteristics, women treated with thrombolytic therapy for acute myocardial infarction have the same mortality and morbidity as men except for a higher incidence of hemorrhagic stroke. The Investigators of the International Tissue Plasminogen Activator/Streptokinase Mortality Study. Circulation 1993;88(5 Pt 1):2097–2103.

64. Stone GW et al. Comparison of in-hospital outcome in men versus women treated by either thrombolytic therapy or primary coronary angioplasty for acute myocardial infarction Am J Cardiol 1995;75(15):987–992.

65. White HD et al. Age and outcome with contemporary thrombolytic therapy. Results from the GUSTO-I trial Global Utilization of Streptokinase and TPA for Occluded coronary arteries trial. Circulation 1996;94(8):1826–1833.

66. Berger AK. Thrombolysis in elderly patients with acute myocardial infarction. Am J Geriatr Cardiol 2003;12(4):251–256; quiz 257.

67. Brass LM et al. Intracranial hemorrhage associated with thrombolytic therapy for elderly patients with acute myocardial infarction: results from the Cooperative Cardiovascular Project. Stroke 2000;31(8):1802–1811.

68. Weaver WD et al. Comparison of primary coronary angioplasty and intravenous thrombolytic therapy for acute myocardial infarction: a quantitative review. JAMA 1997;278(23):2093–2098.

69. Grines CL et al. A comparison of immediate angioplasty with thrombolytic therapy for acute myocardial infarction. The Primary Angioplasty in Myocardial Infarction Study Group. N Engl J Med 1993;328(10):673–679.

70. The Global Use of Strategies to Open Occluded Coronary Arteries in Acute Coronary Syndromes (GUSTO IIb) Angioplasty Substudy Investigators. A clinical trial comparing primary coronary angioplasty with tissue plasminogen activator for acute myocardial infarction. N Engl J Med 1997;336(23):1621–1628.

71. Mehilli J et al. Sex-based analysis of outcome in patients with acute myocardial infarction treated predominantly with percutaneous coronary intervention. JAMA 2002;287(2):210–215.

72. De Luca G et al. Sex-related differences in outcome after ST-segment elevation myocardial infarction treated by primary angioplasty: data from the Zwolle Myocardial Infarction study. Am Heart J 2004;148(5):852–856.

73. Guagliumi G et al. Outcome in elderly patients undergoing primary coronary intervention for acute myocardial infarction: results from the Controlled Abciximab and Device Investigation to Lower Late Angioplasty Complications (CADILLAC) trial. Circulation 2004;110(12):1598–1604.

74. Holmes DR Jr et al. Effect of age on outcome with primary angioplasty versus thrombolysis. J Am Coll Cardiol 1999;33(2):412–419.

75. Hochman JS et al. Outcome and profile of women and men presenting with acute coronary syndromes: a report from TIMI IIIB TIMI Investigators. Thrombolysis in Myocardial Infarction. J Am Coll Cardiol 1997;30(1):141–148.

76. Malenka DJ et al. Gender-related changes in the practice and outcomes of percutaneous coronary interventions in Northern New England from 1994 to 1999. J Am Coll Cardiol 2002;40(12):2092–2101.

77. Chiu JH et al. Impact of female sex on outcome after percutaneous coronary intervention. Am Heart J 2004;148(6):998–1002.

78. Farouque HM et al. Risk factors for the development of retroperitoneal hematoma after percutaneous coronary intervention in the era of glycoprotein IIb/IIIa inhibitors and vascular closure devices. J Am Coll Cardiol 2005;45(3):363–368.

79. Piper WD et al. Predicting vascular complications in percutaneous coronary interventions. Am Heart J 2003;145(6):1022–1029.

80. Konstance R et al. Incidence and predictors of major vascular complications after percutaneous coronary intervention in the glycoprotein IIb/IIIa platelet inhibitor era. J Interv Cardiol 2004;17(2):65–70.

81. Peterson ED et al. Effect of gender on the outcomes of contemporary percutaneous coronary intervention. Am J Cardiol 2001;88(4):359–364.
82. Lincoff AM et al. Bivalirudin and provisional glycoprotein IIb/IIIa blockade compared with heparin and planned glycoprotein IIb/IIIa blockade during percutaneous coronary intervention: REPLACE-2 randomized trial. JAMA 2003;289(7): 853–863.
83. Klein LW. Percutaneous coronary intervention in the elderly patient (part I of II). J Invasive Cardiol 2006;18(6):286–295.
84. Kinnaird TD et al. Incidence predictors and prognostic implications of bleeding and blood transfusion following percutaneous coronary interventions. Am J Cardiol 2003;92(8):930–935.
85. Eagle KA et al. ACC/AHA 2004 guideline update for coronary artery bypass graft surgery: a report of the American College of Cardiology/American Heart Association Task Force on Practice Guidelines (Committee to Update the 1999 Guidelines for Coronary Artery Bypass Graft Surgery). Circulation 2004;110(14):e340–437.
86. Vaccarino V et al. Gender differences in recovery after coronary artery bypass surgery. J Am Coll Cardiol 2003;41(2):307–314.
87. Aldea GS et al. Effect of gender on postoperative outcomes and hospital stays after coronary artery bypass grafting. Ann Thorac Surg 1999;67(4):1097–1103.
88. Graham MM et al. Quality of life after coronary revascularization in the elderly. Eur Heart J 2006;27(14):1690–1698.
89. Hogue CW Jr et al. Sex differences in neurological outcomes and mortality after cardiac surgery: a society of thoracic surgery national database report. Circulation 2001;103(17):2133–2137.
90. Vaccarino V et al. Sex differences in hospital mortality after coronary artery bypass surgery: evidence for a higher mortality in younger women. Circulation 2002; 105(10):1176–1181.
91. Utley JR et al. Intraoperative blood transfusion is a major risk factor for coronary artery bypass grafting in women. Ann Thorac Surg 1995;60(3):570–574; 574–575.
92. Hammar N et al. Comparison of early and late mortality in men and women after isolated coronary artery bypass graft surgery in Stockholm Sweden 1980 to 1989. J Am Coll Cardiol 1997;29(3):659–664.
93. O'Connor GT et al. Differences between men and women in hospital mortality associated with coronary artery bypass graft surgery. The Northern New England Cardiovascular Disease Study Group. Circulation 1993;88(5 Pt 1):2104–2110.
94. Loop FD et al. Coronary artery surgery in women compared with men: analyses of risks and long-term results. J Am Coll Cardiol 1983;1(2 Pt 1):383–390.
95. Bhatt DL et al. Utilization of early invasive management strategies for high-risk patients with non-ST-segment elevation acute coronary syndromes: results from the CRUSADE Quality Improvement Initiative. JAMA 2004;292(17):2096–2104.
96. Hochman JS, Tamis-Holland JE. Acute coronary syndromes: does sex matter? JAMA 2002;288(24):3161–3164.
97. Krumholz HM et al. Selection of patients for coronary angiography and coronary revascularization early after myocardial infarction: is there evidence for a gender bias? Ann Intern Med 1992;116(10):785–790.
98. Vaccarino V et al. Sex differences in 2-year mortality after hospital discharge for myocardial infarction. Ann Intern Med 2001;134(3):173–181.

99. Maynard C et al. Gender differences in the treatment and outcome of acute myocardial infarction. Results from the Myocardial Infarction Triage and Intervention Registry. Arch Intern Med 1992;152(5):972–976.
100. Dittrich H et al. Acute myocardial infarction in women: influence of gender on mortality and prognostic variables. Am J Cardiol 1988 62(1):1–7.
101. Goldberg RJ et al. A communitywide perspective of sex differences and temporal trends in the incidence and survival rates after acute myocardial infarction and out-of-hospital deaths caused by coronary heart disease. Circulation 1993;87(6): 1947–1953.
102. Greenland P et al. In-hospital and 1-year mortality in 1,524 women after myocardial infarction. Comparison with 4,315 men. Circulation 1991;83(2):484–491.
103. Fiebach NH, Viscoli CM, Horwitz RI. Differences between women and men in survival after myocardial infarction. Biology or methodology? JAMA 1990;263(8): 1092–1096.
104. Vakili BA, Kaplan RC, Brown DL. Sex-based differences in early mortality of patients undergoing primary angioplasty for first acute myocardial infarction. Circulation 2001;104(25):3034–3038.
105. Chandra NC et al. Observations of the treatment of women in the United States with myocardial infarction: a report from the National Registry of Myocardial Infarction–I. Arch Intern Med 1998;158(9):981–988.

21
Acute Coronary Syndrome in African Americans and Hispanic Americans

Tseday Sirak, Simbo Chiadika, Matthew Daka,
and Claude Simon

Among African Americans and Hispanics in the United States, coronary heart disease (CHD) is highly prevalent and is the single most frequent cause of myocardial infarction and death in that population [1]. However, multiple factors contribute to overall poorer care and worse outcomes among African Americans and Hispanics when compared with whites. These factors include difference in disease manifestation, socioeconomic status, access to care, patient perception of the health care system and of providers, attitudes of health care providers toward minority patients, therapeutic modalities and responses to treatment, and patient education.

Although race-specific CHD data are sparse among black and Hispanic persons, rates of death among African Americans are among the highest in the industrialized world. This may be due to the complexities of race as a health factor or to controversies regarding whether health issues should even be considered in terms of race, as race is inextricably linked with socio-economic status in the United States. Nevertheless, current data indicate that there are increasing disparities in cardiovascular health care among African Americans and Hispanics [1–3]. Compared with whites, African Americans are more likely to present with CHD at an earlier age, have higher out-of-hospital coronary death rates, and are more likely to have sudden cardiac death as the initial clinical presentation of CHD. Although the reasons for these differences are not well understood, it is possible that these health consequences are explained by significant heterogeneity in acute coronary syndrome manifestation among African Americans. A high prevalence of certain coronary risk factors, delays in identification and treatment of high-risk individuals, limited access to cardiovascular care, and lack of compliance and trust in the health care system appear to contribute to the burden of CHD among African Americans.

Coronary Risk Factors

African Americans are 1.5 times more likely to have multiple risk factors than whites [4, 5]. This clustering of risk factors synergistically increases the prevalence of CHD. Although the relationship between the incidence of coronary heart disease and standard risk factors, including low-density lipoprotein (LDL) cholesterol level, high-density lipoprotein (HDL) cholesterol level, high blood pressure, smoking, and diabetes are well described and established in several populations, the risk of sequelae attributable to some risk factors (i.e., hypertension, diabetes, smoking, obesity, and physical inactivity) is greater for African and Hispanic Americans [6, 7].

Hypertension

Although both systolic and diastolic blood pressures are risk factors for CHD mortality, systolic blood pressure is a better predictor of CHD, stroke, heart failure, end-stage renal disease, and overall mortality [8]. Hypertension is known to cause left ventricular hypertrophy (LVH), endothelial dysfunction leading to atherosclerosis, and decrease in compliance of large arteries and overall left ventricular dysfunction. Greater disease severity is associated with LVH and higher mortality rate [6]. At any given blood pressure level, African Americans appear to have greater cardiovascular and renal damage compared with whites [9–11]. In African Americans, hypertension is more prevalent, develops at younger ages, and is associated with 3 to 5 times higher cardiovascular mortality than whites [12–14]. Between the ages of 35 to 54 years, blacks died 6 to 10 times as frequently from hypertensive diseases according to a 1973 statistic [15], an excess far out of proportion to the approximate 2 to 3 times excess of prevalence of hypertensive blacks. After the age of 55 years, the excess mortality is more nearly proportionate to the prevalence, especially in older age groups [9, 15]. Overall, African Americans die 3 times as frequently as whites from hypertension-related diseases in the United States [15].

Left Ventricular Hypertrophy

As a manifestation of the end-organ effects of hypertension, LVH represents a particularly important index of preclinical disease that carries incremental prognostic value beyond that afforded by traditional coronary risk factors [16]. In African Americans, LVH is highly predictive of ischemic heart disease morbidity and mortality and seems to be a stronger risk factor than hypertension itself, cigarette smoking, or hypercholesterolemia [6, 17]. Patients with LVH have a two- to four-fold higher incidence of CHD, myocardial infarction, stroke, heart failure, or other cardiovascular diseases, [6, 14, 10] possibly as a result of increased susceptibility of the hypertrophied heart to subendocardial hypoperfusion especially during exertion. Earlier studies have found left ventricular relative wall thickness (RWT) to be higher in black normotensive [18, 19] and hypertensive [19–22] subjects compared with whites. Whatever the cause for the ethnic differences in LV mass and geometry, these findings have potentially far-reaching implications, hence the importance of screening in this population. Because electrocardiography is insensitive and less specific in black individuals than in whites for detection of LVH, echocardiographic evaluation is especially valuable in these individuals [23].

The Metabolic Syndrome and Diabetes

Obesity, especially visceral obesity, is a major component of the metabolic syndrome and is associated with an increased risk of cardiovascular disease morbidity and mortality [24, 26]. Other components of the metabolic syndrome include insulin resistance, hypertriglyceridemia, reduced HDL cholesterol, and hypertension. Although the prevalence of obesity among African-American men is similar to that among white men, in African-American women, obesity is twice as prevalent and the visceral pattern is more common than in their white counterparts [27–29].

Diabetic patients have at least two- to four-fold higher risk for vascular disease than nondiabetics [30, 31]. Cardiovascular disease is responsible for approximately 80% of all deaths and more than 75% of all hospitalizations in patients with diabetes [31]. The prevalence of type II diabetes has tripled in the past three decades and is 2 to 3 times higher in African Americans than in whites [32, 33]. Diabetic African-American and Hispanic patients have similar complications as their white counterparts, but they are more likely to have a more aggressive clinical course and far more complications at presentation than whites.

Smoking

African Americans in the Coronary Artery Surgery Study (CASS) had a higher mortality rate during 16 years of follow-up, regardless of whether they received medical or surgical therapy. The increased mortality was attributed entirely to cigarette smoking [34]. Although African-American women smoke at comparable rates as white women, there is a greater prevalence of tobacco smoking among African-American men compared with white men [34, 35].

Biologic, Biochemical, and Biomarker Differences

The greater mortality from CHD and the acute coronary syndromes [36–38] in African Americans compared with whites has been attributed to a greater clustering of risk factors such as hypertension, LVH, diabetes, and tobacco smoking

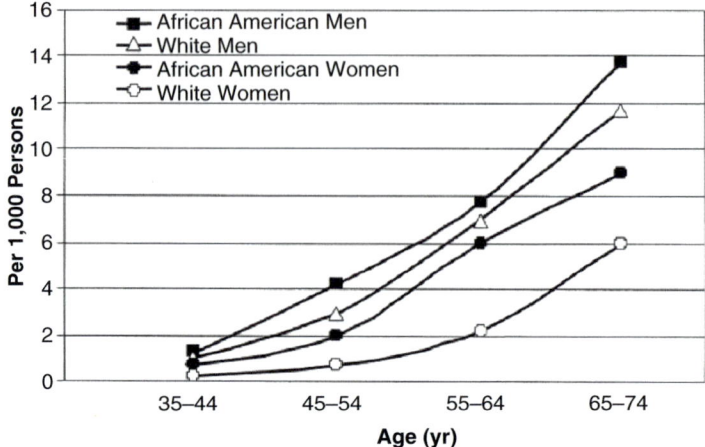

Figure 21.1. Annual rate of first myocardial infarction by age among African-American and white men and women. (Adapted from American Heart Association. 1998 Heart and Stroke Statistical Update. Dallas, TX: American Heart Association; 1998. [43].)

[14, 23, 38–41] in addition to inadequate screening and suboptimal use of evidence-based treatment of this group in clinical practice [42]. There is a definite difference between African Americans and whites of both genders with regard to rates of first myocardial infarction by age (Fig. 21.1) [43]. It is unclear to what extent inherent biologic factors and biochemical differences contribute to these more adverse outcomes in African Americans and Hispanics.

Lipid Profiles

Data from the Insulin Resistance Atherosclerosis Study (IRAS) [44] on lipid profiles (Tables 21.1 and 21.2) by ethnicity indicate that African Americans have higher HDL, lower triglycerides, and greater LDL size than other ethnic groups. At each level of serum total cholesterol, however, African-American men had a lower reported incidence of coronary artery disease (CAD) than white men. This differing impact of serum cholesterol on CAD occurrence among the races

Table 21.1. Pathophysiologic factors related to cardiovascular disease that may differ in black patients.

Unfavorable	Favorable	No effect	Not well-established
↑ Risk-factor prevalence	↑ Fibrinolysis	↑ Lipoprotein(a)	↓ Coronary flow reserve
↑ Risk-factor clustering	↑ HDL cholesterol		↑ Platelet survival
↑ Left ventricular mass	↓ LDL cholesterol		↑ Hematologic parameters*
↓ Vasodilatation (peripheral)			↓ Insulin sensitivity

Source: Adapted from Haffner SM, D'Agostino R Jr, Goff D, et al. LDL size in African Americans, Hispanics, and non-Hispanic whites the Insulin Resistance Atherosclerosis Study. Arterioscler Thromb Vasc Biol 1999;19:2234–2240.
*Hematologic parameters include fibrinogen, factor VIII, von Willebrand factor, and antithrombin III.

TABLE 21.2. Lipid profiles by ethnic group in the Insulin Resistance Atherosclerosis Study (IRAS).

	African American (n = 462)	Hispanic (n =546)	Non-Hispanic white (n = 612)
Total cholesterol (mg/dL)	212.5	211.1	213.2
LDL cholesterol (mg/dL)	143.8	139.4	140.7
HDL cholesterol (mg/dL)*	47.0	42.3	44.0
Triglycerides (mg/dL)*	102.1	147.7	134.0
LDL size (Å)*	262.1	257.6	259.2

Source: Adapted from Haffner SM, D'Agostino R Jr, Goff D, et al. LDL size in African Americans, Hispanics, and non-Hispanic whites the Insulin Resistance Atherosclerosis Study. Arterioscler Thromb Vasc Biol 1999;19:2234–2240.
*$P < 0.001$ for all.

highlights the importance of cholesterol subfractions as more accurate determinants of risk and mediators of atherosclerosis.

Lipoprotein(a)

A disparity between levels of lipoprotein(a) in adult African Americans compared with whites is evident. Lipoprotein(a) has been shown to be a leading independent risk factor for CAD, stroke, and peripheral vascular disease in non-black men [45]. However, despite the finding that lipoprotein(a) levels are in general twice as high among African Americans, this finding does not impart a higher risk of CAD or atherosclerosis for African Americans [46].

High-Sensitivity C-reactive Protein

There are emerging data showing racial/ethnic variations in the levels of high-sensitivity C-reactive protein (hs-CRP), an inflammatory marker associated with increased CAD risk [47]. A Canadian study showed that the proportions of groups with hs-CRP levels above the high-risk level of 3 mg/L were 54% in Aboriginals, 28.5% in South Asians, 24.8% in Europeans, and 6% in Chinese [48].

Higher levels are found in African Americans than in whites. Assessment of hs-CRP levels among 24,455 white, 254 Hispanic, 475 African-American, and 357 Asian women in the U.S. Women's Health Study showed median hs-CRP levels of 2.02 mg/L in whites, 2.06 mg/L in Hispanics, 2.96 mg/L in African Americans, and 1.12 mg/L in Asians ($P < 0.001$). As expected, levels of hs-CRP were higher in women receiving hormone replacement therapy, but the pattern of differences among the ethnic groups was similar among users and nonusers, with African-American women having the highest levels in both categories. Hispanic women had the second highest levels [49].

Endothelial Dysfunction and Vasodilatation

There has recently been considerable research on the role of the vascular wall in the pathogenesis of hypertension and angina-like chest pain with angiographically normal coronary arteries. Attenuated forearm blood flow responses in healthy African Americans to nitric oxide–dependent and –independent vasorelaxation have been demonstrated in well-designed experimental studies, suggesting a possible explanation for the pathogenesis of hypertension [50]. Similar studies have sought to explain the frequent occurrence in African Americans of angina-like chest pain with angiographically normal coronary arteries [51].

In a study of 80 African-American and white patients with minimal CAD and chest pain, no racial differences in coronary vascular relaxation were found, regardless of hypertension or LVH [52].

African Americans are reported to respond less well to angiotensin-converting enzyme (ACE) inhibitors and are at increased risk of cardiovascular (CV) disease progression. In the ALLHAT study, African-American patients receiving lisinopril had significantly increased risks for stroke and combined CHD, along with a trend for increased heart failure risk and reduced blood pressure–lowering effect when compared with non–African-American patients receiving lisinopril [53]. In African Americans with diabetes, persistent microalbuminuria despite ACE inhibitor therapy may be associated with poor prognosis for cardiovascular disease and mortality. African-American type II diabetics with persistent microalbuminuria have severely impaired flow mediated vasodilation and nitroglycerin-dependent dilation (NDD) when compared with matched patients who had microalbuminuria that was eliminated by ACE inhibitors. This may explain the poor prognosis for cardiovascular disease in patients who have persistent microalbuminuria. Alternative strategies for reducing microalbuminuria in high-risk patients who do not respond adequately to ACE inhibitor therapy such as African Americans are needed [54].

Thrombosis, Fibrinolysis, and Other Hemostatic Correlates

A vital difference between African Americans and whites with acute coronary syndromes may exist in the balance between thrombosis and the fibrinolytic system. The implications of this finding are integral to understanding the development of acute coronary syndromes and the response to treatment. Studies performed predominately in black Africans have demonstrated enhanced endogenous fibrinolytic activity compared with white races in Africa, Europe, and the United States [55, 56]. The proposed mechanisms responsible for this increased fibrinolysis are speculative but include reduced inhibition or enhanced susceptibility to fibrinolysis. These findings are particularly relevant when interpreting the response of black Americans in fibrinolytic therapy trials.

Fibrinogen has been postulated to be associated with increased atherosclerotic cardiovascular risk. When fibrinogen was measured in 4,193 participants in the Coronary Artery Risk Development In young Adults (CARDIA) study, levels were higher in African Americans compared with whites [57]. Population-based surveys adjusting for age and sex have demonstrated potentially important racial differences in hemostatic factors, with African Americans having higher levels of factor VIII, von Willebrand factor, and antithrombin III than whites [58].

These racial differences are thought-provoking and hypothesis-generating for ongoing research. Their direct impact on the acute coronary syndromes in African Americans and Hispanics is still being elucidated.

Response to Antithrombotic Therapy and Fibrinolysis

More evidence for the biologic distinctions between African Americans and whites with respect to thrombosis and fibrinolysis has been gained from some pivotal trials of antithrombin and fibrinolytic agents. Analysis of the TIMI-II and TAMI-I trials revealed significant clinical and hematologic differences between African Americans and whites after receiving tissue plasminogen activator (tPA) [59, 60].

TIMI-II compared 2,564 whites and 174 African Americans receiving tPA for suspected MI [60]. African Americans were found to have a more pronounced reduction in plasma fibrinogen levels after fibrinolytic therapy. However, infarct artery patency at 18 to 48 hours and 1-year outcomes were similar between the races. In contrast, analysis of a smaller subgroup from the TAMI-I trial revealed important differences between 352 white and 24 black patients treated with tPA [59]. In this report, African Americans displayed a significantly lower nadir of plasma fibrinogen levels, a greater fall in fibrinogen levels, and increased levels of fibrinogen degradation products. The enhanced sensitivity to tPA in African Americans was manifested by improved infarct-related artery patency at 90 minutes and increased transfusion requirements. Survival at hospital discharge did not differ in this small study between African Americans and whites.

The Global Utilization of Streptokinase and t-PA for Occluded Arteries (GUSTO) trial and the GUSTO Angiographic substudy provide the largest available database for examining race-dependent differences in response to fibrinolytic therapy [61, 62]. The GUSTO trial included 41,021 patients, of whom 1,157 were African Americans. The angiographic substudy included 2,431 patients, of whom 103 were African Americans [63]. In this trial, the efficacy of reperfusion appeared better in African Americans than in whites. Among all patients undergoing angiography (n = 18,791), the rate of TIMI grade 3 flow was 54.8% in African-Americans patients and 47.6% in white patients ($P = 0.002$) [63].

These differences existed despite African Americans receiving fibrinolytic therapy on the average 18 minutes later than whites, a factor known to worsen reperfusion and survival outcomes, but occurred at the cost of increased bleeding complications. Similar findings of fewer myocardial but more cerebral events among African Americans with acute coronary syndromes (unstable angina and non–Q-wave MI) randomly assigned to heparin or hirudin (GUSTO II) or eptifibatide or placebo (Platelet Glycoprotein IIb/IIIa in Unstable Angina: Receptor Suppression Using Integrilin [PURSUIT] trial) have also been reported [64].

Differences in Presentation

It is notable that African Americans with CAD often present differently than others. As earlier noted, there is a clustering of CAD risk factors in this group. These patients are 1.5 times more likely to have multiple risk factors than whites [65], and these multiple risk factors work synergistically to increase the risk of CAD.

The majority of African Americans with acute coronary syndromes present with typical chest pain symptoms as in whites. However, the incidence of silent ischemic episodes and atypical symptoms is higher in African Americans than in whites [66, 67]. It has been hypothesized that this may be due in part to the high prevalence of hypertension and diabetes in African Americans. Diabetes, in particular, has been associated with atypical presentations of coronary ischemia. This may account for some of the delay in disease recognition and in seeking medical care seen among African Americans [68].

African Americans with acute chest pain syndromes suggestive of coronary artery disease are more likely to have minimal or no angiographic coronary artery disease than are whites [51, 69–71]. Paradoxically however, when significant coronary artery disease is present on angiography, they tend to have much more extensive burden of atherosclerosis than is observed in whites [72].

African Americans are more likely to present with non–ST-elevation myocardial infarction, or unstable angina, whereas ST-elevation myocardial infarction is seen in higher frequency in whites [68]. Despite this, however, they have poorer overall outcomes than do whites [73]. African Americans tend to present with acute coronary syndromes at younger ages and have higher mortality rates at younger age than in whites [1, 2, 17]. This higher mortality rate seen at an earlier age in this group has been speculated to be due to the greater prevalence of coronary artery disease risk factors such as hypertension, cigarette smoking, and diabetes [63, 74]. In the fibrinolytic era, this less definite presentation of acute coronary syndrome in African Americans may account for why they tended to get fibrinolytic therapy less frequently and much later than whites [66, 75–76]. In addition to such poor short-term prognosis, worse long-term prognosis when compared with whites has also been documented [63]. In the

GUSTO trial of fibrinolytic therapy for myocardial infarction, the 1-year unadjusted all-cause mortality among black patients was 11.6% compared with 9.7% for whites ($P = 0.03$) [63].

There is a significantly higher incidence of out-of-hospital sudden cardiac death as the first manifestation of coronary heart disease in African Americans compared with whites. Sudden cardiac death rates have been reported to be 3 times higher in black men than in white men, even after adjusting for age, socioeconomic status, and access to care [77–79].

Factors Contributing to Delay in Diagnosis and Access to Care

There is a vast disparity in treatment of acute myocardial infarction in African Americans compared with whites [37, 80–82]. This difference has been demonstrated to be even greater in African-American women compared with white men and women. In an analysis of sex and racial differences in 598,911 patients treated for myocardial infarction in the National Registry of Myocardial Infarction (NRMI) between 1994 and 2002, Vaccarino et al. noted that the rates of reperfusion therapy and coronary angiography were significantly less for African Americans compared with whites; the rates of reperfusion, coronary angiography, and coronary artery bypass surgery were lowest in African-American women; African-American women had the highest rate of adjusted mortality across all sex and racial groups [82]. While the use of more traditional treatments (e.g., aspirin and beta-blockers) were similar between African Americans and whites in general in the NRMI registry, still African-American women had significantly lower use of such treatments when compared with white men (risk ratio: 0.94 for aspirin, 0.96 for beta-blockers; $P < 0.001$) [82]. These differences in care could not be accounted for by patient preferences with respect to reperfusion therapy because there were few refusals documented across all age and gender groups.

However, access to care and delay in diagnosis may play a role. African-American patients who present to the emergency department with chest pain are less likely to undergo electrocardiograms than are white patients and as such have a relative delay in diagnosis of acute coronary ischemia [83].

Health Care Systems

In their analysis of the Cardiac Access Study from three urban hospitals, LaVeist et al. found that the racial disparity in obtaining coronary angiography was in part due to the health care system context in which African American and white patients obtain their care, combined with the specific clinical characteristics of the patients [84]. The need for transfer to another hospital for coronary angiography or admission to a hospital without in-house catheterization was important barriers to angiography in African Americans [84]. Although African

Americans are more likely to be treated in large academic hospitals [37] and more likely than whites to reside in areas with advanced-technology cardiac services [85], when such services are not available, they are less likely than whites to travel the distance to obtain advanced-technology cardiac services at the time of acute myocardial infarction [85]. This may account for some of the disparities in obtaining invasive procedures when unavailable to them. Even after adjusting for provider type, number of hospital beds, geographic region, hospital services, and hospital academic status, Sonel et al. found that differences in care still persisted [37]. Bradley et al. found that a substantial portion of the disparity in time to acute reperfusion therapy (door to drug, door to balloon) in patients hospitalized with ST-segment elevation myocardial infarction was accounted for by the specific hospital to which patients were admitted, not to differential treatment by race within a given hospital, according to NRMI data. Therefore, hospital-to-hospital differences in time to reperfusion by race was not attributable to quality assurance factors such as hospital volume, teaching status, or urban/rural location [86]. African Americans visit hospitals that have lower rates of evidence-based medical treatment, higher rates of cardiac procedures, and worse risk-adjusted mortality after acute myocardial infarction [87].

Certain physician characteristics have also been linked to barriers to optimal care in African Americans. African Americans are significantly less likely to obtain specialty cardiac care and less likely to see a board-certified physician [84, 88]. In addition, physicians themselves may carry certain detrimental expectations in that they may assume that African-American patients in general are less willing to pursue more invasive treatments [84].

Patient characteristics such as socioeconomic economic status, income, insurance factors, and education also play a role in the disparity of care [89, 90]. Even after adjustment for insurance factors, disparities were still observed [37]. According to a Veterans study by Whittle et al. [91], when financial incentives for physicians were absent, whites were still more likely than African Americans to undergo invasive procedures. Furthermore, because of differences in attitudes from whites about procedural risk, African Americans are generally less willing to undergo invasive procedures [92]. Also, a patient's level of education seems to play a role in his or her willingness to accept a physician's recommendation to undergo cardiac catheterization. Schecter et al. showed that coronary care unit patients who attended high school or higher levels of education were more likely to be white and more likely to undergo cardiac catheterization [93].

African Americans are as likely as whites to receive older well-established medical regimens (aspirin, beta-blockers, ACE inhibitors) in the setting of an acute coronary syndrome; however the use of newer medical therapies (e.g., glycoprotein IIb/IIIa inhibitors, clopidogrel, and statins) is much lower [37]. Finally, Sonel et al. speculated that the underrepresentation of African Americans in clinical trials of newer therapies may account in part for the different expectations of the impact of administering such therapies [37].

Compliance and Barriers to Treatment and Trust Issues

African Americans in general appear to be less likely than whites to comply with prescribed medications. In a retrospective study comparing medication compliance among Medicaid-insured patients who were given first-time prescriptions for oral antidiabetic agents, African Americans had a 12% lower adherence rate than whites [34]. Such low rates of adherence may be related to lower socioeconomic status and to lower levels of education. A study published by the Institute of Medicine in 2002 found that African Americans, Hispanics, and Native Americans have a burden of illness and mortality from diabetes that is between 50% and 100% higher than that among whites and that some of the disease burden may be attributed to medication noncompliance.

To assess whether disparities in outcomes were related to medication compliance, Shenolikar and colleagues at Wake Forest in Winston-Salem, North Carolina, examined a group of Medicaid-insured patients with a new, first-time oral prescription for diabetes. The cohort included 1,527 African Americans, 1,128 white patients, and 514 patients of other racial/ethnic backgrounds. Medication adherence was determined by assessing the ratio between prescriptions and refills, with the assumption that a refill implies that the patient had taken the prescribed drug. The outcome was expressed as a medication possession ratio, calculated as the number of days that the patient possessed a prescription divided by the number of days between refills. Multivariate regression analyses were used to determine the difference in adherence rates, adjusting for other covariates, including demographic characteristics (such as age and gender), clinical confounders (such as use of health care services over the previous 12 months), type of therapy, total number of medications, and number of comorbidities. They found that whites had significantly higher adherence rates than African Americans (0.59 [SD = 0.31] vs. 0.54 [SD = 0.31]; $P < 0.05$). Whites took their medication 59% of the time, compared with African Americans, who took their medications 54% of the time. In multivariate analyses, the difference translated into a 12% lower compliance rate among African Americans after adjustment for covariates [94].

In addition to generally lower socioeconomic status and lower education levels, lack of trust in the health care system may also contribute to noncompliance and barriers to treatment in the African-American population as a whole. The legacy of the Tuskegee experiment, which was created purportedly to improve the health status of African Americans but ethically violated and failed to educate and treat its study participants, has also laid the foundation for today's pervasive sense of African-American distrust in health professionals and public health systems in general [95].

It is clear that patterns of trust in our healthcare system differ by race. Although the Tuskegee experiment may have contributed largely to this mistrust of medical care, other broader historical and personal experiences should not be excluded. Improved understanding of these factors is essential for enhancing patient access to and satisfaction with the health care system. Hence, to help improve the health of our African-American and Hispanic patients, we must rebuild their trust by being staunch advocates for their well-being and holding ourselves to the highest ethical and moral standards.

Conclusion

When compared with whites in the United States, African Americans and Hispanics appear to have greater morbidity and mortality secondary to CHD. This is due to higher prevalence and increased clustering of risk factors, occurrence at younger ages, atypical presentations, a higher incidence of out-of-hospital sudden cardiac death as the initial presentation, delays in disease recognition and in presentation for medical treatment, more extensive atherosclerotic burden at presentation, disparity in treatment and access to care, perception biases, greater noncompliance, and generally lower socioeconomic status and education.

References

1. Gillum RF, Mussolino ME, Madans JH. Coronary heart disease incidence and survival in African-American women and men. The NHANES I epidemiologic follow-up study. Ann Intern Med 1997;127:111–118.
2. Gillum RF. Sudden cardiac death in Hispanic Americans and African Americans. Am J Public Health 1997;87:1461–1466.
3. Traven ND, Kuller LH, Ives DG, et al. Coronary heart disease mortality and sudden death among the 35–44 year age group in Allegheny County, Pennsylvania. Ann Epidemiol 1996;6:130–136.
4. Rowland ML, Fulwood R. Coronary heart disease risk factor trends in blacks between the First and Second National Health and Nutrition Examination Surveys, United States, 1971–1980. Am Heart J 1984;108:771–779.
5. Hutchinson RG, Watson RL, Davis CE, et al. Racial differences in risk factors for atherosclerosis. The ARIC study. Angiology 1997;48:279–290.
6. Liao Y, Cooper RS, McGee DL, et al. The relative effects of left ventricular hypertrophy, coronary artery disease, and ventricular dysfunction on survival among black adults. JAMA 1995;273:1592–1597.
7. Gavin JR III. Diabetes in minorities:reflections on the medical dilemma and the healthcare crisis. Trans Am Clin Climatol Assoc 1995;107:213–223.
8. Kannel WB. Historic perspectives on the relative contributions of diastolic and systolic blood pressure elevation to cardiovascular risk profile. Am Heart J 1999;138: 205–210.
9. Heyman A, Fields WS, Keating RD. Joint Study of Extracranial Arterial Occlusion VI. Racial differences in hospitalized patients with ischemic stroke. JAMA 1972; 222:285.
10. Dustan H. Growth factors and racial differences in severity of hypertension and renal diseases. Lancet 1992;339:1339–1340.
11. Whittle JC, Whelton PK, Seidler AJ, et al. Does racial variation in risk factors explain black-white differences in the incidence of hypertensive end-stage renal disease? Arch Intern Med 1991;151:1359–1364.

12. McCord C, Freeman HB. Excess mortality in Harlem. N Engl J Med 1990;322: 173–177.
13. U.S. Department of Health and Human Services. Report of the Working Group on Research in Coronary Heart Disease in Blacks. Bethesda, MD: U.S. Public Health Service, National Institutes of Health; 1994.
14. Gillum RF, Grant CT. Coronary heart disease in black populations. II. Risk factors. Am Heart J 1982;104:852–864.
15. Vital Statistics of the United States, 1973, Vol. II. Mortality, Part A. Washington, DC: U.S. Department of Health, Education and Welfare, Public Health Service, National Center for Health Statistics; 1977.
16. Levy D, Garrison RJ, Savage DD, et al. Prognostic implications of echocardiographically determined left ventricular mass in the Framingham Heart Study. N Engl J Med. 1990;322:1561–1566.
17. Thomas J, Thomas DJ, Pearson T, et al. Cardiovascular disease in African-American and white physicians: the Meharry Cohort and Meharry-Hopkins Cohort Studies. J Health Care Poor Underserved 1997;8:270–283.
18. Lorber R, Gidding SS, Daviglus ML, et al. Influence of systolic blood pressure and body mass index on left ventricular structure in healthy African-Americans and white young adults: the CARDIA study. J Am Coll Cardiol 2003;41:955–960.
19. Chaturvedi N, Athanassopoulos G, McKeigue PM, et al. Echocardiographic measures of left ventricular structure and their relation with rest and ambulatory blood pressure in blacks and whites in the United Kingdom. J Am Coll Cardiol 1994;24: 1499–1505.
20. Gottdiener JS, Reda DJ, Materson BJ, et al. Importance of obesity, race and age to the cardiac structural and functional effects of hypertension. J Am Coll Cardiol 1994;24:1492–1498.
21. Gardin JM, Wagenknecht LE, Anton-Culver H, et al. Relationship of cardiovascular risk factors to echocardiographic left ventricular mass in healthy young black and white adult men and women. The CARDIA Study. Circulation 1995;92:380–387.
22. Koren MJ, Mensah GA, Blake J, et al. Comparison of left ventricular mass and geometry in black and white patients with essential hypertension. Am J Hypertens 1993; 6:815–823.
23. Lee DK, Marantz PR, Devereux RB, et al. Left ventricular hypertrophy in black and white hypertensives. Standard electrocardiographic criteria overestimate racial differences in prevalence. JAMA 1992;267:3294–3299.
24. Wilson PW. Established risk factors and coronary artery disease: the Framingham study. Am J Hypertens 1994;7(7 Pt 2):7S–12S.
25. Manson JE, Colditz GA, Stampfer MJ, et al. A prospective study of obesity and risk of coronary heart disease in women. N Engl J Med 1990;322:882–889.
26. Banerji MA, Lebowitz J, Chaiken RL, et al. Relationships of visceral adipose tissue and glucose disposal in independent of sex in black NIDDM subjects. Am J Physiol 1997;273:E425–432.
27. Kumanyika S. Searching for the association of obesity with coronary artery disease [editorial]. Obes Res 1995;3:273–275.
28. Svec F, Rivera M, Huth M. Correlation of waist to hips ratio to the prevalence of diabetes and hypertension in black females. J Natl Med Assoc 1990;82:257–261.
29. Clark LT, Karve MM, Rones KT, et al. Obesity, distribution of body fat and coronary artery disease in black women. Am J Cardiol 1994;73:895–896.

30. Kannel WB, Wilson PW. An update on coronary risk factors. Med Clin North Am 1995;79:951–971.
31. Harris MI, Flegal KM, Cowie CC, et al. Prevalence of diabetes, impaired fasting glucose, and impaired glucose tolerance in US adults. The Third National Health and Nutrition Examination Survey, 1988–1994. Diabetes Care 1998;21:518–524.
32. Carter JS, Pugh JA, Monterrosa A. Non-insulin-dependent diabetes mellitus in minorities in the United States. Ann Intern Med 1996;125:221–232.
33. Brancati FL, Kao WHL, Folsom AR, et al. Incident type 2 diabetes mellitus in African American and white adults. The Atherosclerosis Risk in Communities study. JAMA 2000;283:2253–2259.
34. Taylor HA, Mickel MC, Chaitman BR, et al. Long-term survival of African Americans in the Coronary Artery Surgery Study (CASS). J Am Coll Cardiol 1997;29: 358–364.
35. Fiore MC, Novotny TE, Pierce JP, et al. Trends in cigarette smoking in the United States. The changing influence of gender and race. JAMA 1989;261:49–55.
36. American Heart Association. Heart Disease and Stroke Statistical Update: 2004 Update. Dallas, TX: American Heart Association; 2003.
37. Sonel AF, Good CB, Mulgund J, et al. CRUSADE investigators. Racial variations in treatment and outcomes of black and white patients with high-risk non-ST-elevation acute coronary syndromes:insights from CRUSADE (Can Rapid Risk Stratification of Unstable Angina Patients Suppress Adverse Outcomes With Early Implementation of the ACC/AHA Guidelines?) Circulation 1994;90:1613–1623.
38. Lenfant C. Report of the NHLBI Working Group on Research in Coronary Heart Disease in Blacks. Circulation 1994;90:1613–1623.
39. Xie X, Liu K, Stamler J, et al. Ethnic differences in electrocardiographic left ventricular hypertrophy in young and middle-aged employed American men. Am J Cardiol 1994;73:564–567.
40. Neaton JD, Kuller LH, Wentworth D, et al. Total and cardiovascular mortality in relation to cigarette smoking, serum cholesterol concentration, and diastolic blood pressure among black and white males followed up for five years. Am Heart J 1984; 108:759–769.
41. Tyroler HA, Knowles MG, Wing SB, et al. Ischemic heart disease risk factors and twenty-year mortality in middle-age Evans County black males. Am Heart J 1984; 108:738–746.
42. Johnson JL, Heineman EF, Heiss G, et al. Cardiovascular disease risk factors and mortality among black women and white women aged 40–64 years in Evans County, Georgia. Am J Epidemiol 1986;123:209–220.
43. American Heart Association. 1998 Heart and Stroke Statistical Update. Dallas, TX: American Heart Association; 1998.
44. Haffner SM, D'Agostino R Jr, Goff D, et al. LDL size in African Americans, Hispanics, and non-Hispanic whites the Insulin Resistance Atherosclerosis Study. Arterioscler Thromb Vasc Biol 1999;19:2234–2240.
45. Sorrentino MJ, Vielhauer C, Eisenbart JD, et al. Plasma lipoprotein (a) protein concentration and coronary artery disease in black patients compared with white patients. Am J Med 1992;93:658–662.
46. Moliterno DJ, Jokinen EV, Miserez AR, et al. No association between plasma lipoprotein(a) concentrations and the presence or absence of coronary atherosclerosis in African-Americans. Arterioscler Thromb Vasc Biol 1995;15:850–855.
47. Ferdinand KC. Coronary Artery disease in minority racial and ethnic groups in the United States. A symposium: the interplay of dyslipidemia and inflammation:

reducing cardiovascular risk in diverse patient populations. Am J Cardiol 2006: 97(2), suppl. 1:12–19

48. Anand SS, Razak F, Yi Q, et al. C-reactive protein as a screening test for cardiovascular risk in a multiethnic population, Arterioscler Thromb Vasc Biol 2004;24: 1509–1515.

49. Albert MA, Glynn RJ, Buring J, et al. C-reactive protein levels among women of various ethnic groups living in the United States (from the Women's Health Study). Am J Cardiol 2004;93:1238–1242.

50. Cardillo C, Kilcoyne CM, Cannon RO, et al. Attenuation of cyclic nucleotide-mediated smooth muscle relaxation in blacks as a cause of racial differences in vasodilator function. Circulation 1999;99:90–95.

51. Simmons BE, Castaner A, Campo A, et al. Coronary artery disease in blacks of lower socioeconomic status:angiographic findings from the Cook County Hospital Heart Disease Registry. Am Heart J 1988;116:90–97.

52. Houghton JL, Smith VE, Strogatz DS, et al. Effect of African-American race and hypertensive left ventricular hypertrophy on coronary vascular reactivity and endothelial function. Hypertension 1997;29:706–714.

53. ALLHAT Officers and Coordinators for the ALLHAT Collaborative Research Group. Major outcomes in high-risk hypertensive patients randomized to angiotensin-converting enzyme inhibitor or calcium channel blocker vs diuretic the Antihypertensive and Lipid-Lowering Treatment to Prevent Heart Attack Trial (ALLHAT). JAMA 2002;288:2981–2997.

54. Jawa A, Nachimuthu S, Pendergrass M, et al. Impaired vascular reactivity in African-American patients with type 2 diabetes mellitus and microalbuminuria or proteinuria despite angiotensin-converting enzyme inhibitor therapy. J Clin Endocrinol Metab 2006;91(1):31–35.

55. Szczeklik A, Dischinger P, Kueppers F, et al. Blood fibrinolytic activity, social class and habitual physical activity. II. A study of black and white men in southern Georgia. J Chron Dis 1980;33:291–299.

56. Barr RD, Ouna N, Kendall AG. The blood coagulation and fibrinolytic enzyme systems in healthy adult Africans and Europeans: a comparative study. Scot Med J 1973;18:93–97.

57. Folsom AR, Qamhieh HT, Flack JM, et al. Plasma fibrinogen: levels and correlates in young adults. Am J Epidemiol 1993;138:1023–1036.

58. Folsom AR, Wu KK, Conlan MG, et al. Distributions of hemostatic variables in blacks and whites: population reference values from the Atherosclerosis Risk in Communities (ARIC) Study. Ethnicity Dis 1992;2:35–46.

59. Sane DC, Stump DC, Topol EJ, et al. Racial differences in responses to fibrinolytic therapy with recombinant tissue-type plasminogen activator. Increased fibrin(ogen)olysis in blacks. Circulation 1991;83:170–175.

60. Taylor HA, Chaitman BR, Rogers WJ, et al. Race and prognosis after myocardial infarction. Results of the thrombolysis in myocardial infarction (TIMI) phase II trial. Circulation 1993;88:1484–1494.

61. The GUSTO Investigators. An international randomized trial comparing four fibrinolytic strategies for acute myocardial infarction. N Engl J Med 1993;329:673–682.

62. The GUSTO Angiographic Investigators. The effects of tissue plasminogen activator, streptokinase, or both on coronary-artery patency, ventricular function, and survival after acute myocardial infarction. N Engl J Med 1993;329:1615–1622.

63. Asher CR, Stebbins AL, Maynard CL, et al. Long-term survival differences between African Americans and caucasians following myocardial infarction: one-year follow-up from the GUSTO-I trial [abstract]. Circulation 1996;94:I-196.

64. Moliterno DM, Asher CR, Califf RM, et al. Less myocardial but more cerebral ischemic events in African Americans than Caucasians with acute coronary syndromes: results from the GUSTO-II [abstract]. J Am Coll Cardiol 1997;29:131A.

65. Rowland ML, Fulwood R. Coronary heart disease risk factor trends in blacks between the First and Second National Health and Nutrition Examination Surveys, United States, 1971–1980. Am Heart J 1984;108:771–779.

66. Ghali JK, Cooper RS, Kowatly I, et al. Delay between onset of chest pain and arrival to the coronary care unit among minority and disadvantaged patients. J Natl Med Assoc 1993;85:180–184.

67. Raczynksi JM, Taylor H, Cutter G, et al. Diagnoses, symptoms, and attribution of symptoms among black and white inpatients admitted for coronary heart disease. Am J Public Health 1994;84:951–995.

68. Clark LT, Ferdinand KC, Flack JM, et al.. Coronary Heart Disease in African Americans. Heart Dis 2001;3(2):97–108.

69. Maynard C, Fisher LD, Passamani ER, et al. Blacks in the Coronary Artery Surgery Study: risk factors and coronary artery disease. Circulation 1986;74:64–71.

70. Freedman DS, Gruchow HW, Manley JC, et al. Black/white differences in risk factors for arteriographically documented coronary artery disease in men. Am J Cardiol 1988;62:214–219.

71. Diver DJ, Bier JD, Ferreira PE, et al., for the TIMI-IIIA Investigators. Clinical and arteriographic characterization of patients with unstable angina without critical coronary arterial narrowing (from the TIMI-IIIA trial). Am J Cardiol 1994;74:531–537.

72. Strong JP, Malcom GT, Oalmann MC, et al. The PDAY study: natural history, risk factors, and pathobiology. Pathobiological Determinants of Atherosclerosis in Youth. Ann NY Acad Sci 1997;811:226–235.

73. Nakamura Y, Moss AJ, Brown MW, et al. Ethnicity and long-term outcome after an acute coronary event. Multicenter Myocardial Ischemia Research Group. Am Heart J 1999;138:500–506.

74. Haywood LJ. Coronary heart disease mortality/morbidity and risk in blacks. I: Clinical manifestations and diagnostic criteria: the experience with the Beta Blocker Heart Attack Trial. Am Heart J 1984;108:787–793.

75. Borzak S, Joseph C, Havstad S, et al. Lower fibrinolytic use for African Americans with myocardial infarction: an influence of clinical presentation? Am Heart J 1999;137:338–345.

76. Maynard C, Litwin PE, Martin JS, et al. Characteristics of black patients admitted to coronary care units in metropolitan Seattle: results from the Myocardial Infarction Triage and Intervention Registry (MITI). Am J Cardiol 1991;67:18–23.

77. Traven ND, Kuller LH, Ives DG, et al. Coronary heart disease mortality and sudden death among the 35–44-year age group in Allegheny County, Pennsylvania. Ann Epidemiol 1996;6:130–136.

78. Becker LB, Han BH, Meyer PM, et al., Racial differences in the incidence of cardiac arrest and subsequent survival. N Engl J Med 1993;329:600–606.

79. Gillum RF. Sudden coronary death in the United States: 1980–1985. Circulation 1989;79:756–765.

80. Chen J, Rathore SS, Radford MJ, et al. Racial differences in the use of cardiac catheterization after acute myocardial infarction. N Engl J Med 2001;344:1443–1449.
81. Hannan EL, van Ryn M, Burke J, et al. Access to coronary artery bypass surgery by race/ethnicity and gender among patients who are appropriate for surgery. Med Care 1999;37:68–77.
82. Vaccarino V, Rathore SS, Wenger NK, et al. Sex and racial differences in the management of acute myocardial infarction, 1994 through 2002. N Engl J Med 2005;353: 671–682.
83. Arnold AL, Milner KA, Vaccarino V. Sex and race differences in electrocardiogram use (the National Hospital Ambulatory Medical Care Survey). Am J Cardiol 2001; 88:1037–1040.
84. LaVeist TA, Arthur M, Morgan A, et al, The cardiac access longitudinal study. A study of access to invasive cardiology among African American and white patients. J Am Coll Cardiol 2003;41:1159–1166.
85. Blustein, Jan, Weitzman, Beth C. Access to hospitals with high-technology cardiac services: How is race important? American Journal of Public Health. Washington 1995;85(3):345–351.
86. Bradley E, Herrin J, Wang Y, et al. Racial and ethnic differences in time to acute reperfusion therapy for patients hospitalized with myocardial infarction. JAMA 2004;292:1563–1572.
87. Barnato AE, Lucas FL, Staiger D, et al. Hospital-level racial disparities in acute myocardial infarction treatment and outcomes. Med Care 2005;43:308–319.
88. Bach PB, Pham HH, Schrag D, et al. Primary care physicians who treat blacks and whites. N Engl J Med 2004;351:575–584.
89. Rathore SS, Berger AK, Weinfurt KP, et al. Race, sex, poverty, and the medical treatment of acute myocardial infarction in the elderly. Circulation 2000;102:642–648.
90. Rao SV, Schulman KA, Curtis LH, et al. Socioeconomic status and outcome following acute myocardial infarction in elderly patients. Arch Intern Med 2004;164: 1128–1133.
91. Whittle J, Conigliaro J, Good CB, et al. Racial differences in the use of invasive cardiovascular procedures in the Department of Veterans Affairs medical system. N Engl J Med 1993;329:621–627.
92. Whittle J, Conigliaro J, Good CB, et al. Do patient preferences contribute to racial differences in cardiovascular procedure use? J Gen Intern Med 1997;12:267–273.
93. Schecter AD, Goldschmidt-Clermont PJ, McKee G, et al. Influence of gender, race and education on patient preferences and receipt of cardiac catheterizations among coronary care unit patients. Am J Cardiol 1996;78:996–1001.
94. Shenolikar RA, Balkrishnan R, Camacho FT, et al. Race and medication adherence in Medicaid enrollees with type-2 diabetes. J Natl Med Assoc 2006;98(7):1071–1077.
95. Boulware LE, Cooper LA, Ratner LE, et al. Race and trust in the health care system. Public Health Rep 2003;118(4):358–365.

22
Coronary Artery Spasm and Chest Pain with Normal Coronary Arteries

Randy E. Cohen, Atul Kukar, Olivier Frankenberger, and Henry H. Greenberg

When evaluating acute chest pain, as in most other aspects of medicine, the foremost concern is with immediate life-threatening conditions; conditions that cannot afford to be missed. Although this role often falls on that of the emergency room physicians, it is essential for all to be aware of this acute differential diagnosis and the means by which to evaluate these conditions. In addition to acute myocardial infarction (AMI), life-threatening chest pain syndromes include aortic dissection, acute pulmonary embolism, tension pneumothorax, and esophageal rupture. Other serious conditions include microvascular disease, hypertrophic cardiomyopathy, aortic stenosis, myocarditis, pericarditis, coronary artery bridging, and coronary artery spasm. These conditions can present with a myriad of symptoms that at times makes them difficult to discern from acute coronary syndromes (ACS).

When coronary arteries are referred to as "normal," it implies that from a luminographic perspective, as seen with routine coronary angiogram, there appears to be no coronary artery disease (CAD). This normal appearance would include a lack of any visible stenosis or ectatic coronary arteries.

To most cardiologists, chest pain syndromes with normal coronary arteries (CPNCOR) represent a diagnostic challenge. Ruling out significant epicardial coronary artery disease is clearly not enough as other fatal syndromes need to be diagnosed and managed rapidly. A thorough investigation of chest pain is indicated in order to define an etiology, initiate goal-directed therapy, alleviate patient fears, and improve functional status [1].

Although there are many methods of classifying the various etiologies of CPNCOR, one intuitive method is anatomical (Table 22.1): coronary versus noncoronary. Coronary causes may be further subdivided into epicardial diseases (including coronary artery spasm, endothelial dysfunction, and myocardial bridging) and cardiac diseases with coronary microvascular dysfunction

TABLE **22.1.** Etiology of chest pain with normal coronary arteries.

1. Coronary
   (a) Epicardial disease
       i. Coronary artery spasm
       ii. Endothelial dysfunction
       iii. Myocardial bridging
   (b) Cardiac disease with coronary microvascular dysfunction
       i. Hypertension
       ii. Cardiomyopathy
       iii. Valvular heart disease
       iv. Diabetes

2. Noncoronary
   (a) Cardiac and vascular diseases
       i. Pericarditis
       ii. Myocarditis
       iii. Large vessel vasculitis
       iv. Aortic dissection
   (b) Noncardiac diseases
       i. Pulmonary
       ii. Gastrointestinal
       iii. Musculoskeletal
       iv. Psychological

(including hypertension, cardiomyopathy, valvular disease, and diabetes). Noncoronary etiologies may be further subdivided into cardiac (including myocarditis, pericarditis, large-vessel vasculitis, and aortic dissection) and noncardiac (including pulmonary, gastrointestinal, musculoskeletal, and psychological).

Epidemiology

Whereas the number of emergency department (ED) visits for chest pain exceeded 4 million (almost 4% of all ED visits) for the year 2003 [2], the percentage of patients with self-described anginal symptoms and normal coronary arteries is less clear. In fact, by definition, patients with CPNCOR have been exposed to the health care system usually more than once, ruled out for epicardial coronary disease by cardiac catheterization, and often discharged home without any definitive diagnosis or management plan. The significance of the problem has been addressed in the cardiology literature, where up to 30% of all patients presenting to cardiac catheterization laboratories for chest pain syndromes end up having normal coronary arteries [3–5]. The exact ethnic, gender, and socioeconomic backgrounds of patients presenting with CPNCOR are less well defined.

Economic Impact

The estimated direct and indirect health care costs for CAD for the year 2006 are in the range of $142 billion [6]. Although the specific direct health care costs as it relates to patients with CPNCOR may be more difficult to define, given the repeated hospitalizations, diagnostic procedures, and therapeutic interventions, it is certainly not insignificant. Similarly, there are sizable indirect costs as it relates to lost productivity, sick time, and worker's compensation.

It has also been observed that despite normal angiographic findings and the favorable event-free survival (99% at 5 years and 98% at 10 years), up to 50% of patients are unable to perform moderate-vigorous activities, and up to 70% continue to experience persistent chest pain symptoms requiring return visits to ED, outpatient centers, and medical offices, further affecting health care resources and expenditures [7].

Etiologies of Chest Pain with Normal Coronary Arteries

Coronary

Epicardial Diseases

Coronary Artery Spasm

Variant angina, traditionally referred to as Prinzmetal angina, is believed to be secondary to spasm in normal or mildly narrowed coronary arteries. It usually does not present with relation to physical exercise and commonly occurs in the setting of a trigger, such as cold temperatures or emotional stress. Although it is a rare cause of CPNCOR, it is associated with an increased risk of AMI, ventricular arrhythmias, and sudden cardiac death.

It needs to be considered in patients with a long history of chest pain and no significant stenosis seen on coronary angiogram. Its pathophysiology remains uncertain but likely has its foundation in endothelial dysfunction, platelet activation, and the subsequent release of vasoconstrictors, abnormal smooth muscle contraction, and diminished nitric oxide levels. It appears to have a relatively higher incidence in Japanese patients and displays a male preponderance.

The pain of coronary spasm is often identical to that of AMI and thus is difficult to distinguish by history. It occurs more commonly in the early hours of the morning. An absence of risk factors should increase suspicion for variant angina, although cigarette smoking is a common risk factor for both. Hypertension and insulin resistance have been associated with a higher incidence of variant angina. Diagnosis remains difficult to make, as angiographic demonstration of spasm is necessary. Although it can occur in a stenotic segment of a coronary artery, it often occurs adjacent to a fixed stenosis. Electrocardiographically, it can present with ST elevations on the ECG, as it is a form of transient total coronary occlusion.

Diagnostic options include a formalized period of hyperventilation preceding treadmill testing, ambulatory ECG monitoring, and chemical provocation during coronary angiography. The results of exercise treadmill testing are highly variable and patients may equally show ST elevations, depressions or no change.

Chemical provocation has been considered to be the diagnostic test of choice in patients. It is contraindicated in patients with fixed coronary artery stenosis, as it may increase the risk of infarction. Ergonovine maleate, an ergot alkaloid, exerts a direct constrictive effect on smooth muscle in the vasculature via stimulation of alpha-adrenergic and serotonergic receptors. Coronary arteries prone to spasm have an abnormal sensitivity to this agent. It is also possible to use methylergonovine maleate, acetylcholine, and even hyperventilation. Absolute contraindications to either ergot derivative include high-grade stenosis anywhere in the coronary tree, severe left ventricular dysfunction, moderate to severe aortic stenosis, pregnancy, and severe hypertension. Nitrates and calcium channel blockers (CCBs) must be held for at least 48 hours prior to the test in order to ensure its validity. Coronary artery spasm will persist throughout systole and diastole and usually resolve with the use of intracoronary nitroglycerin.

The mainstay of medical therapy for coronary vasospasm includes the use of oral nitrates and CCBs. Long-acting nitrates help reduce the frequency of attacks, and short-acting nitrates are used as the mainstay of therapy for acute episodes of angina and myocardial ischemia. Nitrates, by acting as an exogenous source of nitric oxide, induce vascular smooth muscle relaxation via stimulation of intracellular cyclic GMP. This leads to direct vasodilation of the coronary arteries and venous capacitance vessels, both resulting in a decrease in myocardial oxygen consumption.

Dihydropyridines (i.e., amlodipine, nifedipine) exert a greater vascular selectivity over non-dihydropyridines (i.e., verapamil, diltiazem), which also inhibit the impulse conduction within cardiac nodal tissue. Both categories of CCBs can be useful in coronary artery spasm because of the ability to directly relax coronary smooth muscle cells and produce coronary vasodilation.

Although beta-blockers may seem an appropriate choice for treatment of the often underlying coronary artery stenosis, they have the potential of allowing unopposed alpha-mediated coronary constriction by blocking beta-induced vasodilation. Thus, unless otherwise indicated for more serious conditions, beta-blockers should be avoided in patients with known or suspected coronary spasm.

Endothelial Dysfunction

The clinical presentation of the patient with isolated endothelial dysfunction can be somewhat similar to that of patients with ACS. Both groups of patients may give a history of chest pain symptoms ranging from typical to atypical, both may have a wide variety of risk factors for CAD, and both may have varying degrees of positive stress tests. The main differentiating factor is the presence of epicardial CAD in one and its absence in the other.

Although the diagnosis of endothelial dysfunction can be made by non-invasive methods (e.g., brachial artery flow-mediated dilation), the gold standard remains the assessment of coronary blood flow (using provocative agents such as acetylcholine) during cardiac catheterization. Under normal conditions when healthy coronary endothelium is exposed to acetylcholine, the vasoconstrictive effects of the drug are counteracted upon by the normal physiologic release of endothelial-derived vasodilators (nitric oxide, prostacyclin). When the integrity of the endothelium is lost (due to, for example, CAD), the intrinsic endothelial-derived vasodilators are unable to counteract the effects of acetylcholine, producing a net decline in coronary blood flow. A positive study is one in which the coronary artery diameter is reduced by >20% in response to acetylcholine challenge.

Despite our ability to accurately diagnose endothelial dysfunction, once the presence of epicardial CAD has been ruled out, if the clinical suspicion exists, there is little additional yield in performing invasive physiologic studies. Because there is no definitive, clinically proven therapy for endothelial dysfunction, focus is directed toward aggressive risk factor modification.

Myocardial Bridging

On rare occasion, a sliver of myocardium grows over the coronary artery during development or a coronary artery may "dive" within the myocardium and exit further along its course to return to its normal epicardial position. This condition is often found incidentally and patients are often asymptomatic, as the majority of blood flow in the coronary arteries occurs during diastole and compression of the artery occurs during systole as the myocardium contracts. The situation may worsen with exaggerated myocardial thickness as seen in the hypertrophied myocardium of hypertensive heart disease. The extrinsic compression may worsen with exercise and cause angina. On occasion, there can be concomitant atherosclerosis of the intramyocardial segment thought to be secondary to the additional stress placed on the artery.

The mainstay of therapy has been beta-adrenergic blocking agents. They function by decreasing heart rate, which increases time for diastolic filling, and decreasing the systolic phase, which is when constriction and symptoms occur. CCBs may also be used as treatment to have the added advantage of treating vasospasm, which has been implicated as a concomitant cause of symptoms [8]. Long-acting nitrates should be avoided, as they may induce vasodilation in nonbridged segments and effectively increase the degree of obstruction. Short-acting nitrates (i.e., sublingual nitroglycerin) may be used for acute pain if felt due to spasm as well. Myotomy of the sliver of myocardium overlying the coronary artery has been successfully performed in medically refractory cases [9].

Cardiac Diseases with Coronary Microvascular Dysfunction

Hypertension

It is not uncommon for patients with a long-standing history of hypertension (HTN) to experience symptoms of chest pain, either typical or atypical in nature. In fact, these patients may present with chest pain symptoms and a spectrum of blood pressure readings ranging from normotensive to hypertensive emergency. Echocardiographic evaluation of these patients often yields findings of concentric left ventricular hypertrophy (LVH), diastolic relaxation abnormalities, elevated filling pressures, or some combination of the above. When patients with long-standing HTN undergo exercise stress testing (with either echo or nuclear imaging) as part of an evaluation for chest pain symptoms, findings may range from normal perfusion and wall motion to significant perfusion defects and localized wall motion abnormalities suggestive of significant epicardial coronary disease. It is, however, not uncommon that many of these patients with abnormal stress tests continue on to have cardiac catheterizations revealing normal epicardial coronary arteries. All too often, patients with this presentation are told that the stress test was falsely positive, discharged home without a clear explanation for their chest pain symptoms, and told to follow up with their primary care physician to purse noncardiac etiologies for their symptoms. However, recent data suggest that there may in fact be a cardiac etiology for hypertensive patients presenting with CPNCOR. One proposed mechanism is a reduction in coronary blood flow due to an increase in microvascular resistance. The pathophysiology behind the increased microvascular resistance involves compression of the microcirculation by either hypertrophied myocardium or by elevated filling pressures [10]. Another possibility is that in patients with HTN and LVH on ECG, there is a reduction in coronary flow reserve that is distinctly different from hypertensive patients without LVH or EKG and with normal controls [11]. If either or both of these potential mechanisms are active, then the stress tests may in fact not be falsely positive but rather consistent with severe microvascular dysfunction in the presence of normal epicardial coronary blood flow. Therefore, if patients have evidence of cardiac end-organ damage (LVH, diastolic dysfunction, elevated filling pressures) from long-standing HTN, present with chest pain symptoms, and have normal epicardial coronary arteries, perhaps consideration of coronary microvasculature dysfunction is warranted.

Despite one's suspicion for microvascular dysfunction as a cause of CPNCOR, however, treatment will nonetheless focus on aggressive blood pressure control, minimizing further end-organ damage from the effects of HTN (both macro and microvascular).

Cardiomyopathy

Although there may be many etiologies for a nonischemic cardiomyopathy, including cardiotoxic substances, valvular and infiltrative diseases, and idiopathic causes, chest pain may be a common symptom and the reason patients seek out medical attention. Once ischemia has been ruled out, attention may be directed to other causes. In patients with dilated cardiomyopathies, chest pain symptoms are thought to be due to an oxygen supply and demand mismatch. One proposed mechanism involves myogenic compression of the microcirculation and/or microvascular endothelial dysfunction leading to a reduced coronary flow reserve (CFR) [12]. Regardless of the exact etiology for the chest pain symptoms, treatment is geared toward optimizing cardiac performance and volume status, as well as managing risk factors such as HTN, diabetes, and hyperlipidemia.

In patients with hypertrophic cardiomyopathies, studies have found evidence of reduced CFR, as well as reductions in the amount of small arterioles [13].

In patients with a cardiomyopathy due to an infiltrative disease such as amyloid, deposits within the tunica media have been associated with reductions in the luminal diameter of the microcirculation leading to ischemia [14].

One form of cardiomyopathy being increasingly described in the literature is stress cardiomyopathy (also known as *Takotsubo*; transient apical ballooning syndrome). Interestingly, these patients often present with chest pain symptoms suggestive of ACS, with dynamic ECG changes, mildly elevated cardiac enzymes, moderate to severely reduced left ventricular function, but normal (or near normal) epicardial coronary arteries. The prevailing hypothesis is that these patients suffer from some acute form of emotional (e.g., death of a family member or close friend; intense fear or anxiety) or physical stress (e.g., recent motor vehicle accident; major surgery; acute illness) leading to supraphysiologic levels of catecholamines. This in turn leads to cellular injury and subsequent microvascular spasm or microvascular endothelial dysfunction. Fortunately, the majority of these patients recover spontaneously with only supportive measures.

Valvular Heart Disease

Although there are many reasons patients with advanced valvular heart disease may present to the hospital, chest pain symptoms can be among the more challenging. Although it is well documented that anginal symptoms are a part of the constellation of problems patients have with severe aortic stenosis, the etiology of the chest pain is not clearly understood. Similarly, anginal pains have been described with other valvular disorders as well. In aortic as well as mitral valve disease, impaired CFR has been proposed as a possible mechanism of ischemia-related chest pain in the absence of epicardial coronary disease [15]. While it is known that chest pain symptoms improve after aortic valve replacement in patients with aortic stenosis, it has been similarly described that CFR improves (and chest pain resolves) after mitral valve replacement for severe mitral regurgitation [16].

Idiopathic

Perhaps one of the more common conditions seen in clinical practice is the patient with recurrent chest pain symptoms, normal (or near normal) epicardial coronary arteries, and the absence of any other preexisting cardiac disease (e.g., cardiomyopathy, valvular, or hypertensive heart disease). When this clinical syndrome is associated with microvascular dysfunction (demonstrated by invasive or noninvasive measures), it is commonly referred to as Syndrome X. Although the exact mechanism is not known, studies have demonstrated the presence of microvascular endothelial dysfunction [17]. Like many of the other causes of chest pain in patients with normal coronary arteries, treatment is directed toward aggressive risk factor management.

Noncoronary

Cardiac and Vascular Diseases

Pericarditis

The pericardium is a fibrous sac that overlies the heart, preventing it from overdistending and restrains it from excessive swinging in the chest. There is normally 15 to 20 mL of pericardial fluid between the visceral and parietal layers. Pericarditis can occur as an isolated entity or as the result of a systemic disease [18]. It is diagnosed in about 5% of patients who present to the emergency room with chest pain.

Its etiology has a wide differential diagnosis, though it is often secondary to a viral infection or idiopathic in origin. Some of the other causes include post–myocardial infarction, postinfectious, secondary to dissecting aortic aneurysms that bleed back into the pericardial space, chest trauma, neoplastic invasion of pericardium, chest radiation, uremia, post–open heart surgery, in association with systemic diseases (autoimmune or inflammatory), and secondary to pharmaceutical agents. It is often difficult to determine the etiology of pericarditis as laboratory examination rarely helps. It is reasonable to send a complete blood count (CBC) and consider an ANA and rheumatoid factor if systemic disease is suspected. Troponin levels can be elevated as well and are believed to be secondary to epicardial inflammation rather than the necrosis that occurs in vascular myocardial injury. Prolonged troponin elevation, greater than 2 weeks, suggests an associated myocarditis, which carries a worse prognosis.

The history of chest pain usually involves a description of sudden onset, sharp and pleuritic pain that worsens with inspiration. Like ischemic pain, it can radiate to the neck, arms, or shoulders. An interesting feature in the presentation of pericarditis is its unique characteristic of radiation to the trapezius ridges, secondary to the phrenic nerve's proximity to the pericardium. Although its absence does not rule out pericarditis, its presence is a sensitive finding. In addition, the pain is often positional in nature, improving when sitting up and leaning forward, and worsening with the recumbent position.

On physical exam, a friction rub is often heard at some point during the course of the disease. Because of its transient nature, patients need to be examined repeatedly. It is best heard with the patient leaning forward at the left sternal border. It can be described as a high-pitched scratchy or squeaky sound. It has three components, corresponding with atrial systole (only if patient is in sinus rhythm), ventricular systole, and early rapid filling during diastole. The rub can be triphasic, biphasic, or monophasic when auscultated. It is often heard at end expiration, which is in sharp contrast with a pleural friction rub, which is heard throughout inspiration and expiration and obviously disappears with cessation of respiration.

Some of the complications include pericardial effusion, pericardial tamponade, recurrent pericarditis, and pericardial constriction. Tamponade is one of the most feared complications and occurs more frequently when pericarditis is secondary to neoplasm, tuberculosis, or acute infection in the pericardial space. Hemodynamically, the rapid increase in pericardial pressure leads to impaired filling and subsequent reduction in cardiac output.

Electrocardiography is useful in helping distinguish pericarditis from other forms of chest pain. The ECG can progress through four phases. During the acute phase of presentation (stage I), there is classically diffuse upward concave ST-segment elevation and PR segment depression (or PR elevation in aVR). In stage II there is normalization of the ST and PR segments. This is followed by widespread T-wave inversions (stage III). The last stage (stage IV) consists of normalization of the T waves. Stage I changes can be seen in up to 80% of patients presenting with acute pericarditis. The ST elevations seen in AMI are usually convex, localize to a coronary artery distribution, occur without PR-segment depression, and occur together with T-wave inversions.

All patients require an echocardiogram in order to help distinguish etiology, determine if there is an underlying wall motion abnormality, and to evaluate for pericardial effusion. Treatment is largely for symptomatic relief and does not usually prevent sequelae. The mainstay of therapy is nonsteroidal anti-inflammatory drugs (NSAIDs). In the presence of CAD or with patients who are high risk, aspirin (in doses up to 2 to 4 g/day) should be the primary agent used. Ibuprofen and indomethacin can be used, with ibuprofen (1,600 to 3,200 mg/day) being the preferred agent because of a lower incidence of side effects. Colchicine (0.6 mg twice daily) is also an acceptable option for therapy and can be used alone or in combination with NSAIDs. It should be used with caution in patients with renal failure. It is the only therapy that has been associated with a lower incidence of recurrent pericarditis [19]. If a patient continues to have chest pain despite therapy with NSAIDs and colchicine, or has contraindications to both or either, glucocorticoids may be used. Steroids may increase the incidence of recurrent pericarditis and have been noted to worsen pericardial injury secondary to viral infections [20]. Thus, its use is usually limited to cases of pericarditis that are believed to be secondary to connective tissue diseases or severe recurrent pericarditis not responsive to traditional therapy.

Myocarditis

Myocarditis is a set of diseases often caused by infectious, toxic, or autoimmune pathologies all leading to the inflammation of the myocardium. It is difficult to study, diagnose, and treat because of the wide variation of its presentation and the diffuse nature of its consequences. Pathophysiologically, it is characterized early on by an infiltration of mononuclear cells and subacutely by cytotoxic T-cells inducing cell lysis.

Its true incidence remains unknown, because it is often asymptomatic. It is often thought to be caused by viruses including coxsackie, influenza, echovirus, EBV, hepatitis C, and CMV to name just a few, but has also been seen with radiation exposure, toxins, and systemic inflammatory conditions. In addition, it may play an etiologic role in sudden cardiac death in young patients and peripartum cardiomyopathy. It may also be secondary to an adverse toxic reaction to drugs (including antibiotics, sulfonamides, AZT, and many others) and environmental toxins such as lead and carbon monoxide. In this setting, eosinophilia and fever are present with eosinophilic infiltrates found on biopsy. Outside of the United States, it is often caused by other infectious etiologies, such as Chagas disease and diphtheria. Acute myocarditis rarely leads to fulminant heart failure and death. On average, one third recover, one third develop some scarring, and one third develop dilated cardiomyopathy with varying degrees of dysfunction.

Most cases are subclinical and rarely present to a physician. An antecedent viral syndrome is often noted on history, and patients may present with fatigue, myalgias, and arthralgias. The chest pain presentation may be similar to that of pericarditis—a sharp, pleuritic pain syndrome or like ischemic chest pain with substernal pressure. On physical exam, patients can present with a myriad of signs ranging from the nonspecific findings of a viral infection to severe heart failure (pulmonary crackles, jugular venous distention, S3 and lower extremity edema). In addition, any physical exam findings may encompass the same findings seen in pericarditis and pericardial effusion as they often occur concomitantly.

Although myocarditis involves direct cardiomyocyte inflammation, it does not necessitate that there will be necrosis and release of troponin, and thus elevations are only seen in a minority of patients. In addition, an elevated white blood cell count and erythrocyte sedimentation rate (ESR) may be seen, though they are not uncommon in myocardial infarction either. As with all chest pain syndromes, an ECG should be performed rapidly upon presentation. Although nonspecific, one may find sinus tachycardia, ST elevation without "reciprocal" depressions, decreased QRS amplitude, and transient block including Mobitz type I, II, or complete heart block.

Echocardiography is usually the test of choice in evaluating these patients and it also has a myriad of nonspecific findings, which may include impaired left ventricular systolic and/or diastolic dysfunction, segmental wall motion abnormalities, impaired ejection fraction, ventricular thrombus, and a pericardial effusion. Magnetic resonance imaging (MRI) appears to be the gold standard as it can show abnormal signal intensity in the affected myocardium.

Though frequently caused by infectious agents, the yield from blood tests and myocardial biopsy is extremely limited. Biopsy yield is low because of the patchy nature of involvement and is only diagnostic in up to 30% of cases. Treatment usually focuses on the untoward effects of the myocarditis. For example, left ventricular dysfunction with heart failure is managed in the same manner as is caused by any other etiology. Direct treatment of the underlying disorder has not led to success in clinical trials. Many studies have focused on attempting to immunomodulate the course of the disease process using such agents as prednisone and cyclosporine with no convincing results. Of note, it is important to avoid sympathomimetics, beta-blocking agents, and NSAIDs, which may worsen or enhance myocardial inflammation and possible subsequent necrosis.

Aortic Dissection

Thoracic aortic dissection is one of the most dreaded underlying causes of chest pain. It is essential to always maintain a high level of suspicion for this clinical entity as anticoagulation therapy for conditions such as myocardial infarction or pulmonary embolism can be fatal. An intimal tear is usually the culprit and creates a connection between the tunica media and the aortic lumen, creating a true and false lumen. The dissection may also begin secondary to bleeding in the tunic media, causing an expanding hematoma between the aortic layers. Lastly, rupture of the vasovasorum in the tunic adventitia may lead to dissection and intra mural thrombus formation.

The dissection usually traverses the aorta and often stops at a branch vessel or plaque. There are three common sites where the dissection begins: the aortic root, 2 cm above the root, and just distal to the subclavian artery. Ascending aortic dissection is the most dangerous and may lead to death from free wall rupture, hemopericardium and tamponade, dissection of the coronary arteries, or acute severe aortic regurgitation—we will focus our discussion on this type of dissection. Other complications include stroke, renal failure, mesenteric and lower limb ischemia, and paraplegia. The mortality rate for ascending dissections is estimated at about 1% per hour without surgery for the first two days [21].

Although the pathophysiology of the actual dissection is not well understood, there are known risk factors. These include hypertension, connective tissue disorders (especially Marfan syndrome), bicuspid aortic valve, arteritis, coarctation of the aorta, pregnancy, cocaine use, and trauma. There are two basic types of classification: the DeBakey and Stanford classification schemes. The three types of dissection in the DeBakey system are

I: involvement of the entire aorta
II: involvement of the ascending aorta only
III: involvement of the descending aorta only
IIIA: dissection remains above the diaphragm
IIIB: dissecting aorta below the diaphragm

The Stanford classification strategy is more basic and a dissection is type A if the ascending aorta is involved and type B if the descending aorta only is involved.

The pain presentation has specific features that may help distinguish it from other chest pain syndromes. For example, it often has a sudden onset with the most severe pain occurring at the beginning of its onset. This is also the case for a pneumothorax and pulmonary embolism. However, ischemic chest pain and esophageal disorders usually have a crescendo presentation. Also, the pain of aortic dissection is usually described as a tearing sensation that radiates between the scapulae. Yet, the elderly and women will not typically present with this pain syndrome.

Physical exam findings are nonspecific, but a few signs may suggest aortic dissection. Pulse deficits in the arms or legs are the most specific sign and can be found in up to 30% of patients [22]. Often quoted, but of poor specificity, is upper extremity blood pressure differential. Although differences are commonly found in the general population, a differential of more than 20 mm Hg serves as an independent predictor of dissection [23].

Specific diagnostic evaluation is a necessity if aortic dissection is suspected. Misdiagnosis is not uncommon if the physician relies on history and physical examination alone. Plain chest radiography is not adequate to rule out an aortic dissection. Options for more definitive diagnosis include transesophageal echocardiography (TEE), spiral CT, aortography, and MRI (only used for hemodynamically stable patients because of time delays). Although CT and TEE are considered to be safe and accurate, use of CT is limited in patients with renal failure because of the use of intravenous contrast dye. In these situations and in order to assess the amount of acute aortic regurgitation, TEE is a suitable alternate. In general, CT is preferred because it has a slightly higher specificity and sensitivity, is not operator-dependent, and does not have the "blind spot" (2 cm proximal to the innominate artery) of a TEE [24]. Aortography usually does not play an active role in acute diagnosis and may be performed in stable patients when coronary anatomy needs to be visualized. However, this need may be reduced as CT scan technology is advancing (i.e., 64-slice spiral CT) and allowing visualization of coronary arteries and pulmonary circulation.

Traditionally, treatment for Stanford type A dissections is acute surgical therapy whereas Stanford type B patients are managed with aggressive blood pressure control [25]. Descending aorta dissections can be intervened on when there is branch vessel compromise with either open repair or fenestration through the dissection to return flow to compromised territories.

Noncardiac Diseases

Esophageal/Gastric Disorders

Esophageal disorders are the most common type of noncardiac chest pain, usually due to gastroesophageal reflux disease (GERD). Clinical symptoms are often unreliable to differentiate esophageal disorders from ischemic chest pain. Thus, this set of disorders is often evaluated after a thorough cardiac evaluation. In addition to GERD, esophageal spasm, Mallory Weiss tear, achalasia, Boerhaave syndrome, and peptic ulcer disease are just a few other disorders that can present with chest pain. Although we will not discuss all these conditions, we chose a few that are seen often and one that is often fatal without prompt recognition.

A diagnostic workup for GERD includes an upper gastrointestinal endoscopy, 24-hour esophageal pH monitoring, and esophageal manometry. However, most patients are initially treated with high-dose acid suppression, usually with a proton pump inhibitor, and lifestyle/diet modification. Typical instructions include refraining from tomato sauce, peppermint, chocolate, alcohol, cigarettes, and, although controversial, spicy food. In addition, patients are instructed to refrain from lying down for up to 2 hours after eating and never eating within a few hours of sleep. If symptoms do not resolve, patients are often referred to a gastroenterologist for further evaluation.

Esophageal spasm is another entity that often mimics the pain syndrome seen in myocardial ischemia. Like coronary pain, it can radiate to the jaw and can be relieved with nitroglycerin. It can also present with globus (the sensation that an object is trapped in the throat), dysphagia, and regurgitation. It can occur in the setting of diffuse esophageal spasm or as an exaggerated response to coordinated esophageal peristalsis as seen in nutcracker esophagus. Although its pathophysiology is poorly understood, it is often associated with GERD and is evaluated with use of esophageal manometry and barium swallow. Treatment options include CCBs, nitrates, tricyclic antidepressants, botulinum toxin, dilatation, myotomy, and esophagectomy in refractory cases.

Mallory Weiss tears and Boerhaave syndrome exist along a continuum and are mainly caused by emesis—usually forceful and excessive—leading to a sharp increase in intraluminal pressure against a closed cricopharyngeus. The tears are nontransmural while the syndrome encompasses a transmural perforation. Diagnosis is difficult because of a lack of classic symptoms, though a recent history of vomiting and recent excessive dietary or alcohol intake is usually present. The pain may radiate to the back or left shoulder and is aggravated by swallowing. Hematemesis is usually seen with tears and not perforation. Shortness of breath is also common with perforation and is due to pleuritic pain and/or pleural effusions. Also, subcutaneous emphysema and pneumomediastinum can occasionally be noted on chest radiography and physical exam (it may sound like a friction rub as it is coincident with each heartbeat). Mallory Weiss tears are treated conservatively with intravenous fluids, nothing per oral (NPO), and careful observation. Surgical intervention is rarely required.

For Boerhaave syndrome, an esophagram or CT scan can help confirm the diagnosis and is performed with Oral Contrast Agents, as barium can induce a chemical mediastinitis. Boerhaave syndrome can be complicated by mediastinitis, sepsis, and shock and is treated with broad-spectrum antibiotics, intravenous fluids, strict cessation of oral intake, and urgent surgery. Without surgical intervention, it carries an excessively progressive and high mortality rate—up to 90% after 48 hours.

Pulmonary Disorders

Pulmonary disorders can present with a myriad of symptoms that can confound the diagnosis of chest pain. Some of the more common etiologies of pulmonary-induced chest pain include pneumonia, pleurisy, pulmonary hypertension, tension pneumothorax, and acute pulmonary embolism. The latter two are the most acutely dangerous and will be the focus of discussion.

Tension pneumothorax occurs with the accumulation of air under pressure, which is confined by the pleural space. This occurs when a "one-way" valve is created that allows air to enter this potential space and prevents its natural escape. As the pressure increases, the ipsilateral lung collapses, causing hypoxia and a shift toward the contralateral side impinging both the lung and the vasculature entering the right atrium. This compromises venous return and leads to progressively worsening cardiac output. Regardless of its cause, tension pneumothorax leads to respiratory distress, cardiovascular collapse, and ultimately death without treatment. Patients often present with chest pain, dyspnea, and anxiety. On exam, hyperresonance and diminished breath sounds on the affected side, tracheal deviation to the contralateral side, hypotension, distended neck veins, and cyanosis may be present. Although a chest x-ray can confirm the diagnosis, there is often not enough time to obtain one. Treatment consists of acute needle decompression followed by the more definitive therapy with tube thoracostomy.

Acute pulmonary embolism (PE) has often been likened to a great masquerader. As per findings in the PIOPED [26] (Prospective Investigation of Pulmonary Embolism Diagnosis), the most common findings were dyspnea (73%), pleuritic chest pain (66%), cough (37%), and hemoptysis (13%).

If left undiagnosed and untreated, it can lead to subsequent death usually as the result of further embolic episodes. It is mainly a consequence of venous thrombosis, which usually arises from the lower extremities though it may also originate in the pelvic, renal, or upper extremity veins or in the right heart itself. Most events are multiple in nature, affect the lower lobes more frequently, and often produce pleuritic chest pain secondary to an inflammatory response.

Although the chest pain may be difficult to distinguish from that of an acute myocardial infarction, the ECG is unlikely to show ischemic changes and the pain does not usually resolve with nitroglycerin. The most common ECG findings include sinus tachycardia and nonspecific ST-T wave changes. The "popular" S1-Q3-T3 pattern of right heart strain is only seen in about 20% of patients with proven PE. An essential part of the diagnosis is based on risk factors for venous thrombosis, including recent surgery, prolonged immobility, pregnancy, oral contraceptive use (especially with concomitant smoking), malignancy, long bone fractures, indwelling venous catheters, and a hypercoagulable state.

Laboratory evaluation plays an important role in the diagnosis of PE. Arterial blood gases are often performed and may show hypoxemia, hypocapnia, and respiratory alkalosis. However, it can also be completely normal and should not be used to make a definitive decision. D-dimer, on the one hand, is an excellent test as a normal result has a high negative predictive value. A positive test, on the other hand, does not help in confirming the diagnosis. As part of a thorough evaluation, deep vein thrombosis is looked for by using lower extremity ultrasound. However, this imaging form is limited in that it can only evaluate the lower extremities up to the femoral veins and will "miss" deep vein thrombosis in the iliac, pelvic, or inferior vena cava.

The diagnosis of PE is often further evaluated with imaging protocols. A ventilation-perfusion (V/Q) scan is often performed, though usually a clear chest x-ray is required for proper interpretation. In addition, the scans are interpreted in reference to the pretest probability, as are most forms of cardiac stress testing. They can be separated into diagnostic (normal or high probability) or nondiagnostic (low or intermediate probability) and are further interpreted based on pretest likelihood. For example, a high-probability study may have a specificity of ~85% and with a high pretest likelihood this may increase to up to 95%.

The preferred imaging modality is the high-resolution spiral CT. This type of imaging has the ability to detect lobar and segmental pulmonary emboli with a sensitivity of greater than 90%. The disadvantages are that it may not detect small subsegmental emboli, it requires the use of intravenous contrast, and the patient must be able to hold their breath for at least 20 to 30 seconds in order to maintain the sensitivity of the test. The gold standard is pulmonary angiography though it is an invasive procedure (i.e., carries a risk of morbidity and mortality) and also requires intravenous contrast dye. Other modalities that are employed include MRI and echocardiography. TEE may be able to detect large central emboli, and TTE is often used to demonstrate right ventricular dysfunction.

Acute respiratory distress is usually secondary to a combination of alveolar dead space, pneumoconstriction, hypoxemia, and hyperventilation. Pulmonary infarction, though uncommon because of bronchial arterial collateral circulation, may ensue, leading to necrosis of the lung tissue. Although regional hypoxemia occurs, systemic arterial hypoxemia is not a given. It is caused by ventilation-perfusion mismatch, intrapulmonary shunts, and reduced cardiac output. Hemodynamically, there is an increase in the pulmonary vascular resistance thereby increasing right ventricular afterload. If severe, right ventricular failure may ensue. Although a healthy lung and heart may be able to handle substantial insult, a patient with poor cardiopulmonary status to begin with, may experience more severe consequences.

There are a few different options for treatment. The mainstay of therapy includes anticoagulation with a heparin and eventual long-term therapy with warfarin sodium. The duration of therapy remains controversial depending on the etiology and other clinical factors of the individual patient, but is usually maintained for at least 6 to 9 months. Thrombolytic therapy is reserved for those patients who are hemodynamically unstable or those with poor underlying cardiopulmonary reserve. An echocardiogram demonstrating right heart strain is often used to help guide therapy because it may herald systemic cardiovascular collapse. In patients who have a contraindication to anticoagulation or in those in which another PE may prove fatal, inferior vena cava filter may be used to help prevent further embolization to the lungs. However, recent studies have shown that these filters may only have a role in acute prevention (i.e., for only a few weeks).

Other etiologies of chest pain with normal coronary arteries include, but are not limited to, postherpetic neuralgia, chronic pain syndromes, psychiatric disorders, and muscular skeletal disorders.

Conclusion

Despite significant advances in the field of medicine, there are still many syndromes that continue to challenge and mystify the practicing physician. One classic example of this is the patient presenting with an unknown chest pain syndrome. The differential can range from the most acute and life-threatening (e.g., aortic dissection) to more chronic and debilitating syndromes such as recurrent chest pain from endothelial or microvascular dysfunction. The initial approach to these patients should focus on history and physical exam, as these two methods alone can diagnose the majority of both acute and life-threatening as well as chronic chest pain syndromes. Once the initial workup is complete and significant obstructive CAD has been ruled out by coronary angiography, other etiologies can be pursed as outlined in our algorithm (Fig. 22.1). Until

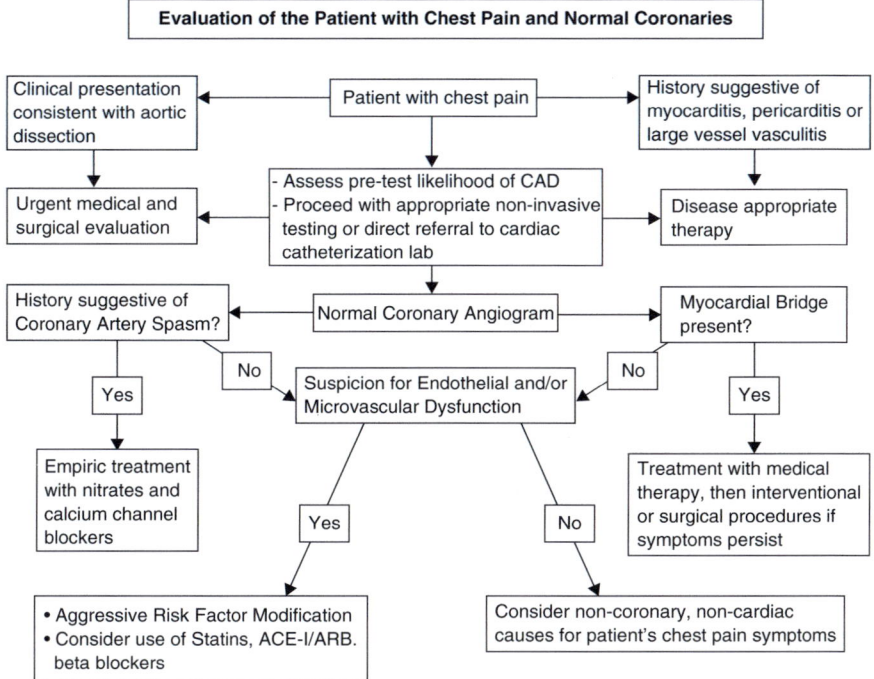

FIGURE 22.1. Approach to the patient with chest pain and normal coronary arteries.

more definitive therapies exist for patients with chest pain and normal coronaries, they will likely continue to present to our medical offices and emergency rooms. Adequate documentation of testing and attempted therapies is key to keep these patients as functional and pain-free as possible.

References

1. Kachintorn U. How do we define non-cardiac chest pain? J Gastroenterol Hepatol 2005;20:S2–S5.
2. National Hospital Ambulatory Medical Care Survey. 2003 Emergency Department Summary. Advance Data, No. 358, Maryland, 2005.
3. Proudfit W, Shirey E. Selective cine coronary arteriography: correlation with clinical findings in 1,000 patients. Circulation 1966;33:901–910.
4. Kemp H, Vokonas P, Cohn P, et al. The anginal syndrome associated with normal coronary arteriograms: report of a six year experience. Am J Med 1973;54:735–742.
5. Ockene I, Shay M, Alpert J, et al. Unexplained chest pain with normal coronary arteriograms: a follow-up study of functional status. N Engl J Med 1980;303:1249–1252.
6. American Heart Association. Heart Disease and Stroke Statistics—2006 Update. Circulation 2006;113;85–151.
7. Papanicolaou M, Califf R, Hlatky M, et al. Prognostic implications of angiographically normal and insignificantly narrowed coronary arteries. Am J Cardiol 1986;58:1181–1187.
8. Teragawa H, Fukada Y, Matsuda K, et al. Myocardial bridging increases the risk of coronary spasm. Clin Cardiol 2003;26:377–383.
9. Joshi S, Blackshear J. 66-year-old man with long-standing intermittent chest pain. Mayo Clin Proc 2003;78:1405–1408.
10. Yang E, Lerman A. Management of the patient with chest pain and a normal coronary angiogram. Cardiol Clin 2005;23:559–568.
11. Hamasaki S, Suwaidi J, Higano S, et al. Attenuated coronary flow reserve and vascular remodeling in patients with hypertension and left ventricular hypertrophy. J Am Coll Cardiol 2000;35:1654–1660.
12. Cannon R, Cunnion R, Parrillo J, et al. Dynamic limitation of coronary vasodilator reserve in patients with dilated cardiomyopathy and chest pain. J Am Coll Cardiol 1987;10:1190–1200.
13. Schwartzkopff B, Mundhenke M, Strauer B. Alterations of the architecture of subendocardial arterioles in patients with hypertrophic cardiomyopathy and impaired coronary vasodilator reserve: a possible cause for myocardial ischemia. J Am Coll Cardiol 1998;31;1089–1096.
14. Saffitz J, Sazama K, Roberts W. Amyloidosis limited to small arteries causing angina pectoris and sudden death. Am J Cardiol 1983;51:1234–1235.
15. Nitenberg A, Foult J, Blanchet F, et al. Coronary flow and resistance reserve in patients with chronic aortic regurgitation, angina pectoris and normal coronary arteries. J Am Coll Cardiol 1988;11:478–486.
16. Akasaka T, Yoshida K, Hozumi T, et al. Restricted coronary flow reserve in patients with mitral regurgitation improves after mitral reconstructive surgery. J Am Coll Cardiol 1998;32:1923–1930.

17. Chauhan A, Taylor G, Petch M, et al. Both endothelial-dependent and endothelial-independent function is impaired in patients with angina pectoris and normal coronary angiograms. Eur Heart J 1997;18:60–68.
18. Lange R, Hillis L. Acute pericarditis. N Engl J Med 2004;351:2195–2202.
19. Adler Y, Finkelstein Y, Guindo J, et al. Colchicine treatment for recurrent pericarditis: a decade of experience. Circulation 1998;97:2183–2185.
20. Kilbourne ED, Wilson CB, Perrier D. The induction of gross myocardial lesions by a Coxsackie virus and cortisone. J Clin Invest 1956;35:362–370.
21. Eggebrecht H, Baumgart D, Herold U, et al. Interventional management of aortic dissection. Herz 2002;27:539–547.
22. Klompas M. Does this patient have an acute thoracic aortic dissection? JAMA 2002; 297:2262–2272.
23. von Kodolitsch Y, Schwartz AG, Nienaber CA. Clinical prediction of acute aortic dissection. Arch Intern Med 2000;160:2977–2982.
24. Gomes AS, Bettmann MA, Boxt LM, et al., for the American College of Radiology. Acute chest pain—suspected aortic dissection. ACR Appropriateness Criteria. Radiology 2000;215(Suppl);1–5.
25. Hagan PG, Nienaber CA, Isselbacher EM, et al. The International Registry of Acute Aortic Dissection (IRAD): new insights into an old disease. JAMA 2000;283: 897–903.

23
Antihypertensive Therapy in the Acute Coronary Syndrome Patient

Lauren Rosenberg, Gurusher Panjrath, Eyal Herzog,
and Franz Messerli

Hypertension is a well-known risk factor for coronary artery disease. It is therefore not uncommon that when patients present with acute coronary syndrome (ACS), hypertension will be an important part of the management. In this short review, we address the initial assessment and management of elevated blood pressure in patients presenting with ACS.

Pathogenesis/Pathophysiology

Myocardial ischemia and infarction occur when the myocardial oxygen demand cannot be met because of a decrease in myocardial blood flow or an increase in myocardial oxygen demand. As a consequence, the goal of therapy in ACS is twofold. The first goal is to increase or at least to maintain coronary flow, and the second is to decrease the overall demand of oxygen by the myocardium. Oxygen demand is determined by several factors among which the most important ones are heart rate, myocardial contractility, myocardial wall tension or stress, and myocardial mass.

Myocardial wall tension is proportional to the aortic pressure, and myocardial oxygen demand doubles when the mean aortic pressure increases from 75 to 175 mm Hg at a constant heart rate and a constant stroke volume. Conversely, lowering the pressure will, in general, reduce myocardial oxygen demand. It stands to reason therefore that treating hypertension in the setting of ACS will, in general, have a beneficial effect. We have to remember though that there are no outcome data attesting to this.

A not uncommon complicating factor of long-standing hypertension is left ventricular hypertrophy (LVH), which has been shown to increase myocardial oxygen demand. LVH is a blood pressure–independent risk factor for myocardial infarction, congestive heart failure, and stroke. Patients with LVH are therefore at a particularly high risk for ACS. The hypertrophied myocardium has been shown to be relatively underperfused making it more prone to ischemia[1].

Similar to blood pressure, an increase in heart rate has been shown to increase myocardial oxygen demand. Conversely, lowering heart rate will diminish oxygen demand.

Clinical Considerations

It must be emphasized that there are currently no outcome studies showing that decreasing blood pressure in hypertensive patients in the setting of ACS is beneficial. Therefore, treatment strategies outlined here are based on the pathogenetic mechanisms of the disorder and on the theoretical advantage of improving myocardial oxygen balance. Several questions need to be considered in the hypertensive patients with ACS. Perhaps the most important one is what the goal blood pressure should be. Although there are no data behind any number or percentage, American College of Cardiology (ACC) guidelines recommend that mean arterial pressure should not be lowered by more than 25%. This recommendation is based on the thought that in lowering blood pressure too abruptly, perfusion pressure may drop and this may have deleterious effects. Indeed, we have shown in the INVEST study [2], in which all 22,000 patients had coronary artery disease and hypertension, that too low a diastolic pressure can be harmful. When diastolic pressure fell below 70 mm Hg, primary outcome doubled. When it fell below 60 mm Hg, it actually quadrupled. The primary outcome was a composite end point of all-cause death, nonfatal stroke, and nonfatal myocardial infarction. The nadir for diastolic blood pressure was 84 mm Hg and the nadir for systolic pressure in INVEST was 119 mm Hg, with a much more shallow curve than for diastolic pressure. Because coronaries are the only vascular bed that is perfused during diastole only, a J-shaped curve between diastolic pressure and coronary events should not be surprising. Of note, however, patients in the INVEST study had chronic, stable coronary heart disease and any extrapolation from this entity to ACS patients is speculative. Nevertheless, we think that, similar to the situation with stable CAD, lowering diastolic pressure below 70 to 80 mm Hg in the setting of ACS should be avoided.

Another issue to consider in a hypertensive patient with ACS is the possibility that the ACS may actually be the result of a hypertensive emergency. The decision, which is the chicken and which is the egg, is a clinical one but not unimportant. The pathogenetic mechanism of disease is different, and as a consequence, therapy may be different as well, particularly with regard to anticoagulation and platelet inhibition.

Treatment

By definition, all antihypertensive drugs lower blood pressure, and there are numerous drug classes available for the treatment of hypertension. For obvious reasons, the therapeutic choices become somewhat restricted. In this chapter, we outline the various agents available and the appropriate dose for their use in the management of hypertension in the setting of ACS. We should remember that patients presenting with ACS often require emergent reperfusion or thrombolytics. A systolic blood pressure above 180 mm Hg or a diastolic above 110 mm Hg is a relative contraindication to the use of thrombolytics. Regardless of whether the patient will go to the cardiac catheterization lab or will be treated with thrombolytics, reperfusion is first priority, and administration of antihypertensive therapy should not be a cause for delay.

Nitroglycerin

Nitroglycerin is an endothelium independent vasodilator with many effects on the cardiovascular system. The primary physiologic action of nitrates is vasodilation of veins, arteries, and arterioles through the relaxation of vascular smooth muscle. It decreases preload by venodilation, therefore causing peripheral pooling and a decrease in myocardial oxygen consumption (MVO_2). Nitrates also reduce afterload via dilation of the arterial system, although to a lesser extent. Nitroglycerin dilates both normal and atherosclerotic coronary arteries and promotes redistribution of coronary blood flow to ischemic regions. Nitroglycerin also has an effect on the systemic arterial circulation, causing decrease in afterload, and therefore a decrease in wall stress and MVO_2.

Dosage and Administration

Patients are often treated initially by EMS or in the emergency department with sublingual nitroglycerin or nitroglycerin paste, which may or may not be effective in decreasing anginal symptoms and blood pressure. However, for the management of hypertension, the intravenous formulation is more appropriate.

Treatment should be initiated with a bolus of 12.5 to 25 µg and should be followed by intravenous infusion at a rate of 10 to 20 µg/min. Patients on intravenous nitroglycerin should be monitored closely with frequent blood pressure measurement and assessment of clinical response. The dose can be increased by 10 µg/min every 3 to 5 minutes if blood pressure or anginal pain has not adequately decreased. Once a partial blood pressure or symptom response is achieved, the dosing increments should be decreased and the time between increasing doses should be lengthened. The maximal dose for intravenous infusion of nitroglycerin is generally thought to be 200 µg/min.

Patients who are treated with nitroglycerin, either by transdermal patch or with intravenous infusion, may develop tolerance to the medication. This has in fact been seen in up to 50% of patients treated with the intravenous formulation [3]. This should be suspected in any patient receiving high doses of nitroglycerin with little clinical response and indicates that another agent may be necessary. To avoid the development of tolerance in patients being treated with transdermal nitroglycerin, we recommend a 6-hour nitroglycerin-free period every 24 hours.

Contraindications

Nitroglycerin should be avoided in patients who have used phosphodiesterase inhibitors such as sildenafil (Viagra, Pfizer, New York) in the previous 24 hours, as they can potentiate the effects of nitroglycerin and cause profound hypotension [4]. Side effects of nitroglycerin include headache and hypotension, and it should be used with caution in patients who are bradycardic (heart rate below 50 beats per minute) or have suspicion of right ventricular infarction.

Beta-Blockers

Beta-blockers have multiple advantageous effects in the setting of ACS. By blocking the effects of circulating catecholamines on cell membrane beta-adrenergic receptors, they have antiarrhythmic, anti-ischemic, and antihypertensive properties. Beta-blockers decrease myocardial oxygen demand and cardiac workload by reducing heart rate and contractility. This contributes in lowering systemic blood pressure. In addition, the effect of increasing diastolic time increases coronary perfusion time.

Multiple trials have shown the advantages of early treatment with beta-blockers. In ISIS-1 [5], more than 16,000 patients were assigned to treatment with atenolol or usual care. Overall mortality from vascular causes was reduced by 15%, and this mortality benefit was still significant at 1 year. In TIMI IIB [6], 1,434 patients who were treated with tissue plasminogen activator (TPA) for ST-elevation myocardial infarction were given either immediate metoprolol followed by daily dosing or a delayed start of metoprolol at days 6 to 8. At 6 days, fewer patients in the immediately treated group had nonfatal reinfarction or recurrent chest pain. There was no mortality difference between these groups, but this may have been due to an overall small number of deaths.

In the COMMIT trial [7], 45,852 patients who presented with an acute myocardial infarction were randomized to receive up to 15 mg of intravenous metoprolol followed by a daily dose of 200 mg metoprolol or placebo. The two primary end points of the study were (1) composite of death, reinfarction, or cardiac arrest; and (2) death from any cause during the scheduled treatment period. Patients were followed up at day of discharge or at 28 days, whichever came first. In this study, there was no significant difference between metoprolol and placebo for the primary end points that were specified. Further analysis showed that a greater number of patients in the placebo group had reinfarction and a greater number had ventricular arrhythmias. This positive effect of metoprolol was counterbalanced by a greater number of patients in the metoprolol-treated group having cardiogenic shock. There was some criticism of this study, because the study included patients in overt heart failure. Some have argued that this inclusion may have caused the increased number of patients that developed cardiogenic shock. In our opinion, the results of this study reinforce that the use of beta-blockers in the setting of acute myocardial infarction should be selective and only given in the appropriate clinical setting.

Dosage and Administration

Beta-blockers should be administered to all high-risk patients intravenously followed by an oral dose. There is no evidence that one agent is superior to another; however, a beta-blocker without sympathomimetic effects should be used. We recommend use of intravenous metoprolol 5 mg every 5 minutes for a total of 3 doses (15 mg total), followed by 25 to 50 mg orally every 6 to 12 hours. This is a general guideline, and heart rate and blood pressure responses should be monitored for optimal dosing with the goal for heart rate between 50 and 60 bpm. Although we describe the use of metoprolol, patients at our institution are generally discharged on either metoprolol succinate or carvedilol.

Contraindications

Beta-blockers should be avoided in patients with symptomatic bradycardia, prolonged first-degree atrioventricular (AV) block, high-grade second-degree block, third-degree block, and in patients in overt heart failure. There is a relative contraindication to beta-blockers in patients with a history of asthma and in patients with a history of severe chronic obstructive pulmonary disease (COPD). Response to beta-blockers in patients with asthma or COPD can be tested with a small dose of a short-acting β_1 selective agent, and if it is tolerated, longer-acting agents can be used.

Calcium Channel Blockers

Calcium channel blockers have antianginal, vasodilatory, and antihypertensive properties. Calcium channel blockers are composed of two groups: dihydropyridine calcium channel antagonists (e.g., nifedipine and amlodipine) and non–dihydropyridine calcium channel antagonists (e.g., verapamil and diltiazem). Both decrease the influx of calcium ions across cardiac and smooth muscle cell membranes. Whereas the dihydropyridines primarily affect the peripheral vascular smooth muscle and cause its relaxation, non-dihydropyridines have more potent cardiac effects, including depression of myocardial contractility, heart rate, and AV node conduction. All of these agents have similar coronary vessel dilation properties.

The calcium channel blocker nifedipine, a dihydropyridine, has been extensively studied in the setting of ACS. In the TRENT study [8], 4,491 patients with suspected myocardial infarction were assigned to receive nifedipine

(10 mg four times daily) or placebo within 24 hours of onset of chest pain. In this study, there was a 7% increase in mortality in the nifedipine group; this increased mortality was a trend, with a non-significant P value. This trend of higher mortality was also seen in the SPRINT II [9] trial in which 1,358 patients received either 20 mg of nifedipine or placebo in the setting of acute myocardial infarction. This trial was terminated early because of a failure to show benefit and a trend toward higher mortality in the nifedipine-treated group.

Nifedipine and other rapid-release, short-acting dihydropyridines are contraindicated in the setting of unstable angina/non–ST-elevation myocardial infarction (UA/NSTEMI) by causing a rapid drop in blood pressure and a reflex activation of the sympathetic nervous system. Clearly, no short-acting calcium antagonist should be used in an ACS patient. Indeed, American College of Cardiology/American Heart Association (ACC/AHA) guidelines strongly recommend against the use of immediate-release dihydropyridine calcium antagonists unless a beta-blocker is administered concurrently. ACC/AHA guidelines recommend the alternative administration of a non–dihydropyridine calcium antagonist to patients with persistent or frequently–recurring ischemia, or in patients with atrial fibrillation or atrial flutter with rapid ventricular response, if a beta-blocker is contraindicated and severe left ventricular dysfunction is absent. An oral, long-acting calcium antagonist such as amlodipine is certainly an acceptable antihypertensive drug in a patient who has been given a beta-blocker.

Angiotensin-Converting Enzyme Inhibitors

There are multiple large, randomized clinical trials that have proved the benefit of administration of angiotensin-converting enzyme (ACE) inhibitors early on in the course of an acute myocardial infarction. They have been shown to reduce LV dysfunction and dilatation and slow the progression to congestive heart failure. Most of these trials suggest benefit within the first 24 hours after presentation, after reperfusion, and once blood pressure has stabilized. In ISIS-4 [10], 58,050 patients were assigned to treatment with captopril (titrated from an initial dose of 6.25 mg) or placebo for 28 days. The study found a 7% reduction in mortality at 35 days and this benefit was also seen at 1 year.

In CONSENSUS II [11], more than 6,000 patients who presented with acute myocardial infarction were treated with intravenous enalapril, followed by oral enalapril or placebo for 6 months. This trial was terminated early because of hypotension that was seen in predominately elderly patients and a high probability that enalapril was not superior to placebo. This adverse effect and the lack of benefit were attributed to the early use of intravenous enalapril. This has been adapted by the ACC/AHA guidelines, and an intravenous ACE inhibitor is relatively contraindicated in the first 24 hours of a ST-elevation myocardial infarction (STEMI), because of the risk of hypotension.

Morphine

Morphine sulfate is commonly used in myocardial infarction for its potent analgesic and anxiolytic properties. Additionally, morphine has beneficial hemodynamic effects, including venodilation and reduction in heart rate and systolic blood pressure. However, no randomized trials have established the unique impact of morphine on myocardial ischemia. Intravenous morphine sulfate administered to relieve anginal symptoms, pulmonary congestion, or anxiety may contribute to reduction of blood pressure. Adverse effects include hypotension, nausea, vomiting, and respiratory depression.

Nitroprusside

Nitroprusside is effective at both arterial and venous dilation and therefore in reducing both preload and afterload. It is rapidly metabolized, its onset of action is very rapid, and it is therefore very easily titrated for the desired hemodynamic effect. It is a commonly used drug in hypertensive emergency for these reasons.

Nitroprusside should not be used in the setting of active ischemia because the dramatic afterload-reducing effects may cause decreased flow in coronary arteries with significant lesions, with an increase in flow through normal vessels.

Hydralazine

The main effect of hydralazine is reduction of afterload by a mechanism that remains unclear. It has a short half-life and may cause a reflex increase in sympathetic nervous system activity. Because of the unpredictable effect of hydralazine on blood pressure and the risk of hypotension, it is contraindicated in the setting of ACS.

References

1. Hamasaki S, Al Suwaidi J, Higano ST, et al. Attenuated coronary flow reserve and vascular remodeling in patients with hypertension and left ventricular hypertrophy. J Am Coll Cardiol 2000;35:1654–1660.
2. Pepine CJ, Handberg EM, Cooper-DeHoff RM, et al. A calcium antagonist vs a non-calcium antagonist hypertension treatment strategy for patients with coronary artery disease: the International Verapamil-Trandolapril Study (INVEST): a randomized controlled trial. J Am Med Assoc 2003;290:2805–2816.
3. Elkayam U, Kulick D, McIntosh N, et al. Incidence of early tolerance to hemodynamic effects of continuous infusion of nitroglycerin in patients with coronary artery disease and heart failure. Circulation 1987;76:577–584.

 4. Cheitlin MD, Hutter AM, Brindis RG, et al. ACC/AHA expert consensus document on the use of sildenafil (Viagra) in patients with cardiovascular disease. American College of Cardiology/American Heart Association. J Am Coll Cardiol 1999;33: 273–282.
 5. ISIS-1 (First International Study of Infarct Survival) Collaborative Group. Randomized trial of intravenous atenolol among 16 027 cases of suspected acute myocardial infarction: ISIS-1. Lancet 1986;2:57–66.
 6. Roberts R, Rogers WJ, Mueller HS, et al. Immediate versus deferred beta-blockade following thrombolytic therapy in patients with acute myocardial infarction: results of the Thrombolysis in Myocardial Infarction (TIMI) II-B Study. Circulation 1991; 83:422–437.
 7. COMMIT Collaborate Group. Early intravenous then oral metopolol in 45,852 patients with acute MI: randomized placebo-controlled trial. Lancet 2005;366: 1622–1632.
 8. Wilcox RG, Hampton JR, Banks DC, et al. Trial of early nifedipine in acute myocardial infarction: the TRENT study. BMJ 1986;293:1204–1208.
 9. Goldbourt U, Behar S, Reicher-Reiss H, et al. Early administration of nifedipine in suspected acute myocardial infarction: the Secondary Prevention Reinfarction Israel Nifedipine Trial 2 Study. Arch Intern Med 1993;153:345–353.
10. ISIS-4 Collaborative Group. A randomized factorial trial assessing early oral captopril, oral mononitrate and intravenous magnesium sulphate in 58,050 patients with suspected acute myocardial infarction. Lancet 1995;345:669–685.
11. Swedberg K, Held J, Kjekshus J, Rasmossen K, et al. Effects of the early administration of enalapril on mortality in patients with acute myocardial infarction. Results of the cooperative New Scandanavian Enalapril Survival Study (CONSENSUS II) N Engl J Med 1992;327:678–684.

24
Hyperglycemia Complicating the Acute Coronary Syndrome: Algorithm for Hyperglycemia Management During ACS

Emad Aziz, Eyal Herzog, and Nicholas H.E. Mezitis

Acute coronary syndrome (ACS) remains one of the most common reasons for hospital admission worldwide. Diabetes mellitus (DM) has reached epidemic proportions in the United States, affecting an estimated 21 million Americans and generating health care expenses in excess of $130 billion annually in the United States [1–2]. It is the fourth most common comorbid condition complicating all hospital discharges, present in 9.5% of all hospital discharges and in 29% of patients undergoing cardiac surgery. Furthermore, diabetic patients after acute myocardial infarction have at least a twofold increased risk of dying compared with the nondiabetic population [3–6]. In addition, the plasma glucose level on admission is predictive of in-hospital mortality after acute ST-elevation myocardial infarction (STEMI). This applies not only to patients with established DM but also to those with so-called stress hyperglycemia [5–9].

The Umpierrez study outcome demonstrated that in-hospital hyperglycemia is a common finding and represents an important marker of poor clinical outcome and mortality in patients with and without a history of diabetes [4]. Patients with newly diagnosed hyperglycemia had a significantly higher mortality rate and a poorer functional outcome than patients with a known history of diabetes or normoglycemia [4].

The American Diabetes Association (ADA) supported an extensive technical review evaluating the relationships between glycemic control and its impact on hospital outcomes [5]. This review became the basis of the 2005 ADA Clinical Practice Guidelines.

Hyperglycemia and Cardiovascular Disease

Review of epidemiologic evidence by Saydah et al. demonstrated the relationship between hyperglycemia and cardiovascular disease (CVD) [6]. Sixteen-year follow-up of 3,092 adults in the second U.S. National Health and Nutrition Examination Survey who underwent an oral glucose tolerance test in the period 1976–1980 showed that diabetes, whether diagnosed from fasting or 2-hour glucose values, was associated with increased mortality [6].

The Finish East-West Study of 1,373 nondiabetic and 1,059 diabetic persons showed the CVD risk of persons with diabetes to be similar to that of persons who had had a myocardial infarction [7].

Among the population of any cardiac care unit (CCU), about 20% of the patients are likely to have type 2 DM. Another 20% may have undiagnosed diabetes and present with hyperglycemia upon admission, while 15% to 20% of patients admitted have impaired glucose intolerance. This suggests that almost 60% of the CCU patient population has glucose intolerance.

The cardiac risk associated with hyperglycemia is significant. In one study by Bolk, the 1-year mortality rate was 19.3% and rose to 44% in patients with glucose levels > 11.1 mmol/L [8]. Mortality was higher in diabetic patients than in nondiabetic patients (40 vs. 16%; $P < 0.05$).

The recent position statement from the ADA [9] recognized hyperglycemia on admission to be attributable to one of three problems:

1. Patients with stress hyperglycemia, whose glucose levels return to normal within 4 to 5 days and who do not require additional care.
2. Patients with admission hyperglycemia, who have some baseline level of insulin resistance, may have undiagnosed diabetes, and develop diabetes after discharge.
3. Patients with hyperglycemia who have diabetes.

All three groups have hospital events related to their glucose levels. Interventions for these patients were validated by findings from the Van den Berghe et al. [10] and the DIGAMI-I [11] trials, which were prospectively conducted clinical trials with patients randomized between tight versus conventional diabetes control.

The Metabolic Effects of Hyperglycemia

Hyperglycemia has been shown to induce proinflammatory cytokines and chemokine genes in monocytes. Certain cytokines, such as tumor necrosis factor-α (TNF-α), impair insulin action in peripheral tissue and have a direct role in obesity-linked insulin resistance. Interleukin-6 (IL-6) also influences glucose metabolism by alteration of insulin sensitivity [12, 13]. The harmful effects of hyperglycemia exceed those of simple inflammation. The biochemistry of the myocardial cell is altered in patients with hyperglycemia because of a radical shift in energy production resulting in fatty acid excess during ischemia, which leads to cell membrane injury and arrhythmias [14]. Studies evaluating the effects of hyperglycemia on the immune system have consistently demonstrated immunosuppression, resulting mainly from phagocyte dysfunction, which can be reversed through normalization of blood glucose levels [15]. Numerous consequences of hyperglycemia-mediated immunosuppression have been observed in the cardiovascular system, including impairment of ischemic preconditioning, reduced coronary blood flow, cardiac myocyte death, blood pressure changes, catecholamine elevations, platelet abnormalities, electrophysiologic changes, as well as hyperglycemia-induced platelet hyperreactivity, which may be responsible for increased thrombotic events [16]. Hyperglycemia-related vascular endothelial cell dysfunction may also be responsible for the poor cardiovascular outcomes.

The Evidence Behind Supporting Tighter Glycemic Control

There is a large body of evidence, both observational and in controlled studies, documenting the relationship between hyperglycemia and outcomes in hospitalized patients. In 1998, Pomposelli et al. [17] evaluated 97 patients with diabetes undergoing general surgery procedures and monitored blood glucose every 6 hours. The investigators observed that a single blood glucose level >222 mg/dL on the first postoperative day was a sensitive (85%) yet relatively nonspecific (35%) predictor of nosocomial infections.

Krinsley observed a close correlation between blood glucose level and in-hospital mortality rates in 1,826 consecutive patients admitted to the ICU [18]. The lowest hospital mortality, 9.6%, occurred among patients with mean glucose values between 80 and 99 mg/dL. Mortality increased progressively as glucose values increased, reaching 42.5% among patients with mean glucose values exceeding 300 mg/dL ($P < 0.001$). In a study by Van den Berghe et al., 1,548 CABG patients admitted to the ICU [19] requiring respiratory support and parenteral glucose infusion were randomized to two groups with glucose targets of 110 versus 180 to 200 mg/dL, respectively. Forty-three percent lower mortality was observed in the intensively treated group (8% vs. 4.5%). Mortality was particularly reduced for those in the ICU >5 days (10.6% vs. 20.2%). The incidence of multiorgan failure, renal failure, bacteremia, critical illness polyneuropathy, and the need for prolonged stay in the ICU were also reduced.

The first Diabetes Mellitus Insulin-Glucose Infusion in Acute Myocardial infarction (DIGAMI 1) study enrolled diabetic patients treated within 24 hours of acute myocardial infarction (AMI). Patients were randomized to intensive diabetes management using intravenous insulin for at least 24 hours with target glucose levels 126 to 196 mg/dL or to standardized therapy. Participants in the intensively treated group had a 30% 1-year and 28% 3.4-year decrease in mortality [20].

DIGAMI 2 was designed to compare three treatment strategies in patients with AMI. Group 1 received an insulin-glucose infusion acutely, followed by insulin-based long-term glucose control. Group 2 also received an initial insulin-glucose infusion followed by standard glucose control, and group 3 received routine metabolic management according to local practice. Unfortunately, this study did not reach recruitment goals and showed no treatment differences. Moreover, the primary treatment goal of fasting blood glucose of 90 to 126 mg/dL was never achieved. Fasting glucose levels (149 mg/dL) and hemoglobin A1C (6.8%) were similar among groups. Thus, if glycemia is predictive of outcomes, no differences would have been expected, and none were observed [21].

In CREATE-ECLA, more than 20,000 patients with ST-elevation myocardial infarction were treated with a 24-hour glucose-insulin-potassium (GIK) infusion or placebo, irrespective of baseline glucose [22]. GIK did not improve mortality; however, the relative hyperglycemia that did result in active therapy patients may have obscured any treatment benefit.

In conclusion, there is a strong clinical rationale for aggressive short-term intensive insulin therapy, which appears to improve outcomes in cardiac as well as critically ill diabetic and nondiabetic patients.

Major Gap Between Recommended Guidelines and Current Practice

Americans do not always receive the care that scientific evidence suggests they should, despite national health care spending approaching 14% of gross domestic product (GDP). Efforts to make evidence-based recommendations available to medical practitioners, through the development and promulgation of clinical practice guidelines, are a necessary step toward solving that problem. Applying those guidelines in practice requires restructuring the environment in which health care is delivered so that "doing the right thing" becomes intuitive. Tools that simplify and embed the recommendations for evidence-based care into the care itself are of particular usefulness.

Inpatient management of hyperglycemia and avoidance of hypoglycemia have become important measures of the quality of health care afforded to hospitalized patients. Translation of clinical trials evidence relating to hyperglycemia management into performance metrics should be useful in inpatient settings throughout the country. Critical care algorithms ("pathways") and management plans for hospitalized patients are becoming increasingly popular, optimizing the quality of care.

Systemic Barriers and Challenges to Improved Hyperglycemia Management

Many of the changes needed to improve the management of the inpatient with hyperglycemia involve changes to culture, long-standing practice patterns, processes of care, and workflow habits. Competing priorities and limited resources can present a major barrier to mobilizing the institutional support that is essential for success. Other barriers include:

- A shortage of skilled nurses further complicated by inadequate support systems. Nurses are essential to successfully implement protocols, order sets, more intensive glucose monitoring, and educational programs targeting enhanced glycemic control.
- Skepticism about the benefits of good inpatient glycemic control, in spite of the preponderance of evidence suggesting it is beneficial. This may be an expression of general resistance to change.

- Fear of hypoglycemia.
- Inadequate knowledge and understanding of diabetes, hyperglycemia, and its management by health care providers and patients alike.
- Lack of integrated information systems that allow comprehensive tracking and trending of glucose values and interventions to permit successful management of glycemia using specialized programs.
- Diabetes and hyperglycemia are prevalent on all services in the hospital, requiring broad educational efforts and process change. Patients frequently move across a spectrum of care providers and geographic locations during a single inpatient stay, entailing numerous transfers, communication challenges, and opportunities for error [23].

Hypoglycemia Concern

According to the American College of Endocrinology's recommendations, the target glucose level within 6 hours of myocardial infarction should be 80 to 110 mg/dL. This goal can be attained; however, hypoglycemia is a major concern for clinicians caring for hospitalized patients with diabetes, and it constitutes a major barrier to aggressive treatment of hyperglycemia, even though the likelihood of its occurrence is low [24].

In one protocol, the incidence of hypoglycemia defined as less than 60 mg/dL was 1.5% with a target range of 70 to 110 mg/dL; when the target range was 125 to 170 mg/dL, the incidence was 0. According to the aggregate of medical literature evaluating more than 10,000 cases, not a single patient has died from hypoglycemia [25].

Implementing Guidelines for Hyperglycemia Control in the Cardiac Patient

Insulin is the most effective agent for achieving glycemic control in hospitalized patients, whether given as a continuous intravenous infusion or subcutaneously. Several insulin infusion protocols have been published, providing algorithms for a safe and effective procedure in the medical ICU. These have resulted in a reduction in errors in managing hyperglycemia [26, 27]. There have been no large studies to investigate the efficacy and safety of different protocols. Furthermore, the limitation inherent in most of these protocols is their complexity for the nonspecialist responsible for the patient's hospital care.

The Pathway of Management of Hyperglycemia in Cardiac Care Units

We sought to address the issues related above by assembling a multidisciplinary group of physicians and nurses from the divisions of cardiology, endocrinology, intensive care medicine, and general internal medicine to develop a simplified protocol for the management of hyperglycemia in the hospitalized patient (Fig. 24.1) [28]. This pathway is comprehensive yet simple and provides guidelines for the treatment of patients in a critical care unit (cardiac, open heart recovery unit, medical ICU, surgical ICU) and for those in a cardiac step-down unit.

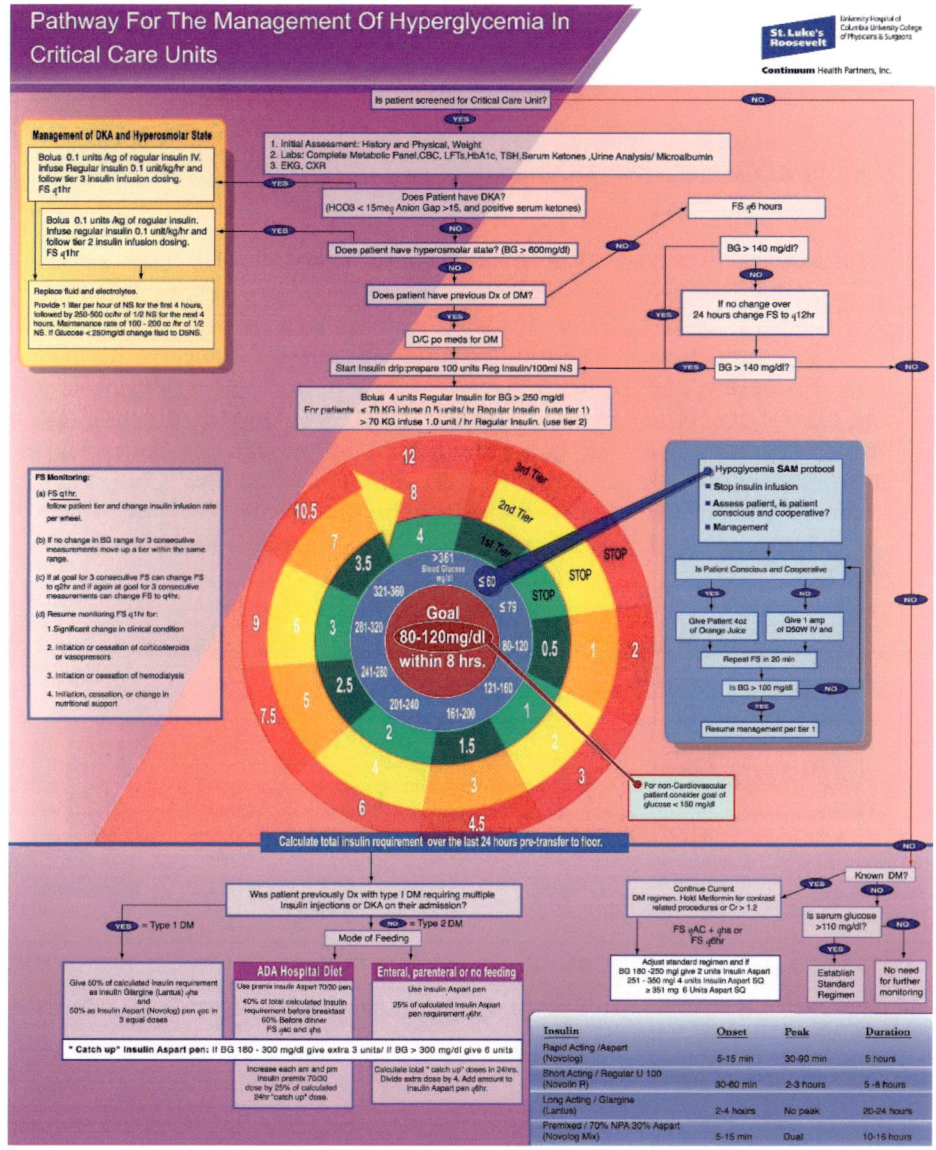

FIGURE 24.1. Pathway for the management of hyperglycemia in critical care units.

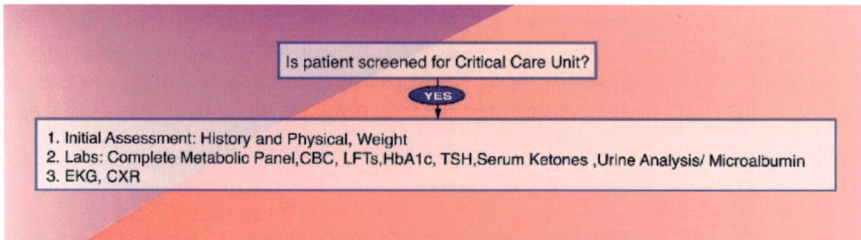

FIGURE 24.2. Initial assessment of patients with hyperglycemia who are screened to a critical care unit.

The Initial Assessment and Management of Patients with Hyperglycemia

Initial assessment of the patient should include history, physical examination, and recording of weight. We have defined a basic laboratory test panel required for all patients (Fig. 24.2). We included patients with diabetic ketoacidosis (DKA) and patients with hyperosmolar state and provided guidelines for their management (Fig. 24.3). Patients managed in this protocol have a diagnosis of DM. If the patient is not known to have DM, capillary blood glucose determinations (BG) every 6 hours will be required. A BG >140 mg/dL qualifies patients for enrollment into our pathway (Fig. 24.4). Initiation of the insulin infusion is achieved by providing a bolus of 4 units of regular insulin for patients with a BG >250 mg/dL and starting an infusion protocol that is based on weight (Fig. 24.5).

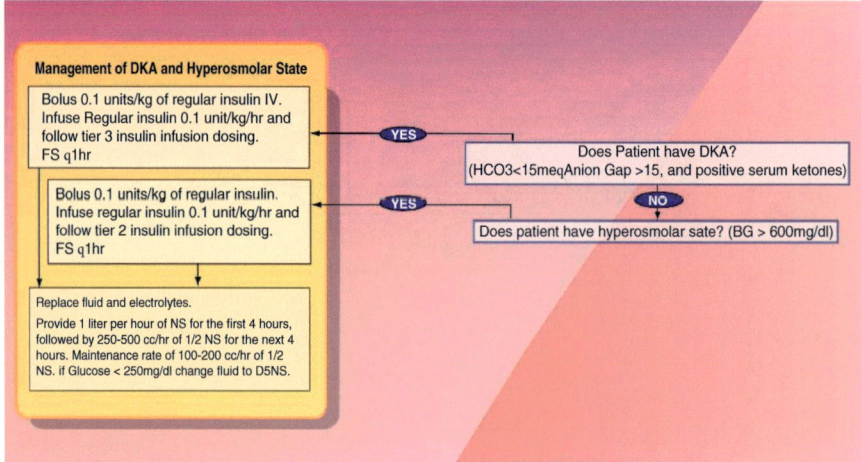

FIGURE 24.3. Management of diabetes ketoacidosis (DKA) and hyperosmolar state.

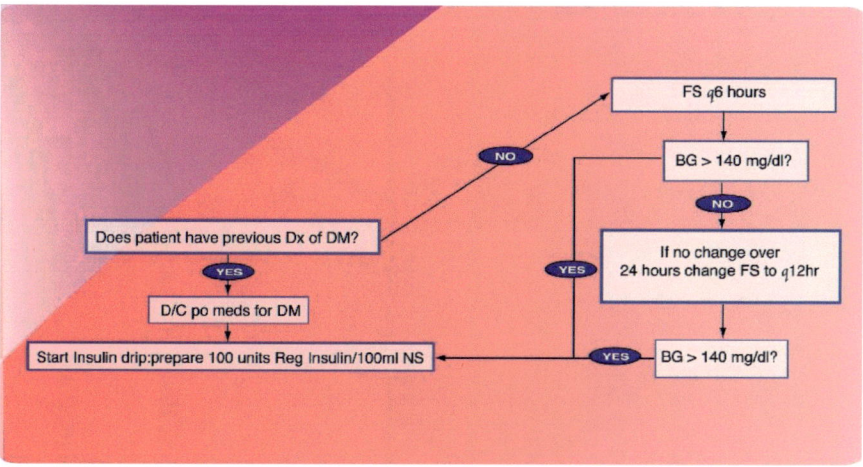

FIGURE 24.4. Blood glucose determination for enrollment into the hyperglycemia pathway.

The Key Feature of the Pathway

The key feature of this pathway is the "wheel," which provides treatment instruction for insulin administration (Fig. 24.6). This wheel features four concentric circles. The innermost circle represents blood glucose ranges. The three outer circles represent three increasing rates of insulin infusion. For patients who weigh less than 70 kg, the insulin infusion rate should be calculated based on tier 1.

For patients who weigh more than 70 kg, the infusion rate is based on tier 2. BG monitoring is performed every hour. The infusion rate is then adjusted according to the instructions corresponding with the BG of the same tier: "dialing up and down the wheel within the tier." If there is *no* decrease in BG range for three consecutive measurements, we move up a tier at the same glucose range.

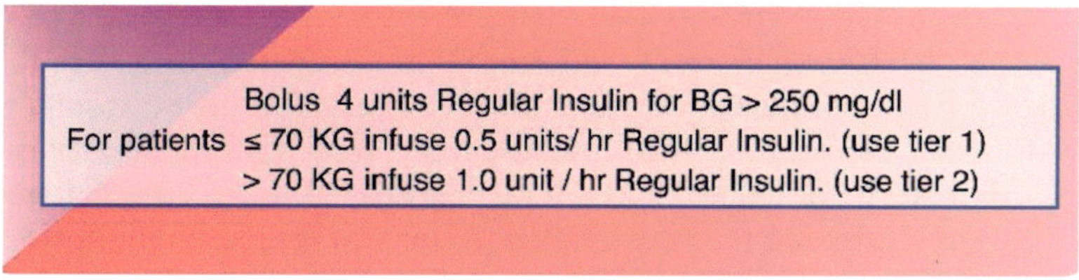

Bolus 4 units Regular Insulin for BG > 250 mg/dl
For patients ≤ 70 KG infuse 0.5 units/ hr Regular Insulin. (use tier 1)
> 70 KG infuse 1.0 unit / hr Regular Insulin. (use tier 2)

FIGURE 24.5. Initiation of insulin infusion protocol.

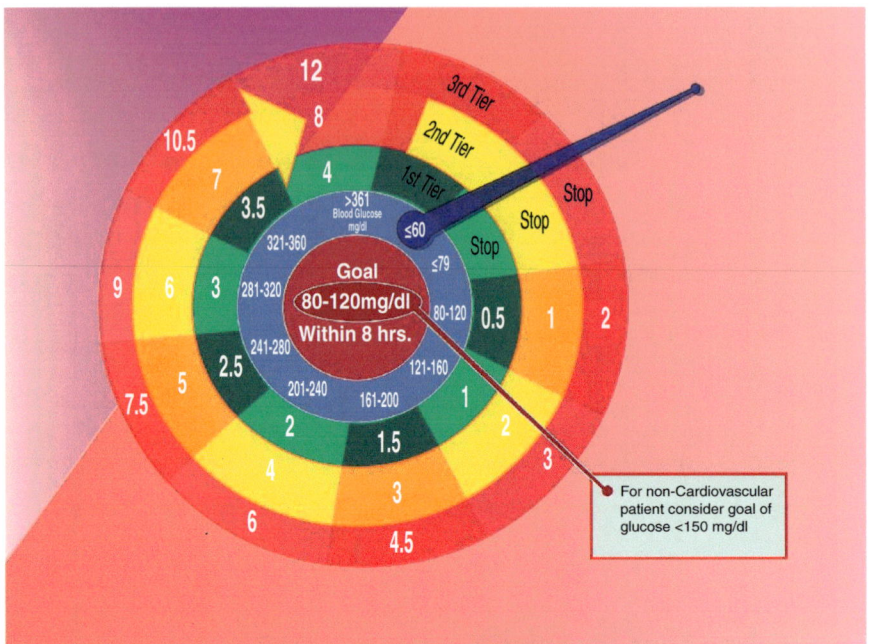

FIGURE 24.6. The "wheel" as a tool for insulin infusion.

Hypoglycemia Protocol

Prevention of hypoglycemia is essential in the aggressive management of hyperglycemia. If a patient is found to be hypoglycemic (BG <60 mg mg/dL), a protocol for management is provided as seen in Figure 24.7. We named this protocol SAM to reflect the key components of treatment: Stop insulin infusion, Assess the patient for consciousness and cooperation, and Manage the patient (with orange juice or D5OW infusion). If a patient's BG exceeds 100 mg/dL, the management using the "wheel" is resumed with the initial insulin infusion rate based on tier 1 and the corresponding BG.

Frequency of Blood Glucose Monitoring

Instructions for frequency of BG monitoring are provided to the health care provider. Initially, all monitoring is performed every hour. If BG results are at goal for three consecutive readings, then the frequency of monitoring is decreased to every 2 hours and again, if there is no change for three consecutive readings, it is decreased to every 4 hours. Return to frequent monitoring (BG every hour) is required for the following conditions: significant change in clinical condition; initiation or cessation of corticosteroids or vasopressors; or initiation, cessation, or change in nutritional support (Fig. 24.8).

Conversion to Subcutaneous Insulin

A protocol was developed to convert from the insulin infusion to subcutaneous insulin injections without sacrificing diabetes control (Fig. 24.9). Calculations are based on the total insulin requirement over the last 24-hour period on insulin infusion. The patients are then divided into two groups.

Group 1

This group is composed of patients with a prior diagnosis of type 1 DM requiring multiple insulin injections or patients with a diagnosis of DKA. Patients receive a combination of long-acting insulin, glargine (Lantus, Bridgewater, NJ) in the evening (bedtime), and rapid-acting insulin Aspart in three equal doses before every meal (Fig. 24.9).

Group 2

For patients with type 2 DM, the mode of feeding determines the insulin injection regimen (Fig. 24.9). Patients who receive a hospital diet are introduced to Premix 70/30 insulin Aspart (Novolog Mix). Forty percent of the calculated dose is given before breakfast and 60% before dinner. For patients who are fasting or on enteral or parenteral feedings, the rapid-acting insulin Aspart is used exclusively with 25% of the calculated total dose given every 6 hours.

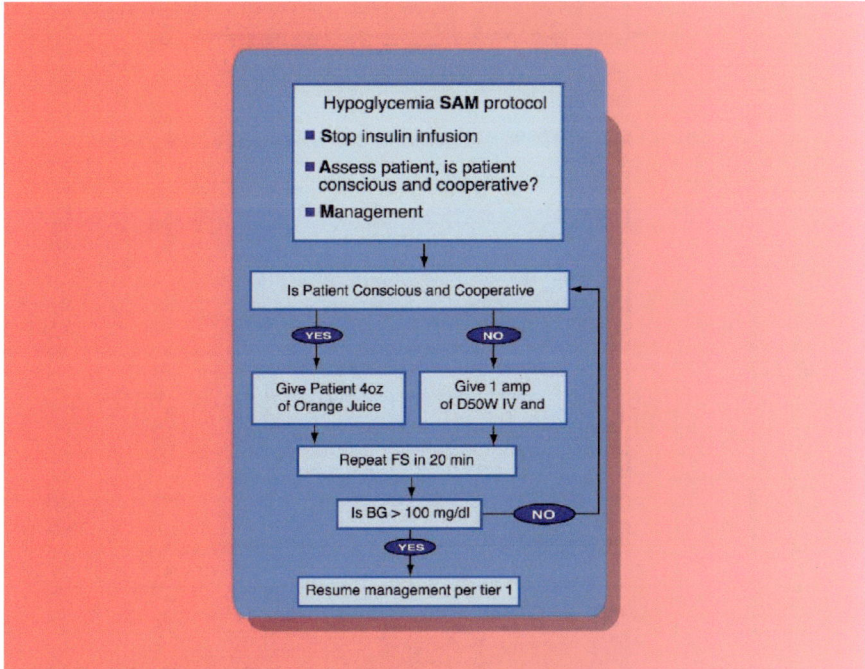

FIGURE 24.7. Management of hypoglycemia.

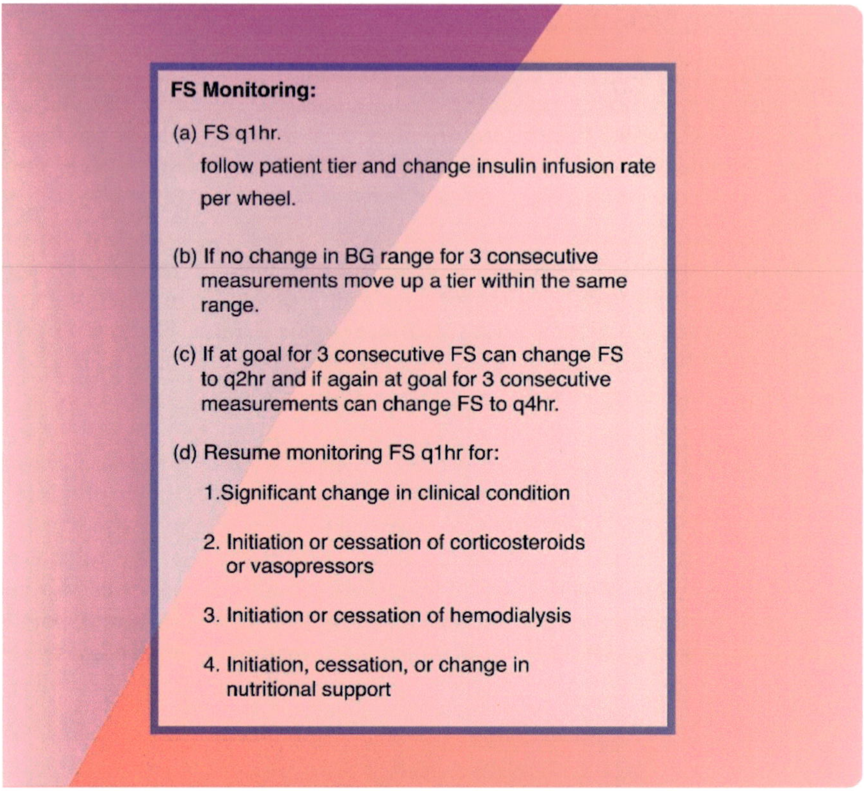

FS Monitoring:

(a) FS q1hr.

follow patient tier and change insulin infusion rate per wheel.

(b) If no change in BG range for 3 consecutive measurements move up a tier within the same range.

(c) If at goal for 3 consecutive FS can change FS to q2hr and if again at goal for 3 consecutive measurements can change FS to q4hr.

(d) Resume monitoring FS q1hr for:

1. Significant change in clinical condition

2. Initiation or cessation of corticosteroids or vasopressors

3. Initiation or cessation of hemodialysis

4. Initiation, cessation, or change in nutritional support

FIGURE 24.8. Guidelines for finger-stick monitoring for patients with hyperglycemia.

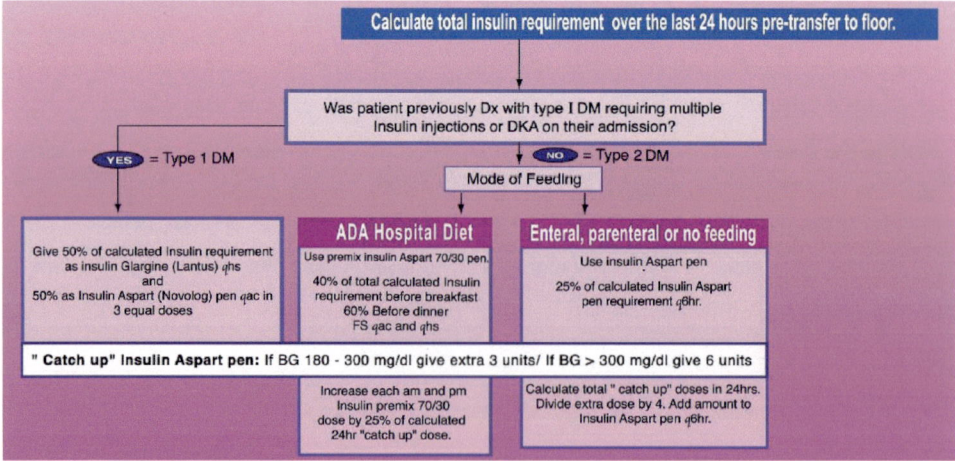

FIGURE 24.9. A protocol for conversion from insulin infusion to subcutaneous injection.

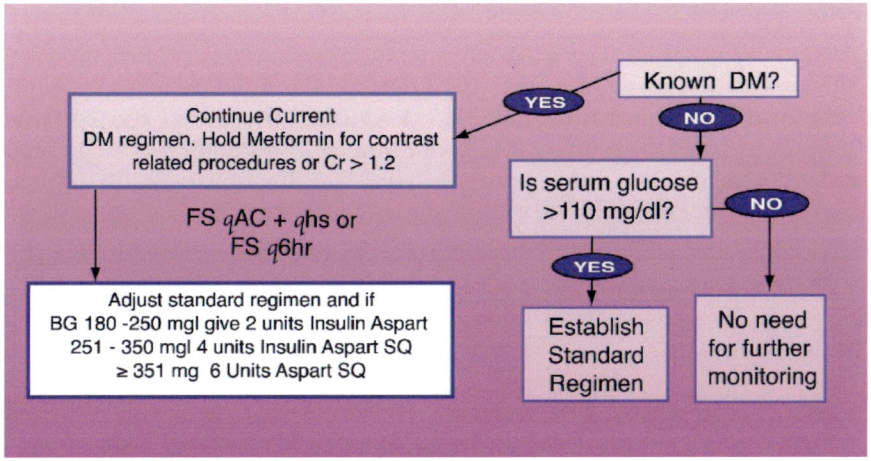

Figure 24.10. Management of diabetes in patients who are not screened to a critical care unit.

The conversion protocol described uses supplemental insulin at two dose levels: 3 units of insulin Aspart are given for BG between 180 and 300 mg/dL and 6 units of the same insulin type are administered for BG >300 mg/dL. This arrangement replaces the conventional "sliding scale." Adjustments in the dose of 70/30 Premix Aspart insulin are made daily to accommodate the supplemental units used over the past 24-hour period. The need for "catchup" insulin doses is hereby gradually reduced.

We have provided a separate algorithm for hyperglycemia management for cardiac care patients managed in areas of the hospital other than the critical care units, as seen in Figure 24.10. Patients with a prior diagnosis of DM continue their current DM regimen with BG monitoring before every meal and every evening. For these patients, a standard regimen is adjusted by using insulin Aspart with three "catch-up" doses as appears in Figure 24.10.

The illustration of our proposed pathway provides detailed reference information about the insulin products used (Fig. 24.11).

Insulin	Onset	Peak	Duration
Rapid Acting /Aspart (Novolog)	5-15 min	30-90 min	5 hours
Short Acting / Regular U 100 (Novolin R)	30-60 min	2-3 hours	5 -8 hours
Long Acting / Glargine (Lantus)	2-4 hours	No peak	20-24 hours
Premixed / 70% NPA 30% Aspart (Novolog Mix)	5-15 min	Dual	10-16 hours

Figure 24.11. Insulin products used in the hyperglycemia pathway.

Conclusion

This comprehensive pathway provides a detailed algorithm for management of hyperglycemia cardiac care units. It introduces 2 new novel concepts: the "wheel", which is the primary tool permitting rapid restoration of euglycemia and is the focus of this pathway, and "catchup" insulin, which permits a simple response to excessive glucose excursions while facilitating adjustments in the basic insulin regimen in anticipation of the patient's discharge from the hospital.

References

1. Talbot TR. Diabetes mellitus and cardiothoracic surgical site infections. Am J Infect Control 2005;33:353–359.
2. Hogan P, Dall T, Nikolov P. Economic cost of diabetes in the US in 2002. Diabetes Care 2003;26:917–932.
3. Rytter IR, Troelsen S, Beck-Nielsen H. Prevalence and mortality of acute myocardial infarctions in patients with diabetes. Diabetes Care 1985;8:230–234.
4. Umpierrez GE, Isaacs SD, Bazargan N, et al. Hyperglycemia: an independent marker of in-hospital mortality in patients with undiagnosed diabetes. J Clin Endocrinol Metab 2002;87:978–982.
5. Clement S, Braithwaite SS, Magee MF. American Diabetes Association Diabetes in Hospitals Writing Committee. Management of diabetes and hyperglycemia in hospitals. Diabetes Care 2004;27:553–591.
6. Saydah SH, Miret M, Sung J, et al. Postchallenge hyperglycaemia and mortality in a national sample of U.S. adults. Diabetes Care 2001;24(8):1397–1402.
7. Haffner SM, Lehto S, Ronnemaa T, et al. Mortality from coronary heart disease in subjects with type 2 diabetes and in nondiabetic subjects with and without prior myocardial infarction. N Engl J Med 1998;339:229–234.
8. Bolk J, van der Ploeg T, Cornel JH, et al. Impaired glucose metabolism predicts mortality after a myocardial infarction. Int J Cardiol 2001;79:207–214.
9. American Diabetes Association. Position Statement. Standards of medical care in diabetes. Diabetes Care 2005;28(Suppl 1):S4–S36.
10. Van den Berghe G, Wouters P, Weekers F, et al. Intensive insulin therapy in critically ill patients. N Eng J Med 2001;345:1359–1367.
11. Malmberg K, for the DIGAMI (Diabetes Mellitus Insulin Glucose Infusion in Acute Myocardial Infarction) Study Group. Prospective randomized study of intensive insulin treatment on long-term survival after acute myocardial infarction in patients with diabetes mellitus. BMJ 1997;314:1512.
12. Shanmugam N, Reddy MA, Guha M, et al. High glucose-induced expression of pro-inflammatory cytokine and chemokine genes in monocytic cells. Diabetes 2003;52:1256–1264.
13. Hotamisligil GS, Shargill NS, Spiegelman BM. Adipose expression of tumor necrosis factor-alpha: direct role in obesity-linked insulin resistance. Science 1993;259:87–91.
14. Stentz FB, Umpierrez GE, Cuervo R, et al. Proinflammatory cytokines, markers of cardiovascular risks, oxidative stress, and lipid peroxidation in patients with hyperglycemic crises. Diabetes 2004;53:2079–2086.

15. Kwoun MO, Ling PR, Lydon E, et al. Immunologic effects of acute hyperglycemia in nondiabetic rats. J Parenter Enteral Nutr 1997;21:91–95.

16. Clement S, Braithwaite SS, Magee MF, et al., on behalf of the Diabetes in Hospitals Writing Committee. Management of diabetes and hyperglycemia in hospitals. Diabetes Care 2004;27:553–591.

17. Pomposelli JJ, Baxter JK III, Babineau TJ, et al. Early postoperative glucose control predicts nosocomial infection rate in diabetic patients. J Parenter Enteral Nutr 1998; 22:77–81.

18. Krinsley JS. Association between hyperglycemia and increased hospital mortality in a heterogeneous population of critically ill patients. Mayo Clin Proc 200378: 1471–1478.

19. Van den Berghe G, Wouters P, Weekers F, et al. Intensive insulin therapy in critically ill patients. N Engl J Med 2001;345:1359–1367.

20. Malmberg K, Ryden L, Egendic S. Randomized trial of insulin-glucose infusion followed by subcutaneous insulin treatment in diabetic patients with acute myocardial infarction (DIGAMI study): effects on mortality at 1 year. J Am Coll Cardiol 1995;26: 57–65.

21. Capes SE, Hunt D, Malmberg K, et al. Stress hyperglycemia and increased risk of death after myocardial infarction in patients with and without diabetes: a systematic overview. Lancet 2000;355:773–778.

22. Mehta SR, Yusuf S, Diaz R. CREATE-ECLA Trial Group Investigators. Effect of glucose-insulin-potassium infusion on mortality in patients with acute ST-segment elevation myocardial infarction: the CREATE-ECLA randomized controlled trial. JAMA 2005;293:437–446.

23. Smith WD, Winterstein AG, Johns T, et al. Causes of hyperglycemia and hypoglycemia in adult inpatients. Am J Health-Syst Pharm 2005;62:714–719.

24. Moghissi E. Hospital management of diabetes beyond the sliding scale. Cleveland Clin J Med 2004;71:801–808.

25. Medical Crossfire. Special Edition. The impact of hyperglycemia on cardiac outcomes in hospitalized patients. Medical Crossfire; Newsletter June 2005, vol. 6; No. 11:1–18.

26. Queale WS, Seidler AJ, Brancati FL. Glycemic control and sliding scale insulin use in medical inpatients with diabetes mellitus. Arch Intern Med 1997;157:545–552.

27. Markovitz L, Wiechmann R, Harris N, et al. Description and evaluation of a glycemic management protocol for diabetic patients undergoing heart surgery. Endocr Pract 2002;8:10–18.

28. Herzog E, Aziz E, Croiter S, et al. Pathway for the management of hyperglycemia in critical care units. Crit Pathways Cardiol 2006;5:2.

25
Transition from Acute Phase to Chronic Phase: Secondary Prevention for Patients with Cardiovascular Disease

Merle Myerson

Algorithm

Step 1. Assess individual risk factors:
- Dyslipidemia
- Hypertension
- Obesity
- Sedentary lifestyle
- Tobacco abuse
- Diabetes

Step 2. Obtain measures:
- Fasting lipid panel (within 24 hours of onset symptoms): review past measures if available
- Blood pressure: assess baseline blood pressure; review past readings if available
- Assess weight, height, body mass index (BMI), waist circumference
- Exercise: assess current activity level and obstacles to participation in an exercise program
- Smoking: assess current tobacco use and willingness to quit

Step 3. Therapeutic plan:
- Lipids: begin high-dose statin; consider use of fibrate for high triglycerides (TG) (if no contraindications)
- Blood pressure: choose medication based on cardiac status
- Diet: instruction by nutritionist or health educator
- Sedentary lifestyle/exercise: referral to cardiac rehabilitation
- Smoking cessation: behavior modification with or without pharmacological therapy

Step 4. Goals for therapy:
Lipids
- LDL cholesterol <70 mg/dL
- TG <150 mg/dL
- HDL cholesterol >40 mg/dL for men and >50 mg/dL for women
Blood pressure
- Goal of <130/80 mmHg

Diet
- BMI <25
- Waist circumference <40 inches for men and <35 inches for women
- Adoption of a heart-healthy diet

Exercise
- Completion of cardiac rehabilitation
- Moderate-intensity aerobic exercise at least 30 minutes 5 times a week

Smoking
- Complete and sustained cessation

Introduction

Prevention can take place at many levels. Primary prevention targets people who may have asymptomatic or preclinical disease or have risk factors for developing disease. Secondary prevention targets people who have clinically manifest cardiovascular disease—myocardial infarction, stroke, or peripheral vascular disease. One may wonder how beneficial secondary prevention is; after all, the patient has already suffered an event. Studies in this area have shown that identifying and aggressively treating risk factors in these patients can significantly impact future morbidity and mortality.

Results from these studies prompted the American Heart Association and the American College of Cardiology in 2006 to release updated guidelines outlining secondary prevention for patients with known cardiovascular disease. The guidelines follow earlier documents but are notable for the major changes with respect to intensity of risk-factor management [1]. The principal author of the guidelines, Dr. Sidney Smith, comments that patients do not receive treatment for risk factors for many reasons. Hospital stays after heart procedures are short, which limits the time during which a patient can be educated. Furthermore, there is often a lack of communication between the cardiologist and the primary care provider [2].

The approach to the patient who presents with an acute coronary syndrome (ACS) begins with the understanding that this patient is at very high risk for having another event simply by virtue of having had an event. Identification of individual risk factors prior to discharge and a specific treatment plan for each risk factor is now considered standard of care.

Lipids

A fasting lipid panel should be obtained preferably within 24 hours of onset of symptoms. Values obtained after this will be artificially low and will not return to baseline for 2–3 months. It is also helpful to see if past lipid panels are available.

The use of statin drugs during or shortly after ACS has been studied. A number of trials (PROVE IT-TIMI 22, MIRACL, ESTABLISH) have shown a benefit although some have shown mixed (A to Z) or negative (SYMPHONY) findings. The statin drugs may have a number of biological actions that have relevance in the acute setting. Some of these pleiotropic effects are believed to include a reduction in plasma viscosity, inflammation, platelet aggregation, thrombin generation, and endothelial dysfunction [3, 4].

Therapeutic plan:

- All patients should receive instruction in a heart-healthy diet. This can be provided by a nutritionist, nurse, or health educator. Educational material should be given to the patient.
- Existing data support the use of a statin after an acute coronary event. Most studies used high doses. There is most likely a class effect.
- Bringing a patient to goal may require use of different classes of lipid-lowering medication; however, statins appear to offer benefits other than lipid-lowering.

Goals for therapy:

- Low-density lipoprotein (LDL) should be less than 70 mg/dL. Statin drugs are generally recommended for the LDL lowering effects as well as the non-LDL lowering (pleiotropic) benefits.
- Triglycerides should be less than 150 mg/dL. This may be accomplished with a statin drug, niacin, fibrate, or fish oil. Fibrates and fish oil specifically target triglycerides. Choice of medication depends on TG level, and levels of LDL and high-density lipoprotein (HDL).
- HDL should be ≥40 mg/dL in men and ≥50 mg/dL in women. Statins and niacin can raise HDL; patients with metabolic syndrome and high TG and low HDL can have an increase of HDL with lowering of TG.

Statin Drugs

Agents and Dose

Lovastatin (Mevacor): 10, 20, 40, 60 mg (Merck, Whitehouse Station, NJ)
Pravastatin (Pravachol): 10, 20, 40, 80 mg (BMS, New York, NY)
Simvastatin (Zocor): 5, 10, 20, 40, 80 mg (Merck, Whitehouse Station, NJ)
Fluvastatin (Lescol): 20, 40, 80 mg (Novartis, Switzerland)
Atorvastatin (Lipitor): 10, 20, 40, 80 mg (Pfizer, New York, NY)
Rosuvastatin (Crestor): 5, 10, 20, 40 mg (Astrazeneca, Wilmington)

Side Effects

- Muscle: myopathy, myalgia, myositis
- Rhabdomyolysis
- Liver: transaminitis, acute liver failure (rare), cholestasis (rare), hepatitis (rare)
- Drug interactions

Absolute Contraindications

- Active or chronic liver disease

Monitoring

- Myopathy and creatinine kinase (CK) elevations

The National Cholesterol Education Program Guidelines recommend an initial CK measurement and evaluation of muscle symptoms. Muscle symptoms should be evaluated at each follow-up visit and a CK level obtained when there is a complaint of muscle soreness, tenderness, or pain. Patients on high doses of statins and on combinations of lipid-lowering agents may be at greater risk for myopathy and elevations of CK.

The incidence of statin-related myopathy is low (0.1% to 0.2%) but mild elevations in CK (less than 3 times the upper limit of normal) with or without muscle soreness are more common but should not preclude the use of statins.

It is important to rule out other causes of muscle soreness or elevated CK (exercise, trauma, strenuous work, hypothyroidism, inflammatory muscle weakness). If CK elevation or symptoms are mild, use of statin with regular monitoring (every 6 to 8 weeks) is recommended. More careful consideration should be given to elevations 3 to 10 times normal. Statins should not be used for elevations greater than 10 times normal without full evaluation.

Statin Liver Effects

The National Cholesterol Education Program Guidelines recommend an baseline evaluation of alanine aminotransferease and aspartate aminotransferase (AST/ALT) and approximately 12 weeks after beginning statin therapy.

Acute liver failure, hepatitis, and cholestasis are relatively rare. Transaminitis, the asymptomatic elevation of AST and ALT greater than 3 times normal, is reported in approximately 1% of patients on statin drugs. This is usually dose-related and occurs within the first 3 to 6 months and is reversible.

Patients with mild elevations (less than 3 times normal) should be evaluated for secondary causes of elevations. If no other cause is found, they may be kept on a statin with routine monitoring. For higher elevations, patients should have the statin dose reduced or stopped and a complete evaluation performed.

Nonalcoholic fatty liver disease may be a cause of elevated liver enzymes. Once diagnosed, statins may be continued in some patients with careful monitoring.

Additional Notes on Statin Drugs

- Metabolized by cytochrome P450 or CYP3A4: lovastatin, simvastatin, atorvastatin.
- Not metabolized, or metabolized to lesser extent by CYP3A4: pravastatin, fluvastatin, rosuvastatin.

- Water soluble: pravastatin.
- Lipid soluble: lovastatin, atorvastatin.
- Best to prevent myopathy: pravastatin is transported in the muscle with a transporter that the muscle does not have. So, there may be fewer muscle side effects.

Blood Pressure

Patients who have just had an acute event may not be at their baseline blood pressure because of impairment of pump function and use of other medications in the acute setting. Blood pressure may need to be monitored and treated as an outpatient. The 2003 Seventh Report of the Joint National Committee on Prevention, Detection, Evaluation, and Treatment of High Blood Pressure defines a blood pressure of less than 120/80 as "normal" and values from 120/80 to 140/90 as a new category, "prehypertension" [5].

There is limited data from large, placebo-controlled, randomized clinical trials to suggest that treatment of prehypertension is beneficial. In the Heart Outcomes Prevention Evaluation (HOPE) trial, treatment based on angiotensin-converting enzyme (ACE) inhibitors compared with a regimen that did not reduced incidence of cardiovascular (CV) events and death from any cause among more than 9,000 high-risk patients with or without elevated BP [6]. In the Comparison of Amlodipine vs. Enalapril to Limit Occurrences of Thrombosis (CMAELOT) Study, 1,991 patients with angiographically documented coronary artery disease and an average baseline BP of 129/78 showed a reduced incidence of CV events by 31% with an amlodipine (10 mg) but not an enalapril (20 mg) based treatment regimen [7]. Whereas a blood pressure goal less than 130/80 mm Hg is recommended.

Lifestyle Modification

Modification	Recommendation	Expected drop SBP
Weight reduction	BMI 18.5 to 24.9	5 to 20 mm Hg/10 kg
DASH diet*	Diet of fruits, vegetables, low-fat dairy, reduced saturated and total fat	8 to 14 mm Hg
Sodium restriction	No more than 100 mEq/L (2.4 g sodium or 6 g sodium chloride	2 to 8 mm Hg
Physical Activity	Aerobic activity at least 30 minutes 3 to 5 days a week	4 to 9 mm Hg
Alcohol modification	Limit to no more than two drinks per day, men; one for women and lighter-weight persons	2 to 4 mm Hg

*Dietary Approaches to Stop Hypertension.
SBP, systolic blood pressure.

TABLE 25.1. Selection of medication.*

Condition	Recommended Drugs
MI	Beta-blocker, ACE inhibitor, aldosterone antagonist
High risk for CAD	Diuretic, beta-blocker, ACE inhibitor
Heart failure	Diuretic, beta-blocker, ACE inhibitor, ARB, aldosterone antagonist
Diabetes	ACE inhibitor, ARB
Chronic kidney	ACE inhibitor, ARB

*Choice of medication should be based on other comorbidities present.

Drug Therapy

General Guidelines for Drug Therapy (Table 25.1)

- Thiazide-type diuretics should be used as initial therapy for most patients with hypertension, either alone or in combination with agent from different class (ACE inhibitors, angiotension receptor blockers [ARBs], beta-blockers, calcium channel blockers [CCBs])
- Most patients with hypertension will require two or more antihypertensive medications to achieve their BP goals. Addition of a second drug from a different class should be initiated when use of a single drug in adequate doses fails to achieve the BP goal.
- When BP is more than 20 mmHg systolic and 10 mmHg diastolic above goal, consideration should be given to initiating therapy with two drugs, either as separate prescriptions or in fixed-dose combinations.

Therapeutic plan:

- All patients should be provided with lifestyle modification counseling.
- Individual class of drugs chosen for cardiac patients is often determined by other needs (see table above)

Goals for therapy:

- Titrate medication to achieve a blood pressure of 130/80 with consideration for <130/80

Diet and Nutrition

The importance of diet cannot be overemphasized. As noted above, diet can impact on blood pressure, lipids, weight, and diabetes. Patients should be seen by a nutritionist or health educator prior to or shortly after discharge [8]. Rather than having a patient go on any particular diet, it is far more preferable for the patient to change his or her eating patterns for a lifetime.

Specific Diets

Mediterranean Diet

Many studies have demonstrated the CV benefits of a Mediterranean style diet. There's no one "Mediterranean" diet but the common Mediterranean dietary pattern has the features listed below. More than half of the fat calories in a Mediterranean diet come from monounsaturated fats (mainly from olive oil). Monounsaturated fat does not raise blood cholesterol levels the way saturated fat does.

- High consumption of fruits, vegetables, bread and other cereals, potatoes, beans, nuts and seeds
- Olive oil is an important monounsaturated fat source
- Dairy products, fish, and poultry are consumed in low to moderate amounts, and little red meat is eaten
- Eggs are consumed 0 to 4 times a week
- Wine is consumed in low to moderate amounts

Very-Low-Fat Diets

Very-low-fat diets consist of less than 15% of total calories from fat. The Pritikin Diet recommends less than 10% of calories come from fat and the Ornish Program recommends 7%. These diets have been shown to lower cholesterol and reduce risk but require a highly motivated individual. Because of the stringent program, the long-term adherence rates for these diets are often poor.

Low-Carbohydrate Diets

Low-carbohydrate diets recommend limiting complex and simple sugars, causing the body to oxidize fat to meet energy requirements. There is a rapid initial weight loss, possibly due to a diuretic effect; however, there are long-term nutritional and CV concerns. These diets are high in protein, high in saturated fat and cholesterol, and low in fruits, vegetables, and whole grains. The Atkins Diet recommends 68% of calories from fat, 27% from protein, and 5% from carbohydrates.

MyPyramid.gov

A federal government-sponsored Website, mypyramid.gov allows individuals to determine their daily caloric requirements and then choose a food "pyramid" that specifies quantities of grains, vegetables, fruits, dairy, protein, sugar, solid fats, and oils allowed per day.

Therapeutic plan:

- Measurement of body weight, height, body mass index, and waist circumference

- Identification, evaluation, and treatment of specific dietary needs (weight reduction, low sodium, low-fat, diabetic) and educational material provided
- Physical activity and exercise recommendations
- Determine the role of medication and surgical approaches

Goals for therapy:

- BMI less than 25
- Waist circumference less than 40 inches for men and 35 inches for women
- Adoption of a heart-healthy eating plan

Physical Activity

Sedentary lifestyle is a risk factor for coronary artery disease. Physical activity and exercise offer numerous benefits including weight loss, lowering of blood pressure and LDL cholesterol and triglycerides, raising HDL cholesterol, improving insulin sensitivity, and improving overall cardiovascular fitness. Patients who have had an acute coronary event should be referred to cardiac rehabilitation programs. In the past, there has been limited reimbursement from Medicare and insurance plans; however, Medicare has recently expanded indications as have private insurers.

Cardiac rehabilitation consists of three phases. Phase I, or inpatient services, focuses on physical therapy to mobilize the patient and preparation for discharge and function at home. Education and activity assessment can also take place at this time. Phase II is a supervised exercise program, generally three sessions a week for 12 weeks to optimize physical fitness. Phase III is an unsupervised exercise program.

Therapeutic plan:

- Patients have a symptom-limited, submaximal treadmill or bicycle exercise stress test prior to beginning cardiac rehabilitation. This test serves to risk stratify the patient and allow for a precise exercise prescription. This can be done before hospital discharge or shortly thereafter [9].
- All patients should be asked about their physical activity or exercise.
- Identify obstacles to participation in an exercise program with attempts to address and work around these obstacles.

Goals for therapy:

- Enrollment in a cardiac rehabilitation program.
- In the event cardiac rehabilitation is not available or not covered by insurance, a symptom-limited stress test should be performed prior to or shortly after discharge to help plan an exercise program. Medically supervised programs are strongly recommended.
- Goal for patient is 30 minutes a day a minimum of 5 days a week of moderate-intensity exercise. Patients may work up to this goal

Smoking Cessation

See Chapter 26.

References

1. Smith SC Jr, Allen J, Blair SN, et al. AHA/ACC guidelines for secondary prevention for patients with coronary and other atherosclerotic vascular disease: 2006 update. Circulation 2006;113:2263–2372.
2. Mitka M. Guidelines update: aggressively target cardiovascular risk factors. JAMA 2006;296:30–31.
3. Wright RS, Murphy J, Bybee KA, et al. Statin lipid-lowering therapy for acute myocardial infarction and unstable angina: efficacy and mechanism of benefit. Mayo Clin Proc 2002;77:1085–1092.
4. Briel M, Schwartz GG, Thompson PL, et al. Effects of early treatment with statins on short-term clinical outcomes in acute coronary syndromes. JAMA 2006;295:2046–2056.
5. The Seventh Report of the Joint National Committee on Prevention, Detection, Evaluation, and Treatment of High Blood Pressure. Available at http://www.nhlbi.nih.gov/guidelines/hypertension/jnc7full.pdf.
6. The Heart Outcomes Prevention Evaluation Study Investigators. Effects of an angiotensin-converting-enzyme inhibitor, ramipril, on cardiovascular events in high-risk patients. N Engl J Med. 2000;342:145–153.
7. Nissen SE, Tuzcu EM, Libby P, et al. Effect of antihypertensive agents on cardioivascular events in patients with coronary disease and normal blood pressure: the CAMELOT study: a randomized, controlled trial. JAMA 2004;292:2217–2225.
8. American Heart Association. Dietary guidelines revision 2000. Circulation 2000;102:2284–2299.
9. American Association of Cardiovascular and Pulmonary Rehabilitation. Guidelines for cardiac rehabilitation and secondary prevention programs. 4th ed. Champaign, IL Human Kinetics; 2004.

26
Smoking Cessation in the Cardiac Patient

Mary O'Sullivan

The most critical issue facing cardiac patients who smoke is that they must understand not only how much the cigarette endangers their survival but also how rapidly and thoroughly stopping smoking will change their course. They must be convinced that they will be able to safely succeed in their efforts, especially under the guidance of the person they trust the most in this regard: their cardiologist. The role of the cardiologist in caring for a smoking patient must focus on several issues that will lead to the patient's success and will bring about a critical change in the patient's prognosis.

First, the physician must teach the patient that much of the effect of smoking on their disease is reversible and that when they stop smoking, within 3 years, their risk for recurrent coronary events becomes that of a nonsmoker [1]. The benefits begin immediately. Within hours, the carbon monoxide that poisons the oxygen delivery system and the adrenergically mediated vasoconstriction that is acutely induced by the cigarette dissipate.

Second, the physician must select a pharmacological cessation plan that will best suit the patient's risks and needs, be it nicotine replacement alone and/or bupropion or varenicline. Encouragement is needed for patients to use such an approach, but if they comply, their chance of success doubles.

Third, the physician must use the simple principles of behavioral modification that significantly enhance the patient's success rate. The key features involved are to:

- Convince the patient that he or she can succeed.
- Have the patient make a concrete plan for what he or she will do when he or she gets a craving.
- Identify and plan for avoidance of triggers such as coffee, alcohol, friends who smoke, and so forth.
- Identify substitutes that the patient likes and can look forward to, (e.g., movies, museums, friends who do not smoke, magazines, etc.).
- Plan to be busy as much as possible, especially immediately after finishing a meal.

- Most important, discuss with the patient the permanence of the addiction and the need to be on guard even years later, especially in situations of stress. Unfortunately, the thought of picking up another cigarette recurs for a very long time, and one puff can lead to full relapse.

How Does Cigarette Smoking Affect the Heart?

Cigarette smoking affects the heart as follows [2]:

- Smoking cigarettes induces a *hypercoagulable state* that is the predominant cause of acute cardiovascular events induced by smoking. It is responsible for 25% to 50% of the link between smoking and coronary artery disease (CAD) [3] and is not reversed by aspirin. It affects both antithrombotic and prothrombotic factors as well as platelet function. This is borne out in multiple clinical situations:
  Smoking increases the risk of myocardial infarction (MI) and sudden death much more than it increases the risk of angina, reflecting the importance of acute thrombus formation [4].
  Similarly, in smokers, the prognosis after thrombolysis is better than in nonsmokers. This reflects the greater share that clot plays in the disease process [5].
  Sudden cardiac death is correlated with the presence of acute thrombosis and not the level of plaque burden [4].
  Smokers who continue to smoke after thrombolysis or angioplasty have a substantially increased risk of reinfarction or reocclusion [6, 7].

At least a part of the thrombotic effects of smoking are induced by even passive smoke [8, 9]. The remarkable sensitivity of the coagulation system to the effect of cigarette smoke [2] mandates that the cardiac patient must cease all smoking, not just cut down their habit, to achieve reversal of these effects. Patients should be taught the seriousness of this issue.

- Carbon monoxide acutely poisons the oxygen delivery system, placing the patient at risk for arrhythmia and MI [4].
- Progression of atherosclerosis by smoking appears to be mediated by free-radical oxidative stress [2, 4] resulting in:
  Diminished nitric oxide, resulting in impaired vasodilatory function at the macrovascular level (e.g., coronary arteries as well as at the microvascular level) [7, 10].
  Inflammatory effects on the vessel wall with recruitment of leukocytes and an increase in multiple inflammatory markers, including C-reactive protein, interleukin-6, and tumor necrosis factor.
  Lipid peroxidation possibly mediated via insulin resistance.
  Genetic predisposition resulting in increased susceptibility. Importance at this time is unknown. Smoking may be a more powerful risk factor for MI

and sudden death in women than in men. In one study, it was the strongest risk factor for sudden death among women [11].

Does Nicotine Play a Role in the Development of Heart Disease?

Nicotine is the severely addicting substance in the cigarette that causes the release of several neurotransmitters (dopamine, γ-aminobutyric acid, norepinephrine, serotonin). The hemodynamic effects of nicotine are adrenergically mediated, including increased cardiac output, heart rate, and blood pressure, and constriction of coronary arteries [12]. However, its role in the development of atherothrombotic disease remains controversial, and it is the free-radical oxidative stress that appears to be the driving force [2, 4].

Is Nicotine Replacement Safe in the Cardiac Patient?

The safety of nicotine replacement therapy in the cardiac patient has long been a concern. The nicotine patch has a slow delivery system and is not associated with increased 24-hour epinephrine excretion or with activation of coagulation [13]. It is the preferred delivery system in this group of patients. Standard doses of nicotine replacement (21 mg patch for a 1-pack per day smoker and 14 mg patch for a 10 cigarette per day smoker) generally result in lower nicotine levels than smoking. Nicotine replacement doubles a person's success rate.

Three randomized controlled clinical trials in patients with stable cardiovascular disease and one in outpatients with cardiac or respiratory disease have been published and support the safety of nicotine replacement in stable cardiac patients [14].

- In the first trial of 156 cardiac patients, symptoms were recorded in daily diaries and some underwent 24-hour ambulatory electrocardiographic monitoring. Transdermal nicotine did not affect the frequency of angina, arrhythmias, or ST-segment depression on electrocardiographic monitoring [15].
- In an outpatient VA trial, 584 patients with at least one cardiovascular disease were randomized to receive the nicotine patch versus placebo [16]. There was no significant difference in the incidence of death, MI, cardiac arrest, or hospital admission for increased angina, dysrhythmia, or congestive heart failure. Concomitant use of the patch and smoking were not associated with an increase in adverse events. The long-term success rate was no better for the patch versus placebo.
- Another small trial of 106 patients with CAD, using transdermal nicotine versus placebo, monitored with repeated ambulatory electrocardiographic monitoring and exercise testing, did not show significant increase in adverse events [17].

These studies support the safety of the use of the patch in cardiac patients. Any risk involved in the use of the patch must be balanced against the need for the patient to be able to succeed in their smoking cessation efforts, and the safety profile shown above supports that use.

These studies do not, however, address the issue of the use of transdermal nicotine in a patient admitted with the acute coronary syndrome. Current recommendations do not support the use of nicotine replacement in patients with unstable angina or MI in the prior 2 weeks because of a lack of data to support the safety of nicotine replacement therapy used in this interval [18]. This issue was addressed in only one study from the Duke University Cardiovascular Databank [19]. After a propensity analysis, two cohorts of 187 patients each were identified that were similar in measured variables (age, sex, race, hypertension, hyperlipidemia, diabetes mellitus, previous heart failure, previous MI, ejection fraction, and acute MI). They found no difference in short- or long-term mortality in patients who did or did not receive patches.

Smoking cessation in the cardiac care unit is recognized as a vital part of the patient's care. Current recommendations do not support the use of nicotine replacement in these patients, and further research is needed to clarify this issue. As with any multifaceted clinical decision, balancing the risks and benefits must be undertaken carefully

Bupropion for Smokers with Cardiovascular Disease

Bupropion, an atypical antidepressant with a structure related to amphetamine, has, like nicotine replacement, been shown to be an effective smoking cessation tool. After approximately 10 days on treatment, the desire to smoke diminishes significantly. In addition, the depression that not uncommonly surfaces in patients stopping smoking is prevented. The contraindications include a seizure history, alcoholism, bipolar disorder, bulimia, and panic attacks. The side effects include dry mouth, headache, agitation, and insomnia, especially if taken late in the day. Hypertension has been described, especially in patients taking both bupropion and the nicotine replacement. The treatment is usually begun at bupropion 150 mg slow release (SR) and subsequently increased to 150 mg SR twice daily. The side effects are dose-dependent, and some patients may obtain an adequate therapeutic benefit with the 150 mg daily dose. The drug is metabolized in the liver, and so dose adjustment is advised with significant liver disease. The drug inhibits the activity of CYP2D6 isoenzyme, which metabolizes beta-blockers, antiarrhythmics, certain antidepressants, selective serotonin reuptake inhibitors, and antipsychotics. In particular, bupropion should not be administered concomitantly with thioridazine secondary to risks of thioridazine toxicity and risk for ventricular arrhythmias.

After the approval of bupropion SR as a smoking cessation aid in the United Kingdom, 18 deaths were reported. The Canadian Adverse Reaction Monitoring Program reported 70 severe adverse cardiovascular reactions to bupropion SR, including nine myocardial infarctions and three cardiac deaths. The contribution of bupropion SR to these deaths is not known, because these case reports could not control for other significant risk factors and therefore contribute little to safety assessment [14].

More recently, in a five-hospital, double-blind, placebo-controlled trial, patients who were admitted with acute cardiovascular disease were randomized to receive either bupropion SR 150 mg twice daily and intensive counseling versus placebo and intensive counseling. Bupropion and placebo groups did not differ in cardiovascular mortality at 1 year, in blood pressure at follow-up, or in cardiovascular events at end-of-treatment or 1 year. Bupropion did improve short-term quit rates but not long-term rates over intensive counseling but did appear to be safe for smokers hospitalized with acute cardiovascular disease [20].

There is one randomized trial for smoking cessation comparing bupropion SR 150 mg twice daily with placebo in outpatients with stable cardiovascular disease [21]. At 1 year, the quit rates were 27% for the bupropion arm versus 11% for the placebo arm. There were no clinically significant changes in blood pressure and heart rate throughout the treatment phase. In studies of bupropion SR being used as an antidepressant in patients with cardiac disease, few adverse cardiac effects were seen. There was occasional hypertension but no effect on cardiac conduction or ejection fraction.

Despite the concern raised by case reports, current evidence suggests that bupropion SR may be a safe and possibly efficacious treatment for smoking cessation for patients with cardiovascular disease. Full evaluation of bupropion SR in patients with cardiac disease is needed. Bupropion may be used in combination with nicotine replacement. The success rate of this combination has not been shown to be statistically superior [22, 23] and has not been evaluated in the cardiac patient. It is suggested that while on combined therapy, blood pressure should be monitored.

Varenicline

Varenicline is a new, effective, non-nicotine agent, developed expressly for smoking cessation. It is a selective nicotinic acetylcholine receptor partial agonist releasing 35% to 65% of the dopamine observed with nicotine. Varenicline also has a competitive antagonist effect on nicotine due to higher affinity for the receptor. It successfully blocks both the desire to smoke and the pleasure of smoking. It appears to have great potential [24]. It has yet to be studied in the cardiac patient.

Conclusion

Smoking cessation in the cardiac patient covers a spectrum of therapy from simple measures of behavioral modification to complex decisions involving pharmacotherapeutic options, for which further research is needed, especially in patients with acute coronary syndrome.

References

1. Kannel WB, Dagostino RB, Belanger AJ. Fibrinogen, cigarette-smoking, and risk of cardiovascular diseases—insights from the Framingham study. Am Heart J 1987; 113:1006–1010.
2. Ambrose JA, Barua RS. The pathophysiology of cigarette smoking and cardiovascular disease, an update. J Am Coll Cardiol 2004;43:1731–1737.
3. Mueller HS, Cohen LS, Braunwald E, et al. Predictors of early morbidity and mortality after thrombolytic therapy of acute myocardial infarction. Analyses of patient subgroups in the Thrombolysis in Myocardial Infarction (TIMI) trial, phase II. Circulation 1992;85:1254–1264.
4. Benowitz NL, Gourlay SG. Cardiovascular toxicity of nicotine: implications for nicotine replacement therapy. J Am Coll Cardiol 1997;29:1422–1431.
5. Barbash GI, Reiner J, White HD, et al. Evaluation of paradoxic beneficial effects of smoking in patients receiving thrombolytic therapy for acute myocardial infarction: mechanism of the "smoker's paradox" from the GUSTO-I trial, with angiographic insights. Global Utilization of Streptokinase and Tissue-Plasminogen Activator for Occluded Coronary Arteries. J Am Coll Cardiol 1995;26:1222–1229.
6. Rivers JT, White HD, Cross DB, et al. Reinfarction after thrombolytic therapy for acute myocardial infarction followed by conservative management: incidence and effect of smoking. J Am Coll Cardiol 1990;16:340–348.
7. Galan KM, Deligonul U, Kern MJ, et al. Increased frequency of restenosis in patients continuing to smoke cigarettes after percutaneous transluminal coronary angioplasty. Am J Cardiol 1988;61:260–263.
8. Glantz SA, Parmley WW. Passive smoking and heart disease: mechanisms and risk. JAMA 1995;273:1047–1053.
9. Barnoya J, Glantz SA. Cardiovascular effects of secondhand smoke: nearly as large as smoking. Circulation 2005;111:2684–2698.
10. Barua RS, Ambrose JA, Eales-Reynolds LJ, et al. Dysfunctional endothelial nitric oxide biosynthesis in healthy smokers with impaired endothelium-dependent vasodilatation. Circulation 2001;104:1905–1910.
11. Talbott E, Kuller LH, Perper J, et al. Sudden unexpected death in women: biologic and psychosocial origins. Am J Epidemiol 1981;114:671–682.
12. Quillen JE, Rossen JD, Oskarsson HJ, et al. Acute effects of cigarette smoking on the coronary circulation: constriction of epicardial resistance vessels. J Am Coll Cardiol 1993;22:642–647.
13. Benowitz NL, Fitzgerald GA, Wilson M, et al. Nicotine effects on eicosanoid formation and hemostatic function: comparison of transdermal nicotine andcigarette smoking. J Am Coll Cardiol 1993;22:1159–1167.
14. Joseph A, Fu S. Safety issues in pharmacotherapy for smoking in patients with cardiovascular disease. Prog Cardiovasc Dis 2003;45:429–441.
15. Working Group for the Study of Transdermal Nicotine in Patients with Coronary Artery Disease. Nicotine replacement therapy for patients with coronary artery disease. Arch Int Med 1994;154:989–995.
16. Joseph AM, Norman SM, Ferry LH, et al. The safety of transdermal nicotine as an aid to smoking cessation in patients with cardiac disease. N Engl J Med 1996;335:1792–1798.
17. Tzivoni D, Keren A, Meyler S, et al. Cardiovascular safety of transdermal nicotine patches in patients with coronary artery disease who try to quit smoking. Cardiovasc Drugs Ther 1998;12:239–244.

18. Fiore MC, Bailey WC, Cohen SJ, et al. Treating tobacco use and dependence, clinical practice guideline. Rockville, MD: U.S. Department of Health nd Human Services, Public Health Service; 2000.

19. Meine T, Patel M, Washam J, et al. Safety and effectiveness of transdermal nicotine patch in smokers admitted with acute coronary syndromes. Am J Cardiol 2005: 95:976–978.

20. Rigotti N, Thorndike A, Regan S, et al. Bupropion for smokers hospitalized with acute cardiovascular disease. Am J Med 2006;119:1080–1087.

21. Tonstad S, Farsang C, Klaene G, et al. Bupropion SR for smoking cessation in smokers with cardiovascular disease: a multicentre, randomized study. Eur Heart J 2003;24:946–955.

22. Jorenby D, Leischow S, Nides M, et al. A controlled trial of sustained-release bupropion, a nicotine patch, or both for smoking cessation. N Engl J Med 1999;340: 685–691.

23. Simon J, Duncan C, Carmody T, et al. Bupropion for smoking cessation. Arch Intern Med 2004:164;1797–1803.

24. Nides M, Oncken C, Gonzales D, et al. Smoking cessation with varenicline, a selective a4B2 nicotinic receptor partial agonist. Arch Intern Med 2006;166:1561–1568.

27
Future Developments

Khashayar Hematpour, Jamshad Wyne, and Mun K. Hong

The optimal "therapy" for acute coronary syndrome (ACS) is undoubtedly the prevention of its occurrence. Multiple primary [1] and secondary prevention trials [2], mainly with statins, have shown their beneficial effects. However, despite their overall reduction in cardiovascular events, statins affecting mainly low-density lipoprotein (LDL) levels have not been shown to significantly affect the coronary heart disease or overall mortality [1]. Furthermore, high-density lipoprotein (HDL) level at the time of ACS presentation, not LDL level or the change in LDL level by statin, predicted the short-term prognosis [3]. Therefore, a new therapeutic target to raise HDL, such as with cholesteryl ester transfer protein inhibitor, was investigated with great hope [4]. The results of this therapy were eagerly anticipated, but the first randomized trial suggested potential increase in mortality with this therapy, possibly related to associated hypertension (unpublished data). Despite this setback, there are other agents in the same class with possibly different side-effect profile that may ultimately improve the lipid profile. In addition, infusion of recombinant HDL may promote regression of coronary atherosclerosis [5] and contribute to stability of the plaques, although this intermittent intravenous infusion would be impractical for most patients. Theoretically, the symbiotic combination of LDL-lowering and HDL-raising therapies could result in the best cardioprotection.

Antiplatelet therapy, especially clopidogrel monotherapy [6] or combination therapy with aspirin [7], has been shown to provide substantial benefit in prevention of secondary cardiovascular events. The hypothesis that dual antiplatelet therapy in high-risk patients, such as diabetics, could provide primary prevention was studied in the CHARISMA trial [8], but ultimately the randomized trial could not provide a definitive answer because of insufficient enrollment of these patients [9]. Novel antiplatelet agents, such as prasugrel [10], may further improve the cardioprotection.

In addition, current emphasis on banning smoking in public, thereby preventing secondhand smoke, improving diet and exercise for children and the general population, and educating the public regarding lifestyle modifications will result in overall reduced risk for developing ACS. Furthermore, in the future it would be ideal to be able to detect patients at risk from their genetic profile [11] and possibly tailor the therapy according to their individual risk [12].

Imaging Modalities to Detect Subclinical Vulnerable Plaques

Even with optimal therapy and compliance with medical therapy and lifestyle modification, there are patients at risk for rupture of the vulnerable plaques and ACS. For these patients, it would be preferable to have a noninvasive imaging modality to detect the subclinical plaques at risk for rupture. Although many different coronary imaging modalities have been investigated for this purpose [13], currently there is no reliable noninvasive methodology. Recently, multislice computed tomographic angiography has gained some acceptance for detecting subclinical coronary artery disease [14]. However, this modality does not address the plaque composition and is similar to traditional invasive coronary angiography in that it is a lumenogram. Furthermore, during ACS, patients with high likelihood would need to go to the catheterization laboratory for definitive diagnosis and subsequent revascularization if needed. There are invasive modalities with potential for detecting vulnerable plaques [15]. Because of their invasive nature, especially in asymptomatic patients, these modalities are not as desirable for detection of vulnerable plaques.

An indirect measure of the presence of vulnerable coronary artery plaques may be the presence of "echolucent" carotid plaques, as reported by Honda et al. [16]. They showed that those patients with echolucent carotid plaques, suggestive of lipid core, had greater frequency of subsequent ACS versus others with similar amount of carotid plaque but without the lipid core. Therefore, increased scrutiny of easily accessible peripheral arteries, such as the carotid or other noncoronary arteries, may provide early clues to the presence of vulnerable plaques.

Laboratory Tests to Facilitate the Diagnosis of ACS

Once patients present with ACS, it is important not to miss this diagnosis. Unfortunately, the rate of missed diagnosis still remains high, between 2% and 4% [17], and missed diagnosis of acute coronary syndrome is associated with a twofold increase in patient mortality rate [18]. This is because initial decision making, which is based on a patient's risk factors, electrocardiogram, and the level of cardiac enzymes, will often be ineffective, especially in patients with initial normal enzyme levels or nondiagnostic electrocardiographic changes.

There have been reports of novel biomarkers, such as resistin [19], albumin cobalt binding test [20], and pregnancy-associated plasma protein A [21]. The potential advantages could be earlier detection of the ACS status, with some of the markers elevated even prior to myocardial necrosis and prior to troponin elevation [20].

Therapies

After the occurrence of ACS, current therapies, including both pharmacological and revascularization options, have greatly improved the survival rates. However, none of the therapies can prevent the reperfusion injury [22], and the amount of myocardial salvage is limited. Therefore, future treatments aimed at preventing reperfusion injury [23] or preserving ischemic myocardium for eventual survival by therapeutic hypothermia [24] could maximize myocardial salvage. In addition, bone marrow infusion could provide progenitor cells for repopulation of the infarcted area and improve myocardial function [25].

References

1. Thavendiranathan P, Bagai A, Brookhart MA, et al. Primary prevention of cardio-vascular diseases with statin therapy: a meta-analysis of randomized controlled trials. Arch Intern Med 2006;166:2307–2313.
2. LaRosa JC, He J, Vupputuri S. Effect of statins on risk of coronary disease: a meta-analysis of randomized controlled trials. JAMA 1999;282:2340–2346.
3. Olsson AG, Schwartz GG, Szarek M, et al. High-density lipoprotein, but not low-density lipoprotein cholesterol levels influence short-term prognosis after acute coronary syndrome: results from the MIRACL trial. Eur Heart J 2005;26:890–896.
4. Barter PJ, Chapman MJ, Hennekens CH, et al. Cholesteryl ester transfer protein. A novel target for raising HDL and inibiting atherosclerosis. Arterioscler Thromb Vasc Biol 2003;23:160–167.
5. Nissen SE, Tsunoda T, Tuzcu EM, et al. Effect of recombinant ApoA-1 Milano on coronary atherosclerosis in patients with acute coronary syndromes: a randomized controlled trial. JAMA 2003;290:2292–2300.
6. CAPRIE Steering Committee. A randomized, blinded, trial of clopidogrel versus aspirin in patients at risk of ischaemic events (CAPRIE). Lancet 1996;348: 1329–1339.
7. The Clopidogrel in Unstable Angina to Prevent Recurrent Events Trial Investigators. Effects of clopidogrel in addition to aspirin in patients with acute coronary syndromes without ST-segment elevation. N Engl J Med 2001;345:494–502.
8. Bhatt DL, Topol EJ, Clopidogrel for High Atherothrombotic Risk and Ischemic Stabilization, Management, and Avoidance Executive Committee. Clopidogrel added to aspirin versus aspirin alone in secondary prevention and high-risk primary prevention: rationale and design of the Clopidogrel for High Atherothrombotic Risk and Ischemic Stabilization, Management, and Avoidance (CHARISMA) trial. Am Heart J 2004;148:263–268.
9. Bhatt DL, Fox KAA, Hacke W, et al. Clopidogrel and aspirin versus aspirin alone for the prevention of atherothrombotic events. N Engl J Med 2006;354:1706–1717.
10. Jernberg T, Payne CD, Winters KJ, et al. Prasugrel achieves greater inhibition of platelet aggregation and a lower rate of non-responders compared with clopidogrel in aspirin-treated patients with stable coronary artery disease. Eur Heart J 2006; 27:1166–1173.
11. Nsengimana J, Samani NJ, Hall AS, et al. Enhanced linkage of a locus on chromosome 2 to premature coronary artery disease in the absence of hypercholesterolemia. Eur J Hum Genet 2007;15:313–319.

12. Smith JD, Topol EJ. Identification of atherosclerosis-modifying genes: pathogenic insights and therapeutic potential. Expert Rev Cardiovasc Ther 2006;4:703–709.
13. Shin JH, Edelberg JE, Hong MK. Vulnerable atherosclerotic plaque: clinical implications. Curr Vasc Pharmacol 2003;1:183–204.
14. Dragu R, Rispler S, Ghersin E, et al. Contrast enhanced multi-detector computed tomography coronary angiography versus conventional invasive quantitative coronary angiography in acute coronary syndrome patients-correlation and bias. Acute Card Care 2006;8:99–104.
15. Kukreja N, Garcia-Garcia HM, Serruys PW. Invasive imaging techniques for the assessment of vulnerable plaque. Minerva Cardioangiol 2006;54:603–617.
16. Honda O, Sugiyama S, Kugiyama K, et al. Echolucent carotid plaques predict future coronary events in patients with coronary artery disease. J Am Coll Cardiol 2004;43:1177–1184.
17. Pope JH, Aufderheide TP, Ruthazer R, et al. Missed diagnoses of acute cardiac ischemia in the emergency department. N Engl J Med 2000;342:1163–1170
18. Welch RD, Zalenski RJ, Frederick PD, et al. Prognostic value of a normal or nonspecific initial electrocardiogram in acute myocardial infarction. JAMA 2001;286:1977–1984.
19. Lubos E, Messow CM, Schnabel R, et al. Resistin, acute coronary syndrome and prognosis results from the AtheroGene study. Atherosclerosis 2007;193:121–128.
20. Immanuel S, Sanjaya AI. Albumin cobalt binding (ACB) test: its role as a novel marker of acute coronary syndrome. Acta Med Indones 2006;38:92–96.
21. Wittfooth S, Qin QP, Lund J, et al. Immunofluorometric point-of-care assays for the detection of acute coronary syndrome-related noncomplexed pregnancy-associated plasma protein A. Clin Chem 2006;52:1794–801.
22. Verma S, Fedak PW, Weisel RD, et al. Fundamentals of reperfusion injury for the clinical cardiologist. Circulation 2002 21;105(20):2332–2336.
23. Asanuma H, Minamino T, Ogai A, et al. Blockade of histamine H2 receptors protects the heart against ischemia and reperfusion injury in dogs. J Mol Cell Cardiol 2006;40:666–674.
24. Hale SL, Kloner RA. Myocardial hypothermia: a potential therapeutic technique for acute regional myocardial ischemia. J Cardiovasc Electrophysiol 1999;10:405–413.
25. Hristov M, Weber C. The therapeutic potential of progenitor cells in ischemic heart disease—past, present and future. Basic Res Cardiol 2006;101:1–7.

Index

Made in the USA
Monee, IL
07 July 2026

56544766R00207